Back Pain and Spinal Manipulation
a practical guide

Back Pain and Spinal Manipulation

A Practical Guide

Second Edition

John Murtagh AM, MB, BS, MD, BSc, BEd, FRACGP

Professor and Head, Department of Community Medicine and General Practice, Monash University, Melbourne

Clive Kenna MB, BS, Cert Orthopaedic Med & Manual Therapy (Paris), FACPM

Consultant, Physical Medicine. Honorary Consultant, Department of Rheumatology, Monash Medical Centre, Melbourne

Illustration and art direction by

Chris Sorrell BA (Hons) Graphic Design

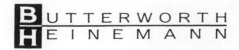
BUTTERWORTH
HEINEMANN

Butterworth-Heinemann
Linacre House, Jordan Hill, Oxford OX2 8DP
225 Wildwood Avenue, Woburn MA 01801-2041
A division of Reed Educational and Professional Publishing Ltd

A member of the Reed Elsevier plc group

OXFORD AUCKLAND BOSTON
JOHANNESBURG MELBOURNE NEW DELHI

First published 1989
Reprinted 1994
Second edition 1997
Reprinted 1999
Transferred to digital printing 2001

British Library Cataloguing in Publication Data
Kenna, Clive
   Back pain and spinal manipulation 2nd ed
   1. Backache   2. Spinal adjustment
   3. Physical therapy
   I. Title   II. Murtagh, John
   617.5'6'0622

Library of Congress Cataloguing in Publicaiton Data
Kenna, Clive
   Back pain and spinal manipulation/Clive Kenna, John Murtagh
   1. Backache   2. Spinal adjustment
   I. Title   II. Murtagh, John
   617.5'64062-dc20   96-19054   CIP

ISBN 0 7506 2185 0

For information on all Butterworth-Heinemann publications
visit our website at www.bh.com

Printed in Great Britain by Antony Rowe Ltd, Eastbourne

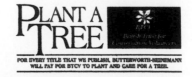

FOR EVERY TITLE THAT WE PUBLISH, BUTTERWORTH-HEINEMANN
WILL PAY FOR BTCV TO PLANT AND CARE FOR A TREE.

Contents

Foreword

The value and status of manipulative therapy in the medical profession has undergone a controversial history. Spinal and joint manipulation has been in medical hands since Hippocrates first compiled his major textbooks in about 400 BC. Subsequently, medical leaders such as Galen, Ambrose Pare, and Avicenna have also taught methods of spinal and joint traction and manipulation.

In the last century most joint diseases were due to infections, especially tuberculosis. Medical opinion then was very largely influenced by John Hilton's book *Rest and Pain*, in which he advocated prolonged, uninterrupted rest for joint diseases. This became standard orthopaedic teaching, followed until recently for the treatment of most musculoskeletal disorders. As a consequence, manipulation fell into considerable disfavour with the medical establishment.

The huge medical vacuum spawned a new breed: bonesetters, osteopaths and finally chiropractors. Some medical voices were raised pointing out this problem. For example, Sir James Paget in 1867 wrote in the British Medical Journal of the 'Cases that Bone-Setters Cure', but his advice – 'to learn by imitating their successes' – went ignored.

In 1934 Mixter and Barr presented their paper on intervertebral disc prolapse and by 1940 surgery was seen as the optimum treatment for sciatic pain, but since back pain was the usual forerunner of the leg pain, why not, it was argued, get in early and operate on those patients with back pain alone? The results of this concept were in general disastrous and meantime patients with low back pain were being treated mainly with pills. The neglect of physical treatments within the profession was counter-balanced only by a handful of practitioners, including orthopaedic medicine specialists such as Cyriax. He used his own particular form of manipulation and taught this widely, especially to physiotherapists. Other schools then flourished, but the major advance occurred when Geoff Maitland in Adelaide initiated a new school of manipulative physiotherapists.

Two Australian doctors who have developed skills in musculoskeletal medicine are the present authors, John Murtagh and Clive Kenna. These medical educators have for many years been involved in teaching with particular reference to manipulative techniques as a part of the total management of musculoskeletal medicine. Their courses, which have been widely acclaimed by the medical profession, are held under the auspices of the Royal Australian College of General Practitioners and it is from these courses that the present work has arisen.

Its content is detailed but its main message is simple.

General practitioners are the first medical practitioners to see these patients. Using their eyes and hands and knowledge of anatomy they can diagnose and assess most of their many patients who present with musculoskeletal conditions. Problem cases can be more easily recognised and so referred on as necessary.

In physical therapy there is no single method, but a multiplicity of approaches. Indeed, the most important point is that the acquisition of this particular manual skill is relatively unimportant in comparison to the more important role of clinical judgement. 'When' and 'when not to' is in fact much more important than 'how'.

The authors are to be congratulated on their innovative and refreshing approach to their subject and those who read this book should enjoy it as a new learning experience.

Brian Corrigan

Preface

The common problem of back pain represents a challenging area of management for the medical profession in terms of diagnosis and of management.

Clinical medicine is both an art and a science and the art of physical therapy for spinal related problems fascinates many members of our scientifically trained profession.

Rural practitioners who work in relative isolation find that physical therapy is a most useful component of their armamentarium for treatment of musculoskeletal disorders, especially spinal problems. For this reason some members of the Royal Australian College of General Practitioners (RACGP) approached the authors to establish a national course on 'back pain and spinal manipulation'. The notes and workshop methods used for the RACGP course, promoted through its official journal *Australian Family Physician* form the basis of this textbook.

This book has been designed, not only as a reference book, but as a basic text for practitioners undertaking a course in this discipline. While advanced theory and detailed techniques are presented in other modes – for example, in workshops (including those conducted by the authors) – this work has had as a primary objective the presentation of a diagnostic approach to back pain. The methods of data gathering and the all-important physical examination receive early attention as vital elements in the establishment of a diagnosis. Then the important physical therapy modalities are outlined: spinal mobilisation, spinal manipulation, muscle energy therapy, exercise prescription and relevant injection therapy.

The reader is invited to complete pre-physical examination questionnaires and to select optimum management plans for a series of actual case histories presented in several chapters.

The authors have different, yet complementary, backgrounds. Clive Kenna, who graduated MB BS from Monash University in 1974, developed a special interest in back pain after working in an industrial medical clinic. He studied a 12 months' course in manipulation therapy and obtained the Graduate Diploma of Manipulative Therapy. He eventually commenced full time practice as a consultant in Physical Medicine which he taught extensively in the educational programmes of the RACGP. In 1987 he pursued further postgraduate training overseas, initially in France with Dr Robert Maigne at the Department of Orthopaedic Medicine at the Hôtel Dieu, Paris. This was followed by further study in Switzerland under Dr Hans Schmid at the Red Cross Hospital, Berne, and the Wilhelm Schulthess Clinic, Zurich, with Dr H Baumgartner and Dr J Dvorak.

John Murtagh, who graduated MB BS from Monash University in 1966, following degree courses in Science and Education, developed a special interest in back pain prior to graduation. He studied and acquired skills in spinal manipulation as a surgical registrar for 12 months at the Bendigo Base Hospital. He subsequently attended the course conducted by James Cyriax in London and has successfully completed an MD thesis 'Back Pain in General Practice' based on 12 years' research. He has given teaching programmes on back pain and spinal manipulation since 1972.

The authors wish to emphasise that administering physical therapy, including spinal manipulation, is not a difficult skill to acquire. The main clinical skills lie in acquiring familiarity with the diagnostic method and in learning the appropriate indications and contra-indications for spinal mobilisation and manipulation (especially for the cervical spine).

The authors have aimed to demystify the subject and to set out the art on a logical basis. The diagnosis is dependent on a very thorough physical examination, which receives considerable emphasis in this work. However, there is no substitute for meticulous 'hands on' practice under supervision, especially in specialist clinics.

The authors acknowledge their many colleagues who have helped in various ways. These include Professor Neil Carson, Dr Brain Corrigan, Dr Lindsay Knight, Dr Rod Kruger, Dr Jill Rosenblatt, Dr Robert Maigne, Dr Hans Schmid, Dr H Baumgartner and Dr J Dvorak for their encouragement and expertise; Terry Oakley for his photography; Chris Sorrell BA (Hons) for his illustrative and graphic design skills; those authors who have granted permission to adapt their artwork: Dr Nikoli Bogduk (Figure 1.4), Professor Rene Cailliet (Figures 1.6, 21.2), Mr Ian Henderson (Figures 2.3, 2.4, 21.2) Dr Terry Little (Figure 6.8), Dr Robert Maigne (Figures 1.9, 4.3), Longmans Cheshire for permission to adapt material from their Health Information Book, *Back Pain*, by John Murtagh; and to the publishers, Butterworth-Heinemann, whose personnel have been of invaluable assistance.

Clive Kenna
John Murtagh

Section 1
General Concepts

1
Patterns of spinal pain

Contents
- [ ] Key checkpoints
- [ ] Anatomical and pathophysiological concepts
- [ ] Disc prolapse and pain patterns
- [ ] The concept of dysfunction
- [ ] Practice tips
- [ ] Summary

Pain experienced in the spine with peripheral extension, such as sciatica, may have one or more of four origins:

- spinal
- vascular
- visceral
- psychogenic.

This book will concentrate on spinal pain which has a multiplicity of causes including various diseases of bone such as tumours and infections. Spinal pain is, however, mainly caused by an alteration in the normal anatomical configuration of the various musculoskeletal structures of the spine, especially the joints, following physical stress. Pain of this type is often referred to as mechanical pain.

Despite profound dogmatism from some teachers about the origin of back pain, the precise cause of the pain in the patient presenting to the clinician is often unknown, so an open mind must be kept as to the possible aetiology.

Following the 'identification' by Mixter and Barr (1934) of lumbar disc protrusion and nerve root compression as the cause of low back pain and nerve root entrapment, a long period referred to as 'the dynasty of the disc' followed. Disc protrusion was considered to be responsible for all types of sciatica, and many explorative laminectomies were performed, often with indifferent results.

Although there is still considerable debate about the exact causes of spinal dysfunction and pain, modern technology and research have opened new horizons in our understanding of this complex area. It does appear that both disc protrusion and injury to the pain-sensitive apophyseal joints, either separately or conjointly, are the dominant causes of back pain, especially low back pain. Injury to the apophyseal joints leads to inflammation, nerve entrapment and reflex muscle spasm.

A detailed knowledge of the structural anatomy of the spine is essential for the clinician to understand the pathogenesis of back pain.

KEY CHECKPOINTS

- Disorders of the intervertebral discs can cause a disorder in the corresponding apophyseal joints.
- The sinuvertebral nerve and the posterior primary ramus are of great clinical importance in the nerve network of the spine.
- Pain usually arises from nociceptive stimulation of the spinal joints or structures juxtaposed to the joints.
- The outer layers of the annulus fibrosus are pain-sensitive.
- The posterior longitudinal ligaments and anterior dura mater are pain-sensitive.
- The usual sequence of sensory events following increasing pressure on a nerve is pain, paraesthesia and anaesthesia.

ANATOMICAL AND PATHOPHYSIOLOGICAL CONCEPTS

The mobile segment of the vertebral column

At each spinal level there are three important joints acting as a single functional element – one anterior (intervertebral disc) joint and two posterior (apophyseal) joints (Figure 1.1). In addition, this mobile segment (described by Junghans in 1956) contains supporting anatomical elements between the vertebrae, namely the anterior longitudinal ligament, the posterior longitudinal ligament, the ligamentum flavum, the interspinous and supraspinous ligaments and the appropriate nerves. (The posterior view of the segment is shown in Figure 1.2.)

Successive layers of these mobile segmental joints form a complex flexible system. Its resistance to injury depends largely on the integrity of the intervertebral disc, because if the disc is injured other structures will inevitably be involved. As Maigne (1986) points out, the proper functioning of the mobile segment requires perfect synergy of the involved muscles. An awkward or unexpected movement may lead to an uncoordinated division of forces and disturb elements of the mobile segment.

Figure 1.1 The mobile segment (Junghans): (A) The mobile segment; (B) Elements of the mobile segment.

1 nucleus pulposus
2 annulus fibrosus
3 vertebral body
4 cartilaginous area
5 apophyseal joint
6 (common) anterior longitudinal ligament
7 (common) posterior longitudinal ligament
8 interspinous and supraspinous ligaments

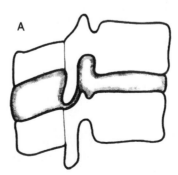
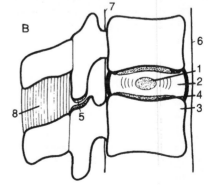

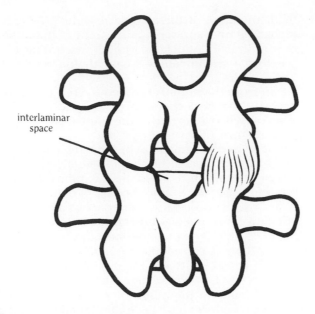

interlaminar
space

Figure 1.2 Posterior view
of the mobile segment:
note how the apophyseal
joint is enveloped by its
capsular ligament.

The intervertebral disc

Until recent times the disc (both annulus and nucleus) was generally believed to be a non-pain-sensitive, and consequently inert, structure. Recently Bogduk (1987) has highlighted the fact that the superficial layer of the annulus fibrosus in the lumbar region has significant innervation from the sinuvertebral nerves and stimulation of these nerve endings can result in pain. Such a stimulus could be produced from a torsional strain of the annulus, from the nucleus pulposus tracking through defects in the annulus to its periphery or by a bulging nucleus straining the overlying annulus. Thus internal disc disruption which can look quite normal on conventional X-rays or CT scan can cause intrinsic disc pain.

However, the disc commonly causes pain by its effect on the pain-sensitive posterior longitudinal ligament and anterior dura mater or by posterolateral prolapse against a nerve root. The anterior dura mater has been shown to be very sensitive to stretching, compression and inflammation.

The apophyseal joints

The apophyseal joints have been clearly shown to be a source of low back pain and referred pain. They are richly innervated from the medial branches of the posterior primary rami. Bradley (1985), who has carefully dissected these nerves, described how the capsule of each joint receives a number of tiny branches from two segmental nerves. For example, the apophyseal joint between the fourth and fifth lumbar vertebrae receives fibres from the third and fourth lumbar nerves.

Being subject to inflammation, like all other synovial joints elsewhere in the body, the apophyseal joints can be a source of pain caused by trauma or arthritis, including degenerative osteoarthritis.

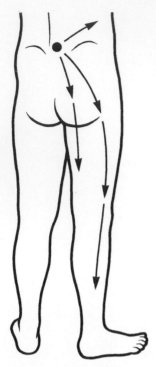

Figure 1.3 Referred pain patterns from an apophyseal joint: illustrating pain radiation pattern from stimulation by injection of the right L4–L5 apophyseal joint (after Brugger, 1962).

Inflammation of these synovial joints produces dull to severe pain, depending on the severity and extent of the inflammation. It can lead to concomitant muscle spasm yet, according to Cailliet, the muscle spasm that accompanies spinal dysfunction is in itself capable of causing pain.

Pain from these joints can be referred to any part of the lower limb (Mooney and Robertson, 1976) as far as the calf and ankle, but most commonly it is referred to the gluteal region and proximal thigh or groin (Figure 1.3).

Bradley and Maigne point out that the medial branch of the posterior ramus, after a course of about 10 mm from its origin, enters and is flattened against the bone in the osseofibrous canal, which is about 6 mm long, located at the inferior border of the transverse process at the root of the articular process. Thus nerve entrapment can occur at this point. Irritation of the medial branch here from arthritic or traumatic joint lesions could refer pain to the structures that it innervates.

Thus there is considerable potential for back pain originating from the apophyseal joints and the medial branch of the posterior ramus.

This important knowledge about the apophyseal joints and the medial branch of the posterior ramus is of clinical significance, since various procedures have been developed to facilitate the diagnosis and the treatment of painful disorders of the back (Figure 1.4).

Local anaesthetic intra-articular diagnostic blocks and subsequent intra-articular corticosteroid injections under X-ray imaging are being employed increasingly in the management of back pain. As a diagnostic and, perhaps, as a therapeutic procedure, the medial branch of the posterior ramus is 'blocked' with local anaesthetic under image intensification. If this nerve block is effective but the pain returns, other methods which block the nerve on a more permanent basis can be performed. This includes cryotherapy (using liquid nitrogen), phenol injections and radio-frequency denervation.

Figure 1.4 Dorsal view of lumbar spine: illustrating techniques of lumbar medial branch blocks and intra-articular apophyseal blocks. The needles on the left are shown adjacent to the medial branches (mb) of the posterior primary rami which innervates the L4–L5 apophyseal joint and those on the right have been introduced into the right L3–L4 and L4–L5 apophyseal joints (courtesy N Bogduk).

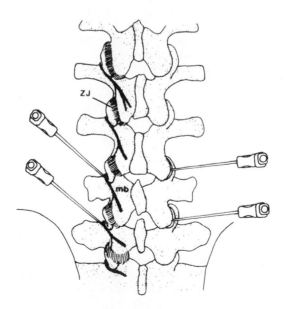

The nervous network of the spine

The various components of the mobile segment are innervated by two main nerves – the posterior primary rami of the spinal nerves and the sinuvertebral nerves (Figure 1.5). The spinal nerve divides outside the intervertebral foramen into anterior and posterior primary rami. The smaller posterior ramus is important within the context of back pain treatment because it innervates accessible components of the posterior compartment, namely the capsule of the apophyseal joints, interspinous ligaments and the fascia and muscle of the back. According to Bradley (1985) and Maigne (1986) the posterior rami innervate all the spinal articulations with the exception of the atlanto-occipital and atlanto-axial articulations, which are innervated by the anterior rami of the corresponding nerves.

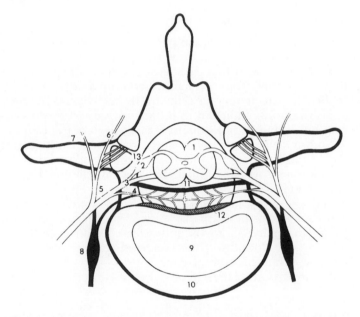

Figure 1.5 The functional unit and nervous network of the spine: showing the relationships of disc, apophyseal joint, spinal cord, nerve roots and the pain-sensitive posterior longitudinal ligament and dura.

1 spinal cord
2 dorsal root ganglion
3 nerve root
4 sinuvertebral nerve
5 posterior primary ramus (PPR)
6 medial branch of PPR
7 lateral branch of PPR
8 sympathetic chain
9 nucleus pulposus
10 annulus fibrosus
11 dura
12 posterior longitudinal ligament
13 apophyseal joint

The posterior primary ramus travels about 6 mm from its origin before dividing into a medial and a lateral branch. The medial branch is important since it supplies branches to the apophyseal joint above and below its course and thereafter innervates the medial group of the posterior spinal muscles and the overlying skin.

The sinuvertebral nerve is formed from branches from a spinal nerve root and the sympathetic truck. The nerve then courses back into the spinal canal through the intervertebral foramen where it divides into a network of fine filaments that fan out in all directions at that level. It supplies the posterior longitudinal ligament, the dura mater and epidural tissues, blood vessels, periosteum, the vertebral body (Stillwell, 1956) and the superficial fibres of the annulus fibrosus (Laxorthes, 1971 and Bogduk, 1983). A summary of the pain-sensitive structures of the mobile segment is illustrated in Figure. 1.6.

Figure 1.6 Pain-sensitive structures of the functional unit: after Cailliet. The tissues labelled (+) are pain-sensitive in that they contain sensory endings that are capable of causing pain when irritated. Tissues labelled (−) are relatively devoid of sensory nerve endings and do not intrinsically cause pain.

IVF = intervertebral foramen containing nerve root (NR)
LF = ligamentum flavum
PLL = posterior longitudinal ligament
ALL = anterior longitudinal ligament
IVD = intervertebral disc
AJ = apophyseal joint
ISL = interspinous ligament
D = dura
VB = vertebral body

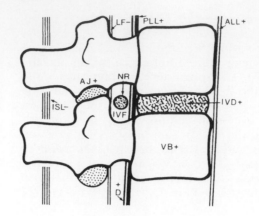

Types of spinal pain

The two basic types of spinal pain are classified simply as radicular pain and non-radicular (or spondylogenic) pain.

Radicular pain is that caused by disorders of spinal nerves and their roots, especially from mechanical compression – for example, sciatica. Radicular pain is very rare in the thoracic spine. If the pain, though appearing to be radicular, is in fact not caused by pressure on a nerve root but is due to reflexogenic reactions, it is pseudoradicular.

Non-radicular or spondylogenic pain is that which originates from any of the components of the vertebrae (spondyles) including joints, the intervertebral disc, ligaments and muscle attachments. An important example of spondylogenic pain is referred pain experienced in an area distal to or removed from the actual source of pain, such as pain experienced in the buttocks from a disorder of an apophyseal joint. Although analogous to visceral referred pain such as appendicitis or renal colic, spondylogenic referred pain must be distinguished clinically from this type of pain.

A comparison of these types of pain is presented in Table 1.1.

Table 1.1 *Comparison of spondylogenic referred pain and radicular pain.*

	ORIGIN	CAUSES	CLINICAL FEATURES
Spondylogenic referred pain	Ligaments Muscles Apophyseal joints Intervertebral discs Dura mater	Inflammation Mechanical compression Mechanical strain	Deep, dull, aching Relieved by rest No localising features No dermatome reference No neurological signs
Radicular pain	Nerve roots Dorsal root ganglia	Mechanical compression Ischaemia	Dermatomal reference Paraesthesia Anaesthesia Neurological signs

Irritation of the primary rami produces changes in the embryo-logical derivatives – the dermatome, myotome and sclerotome of the nerve, manifested respectively in the skin, muscles and periosteum. The affected tissues tend to feel sensitive, thickened and grainy. Hence the importance of palpation of the tissues which can occupy quite separate anatomical locations despite the same innervation.

DISC PROLAPSE AND PAIN PATTERNS

Disc bulging against the posterior ligament and the dura

When a prolapsed disc exerts pressure on the posterior ligament and the dura the consequence is spondylogenic referred pain which is usually experienced in the neck (if of cervical origin) or the low back (lumbar origin) but can be referred over a wider area.

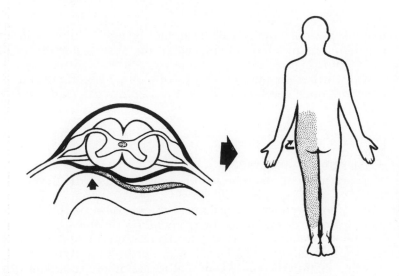

Figure 1.7 Referred pain pattern caused by the disc bulging against the posterior longitudinal ligament and dura. The shaded area indicates possible sites of referred pain.

The pain is usually dull, deep and poorly localised. The dura has no specific dermatomal localisation – for example, in the cervical region the pain is commonly referred to the head, neck, shoulder and mid scapular region. In the lumbar region the pain is usually experienced in the low back, sacro-iliac area and buttocks (Figure 1.7). Less commonly it can be referred to the coccyx, abdomen, groins, and both legs to the calves. It is not referred to the ankle or the foot.

Disc bulging posterolaterally against nerve root

This is a natural route because the annulus fibrosus is no longer reinforced by the posterior ligament. According to Cyriax (1980) and Cailliet (1986), if the disc exerts pressure on the dural sleeve of the nerve root only, the radicular pain is experienced along the course of

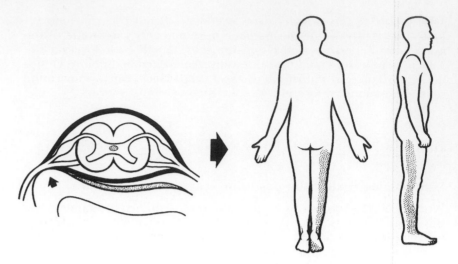

Figure 1.8 Radicular pain pattern caused by the disc bulging against the nerve root. The L5 nerve root is shown in this illustration.

the nerve root, the classic example being sciatica. Pain can be experienced, therefore, in any part of the dermatome of the affected nerve root (Figure 1.8).

With further pressure on the nerve parenchyma there is usually no pain and since conduction down the nerve is affected the following eventuates:

- motor weakness
- absent or sluggish reflexes
- paraesthesia or anaesthesia in the distal end of the dermatome.

The clinical effect of mechanical compression on a nerve root can have a variety of manifestations depending on the state of the nerve (whether normal or damaged), the degree and site of the compression, the types of nerve fibre affected by the pressure and the development of inflammation. Compression of a normal nerve root does not cause pain; however, damaged nerve roots or dorsal root ganglia can be a focus of pain (Table 1.2).

Compression of motor fibres in the nerve will cause weakness of muscles in the corresponding myotomal distribution. Compression of sensory fibres will cause paraesthesia distally with no clear-cut edges and – with increasing pressure – anaesthesia.

In the real world of the clinical presentation of patients with peripheral pain, it is often impossible to delineate the affected nerve root because of overlapping and variations of the classical dermatomal boundaries of nerve roots.

An important consideration is the ability to diagnose rapidly the rare surgical emergency of spinal cord compression. This is characterised by no pain and by distal anaesthesia which may be bilateral. Compression of the cauda equina, on the other hand, can cause pain manifesting as bilateral sciatica, as well as perineal paraesthesia and/or anaesthesia.

Table 1.2 *Pressure effect on neurological structures.*

Spinal cord	No pain
	Distal anaesthesia (can be bilateral)
	Evidence of upper motor neurone lesion
	  – extensor plantar response
	  – spastic gait

Dura	Pain (no dermatome reference)
Dural sleeve of nerve root	Pain (any part of dermatome)
Normal nerve root	No pain Paraesthesia distally (no edge) Anaesthesia (with increased pressure) Motor weakness Sluggish or absent reflexes
Small nerve	No pain Numbness Localised paraesthesia

The minor intervertebral derangement theory of Maigne

An attractive theory has been advanced by Maigne, who proposes the existence, in the involved mobile segment, of a minor intervertebral derangement (MID) which is usually reversed by manipulation. He defines it as 'isolated pain in one intervertebral segment, of a mild character, and due to a minor mechanical cause'.

It is independent of radiological and anatomical disturbances of the segment. The most common clinical situation occurs where a vertebral level is found to be painful and yet to have a normal static and radiological appearance.

The MID always involves one of the two apophyseal joints in the mobile segment, thus initiating nociceptive activity in the posterior primary dermatome and myotome. The overlying skin is tender to pinching and rolling, while the muscles are painful to palpation and feel cordlike and 'grainy'.

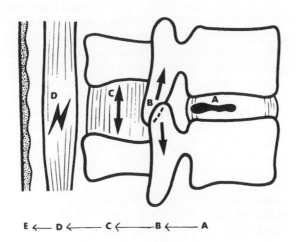

Figure 1.9 Reflex activity from MID in a mobile segment. Apart from the local effect caused by posterior bulging of the disc (A) (which can, per se, be symptomatic or asymptomatic) interference can occur in the apophyseal joint (B) and interspinous ligament (C) leading possibly to muscle spasm (D) and skin changes (E) via the posterior rami.

Maigne points out that the functional ability of the mobile segment depends intimately upon the condition of the intervertebral disc. Thus, if the disc is injured, other elements of the segment will be affected. Even a minimal disc lesion can produce apophyseal joint dysfunction which is a reflex cause of protective muscle spasm and pain in the corresponding segment, with loss of function (Figure 1.9).

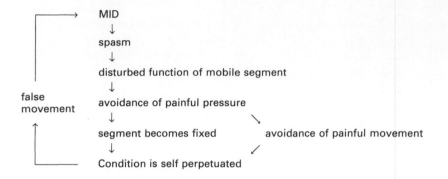

Figure 1.10 Summary of the chain of events initiated by an MID.

In all MIDs there is an element of muscle spasm. The end result is avoidance of painful pressure or movement of the involved segment. This becomes fixed and the condition tends to be self-perpetuating. Similarly, any movement causing a false movement in that segment will re-initiate the process (see Figure 1.10).

THE CONCEPT OF DYSFUNCTION

The therapeutic modalities used in physical therapy of the spine basically treat dysfunction rather than pathology. This normalisation of function is a fundamental principle in musculoskeletal medicine. The dysfunction applies to the joints and often may be regarded as synonymous with mechanical dysfunction. Changes in function may cause profound clinical changes in the absence of any pathology that can be detected by investigation or indeed at surgical exploration.

This joint dysfunction may simply manifest as stiffness, and a stiff joint is a painful joint. Relieving stiffness thus restores function and alleviates pain. According to Professor Karel Lewit of the Neurologic Clinic, Charles University, Prague, 'Function is the result of the correlation and interplay of numerous structures, frequently at distant places in the motor system. Our task, therefore, is to uncover a chain of changes and, if possible, to find the most important link, or links, at any given moment of the "pathogenic chain". It is important to realise that the central nervous system only knows about function, not about structure'.

Because changes in function are reversible in nature it can be expected that, if they are adequately treated, the effect of treatment is immediate, giving the impression of a 'miracle cure'.

It is this concept of spinal dysfunction with which the medical profession has had difficulty coming to terms. This is because one is not treating a pathological condition but a biomechanical abnormality that produces a neurophysiological disorder.

PRACTICE TIPS

- The intervertebral disc is a pain-sensitive structure and internal disruption of the disc can cause intrinsic pain.
- Damage to the dorsal root ganglia by compression can cause a burning pain.
- The clinical effects of the significant protrusion of the nucleus pulposus are usually delayed, occurring, for example, 12 to 24 hours from the time of the injury.
- Torn spinal muscles are rare. Muscular pain is usually due to spasm following injury to the underlying joints.
- Anaesthetic blocks under X-ray control are effective diagnostic techniques for apophyseal joint disorders.
- Spinal manipulation will fail and should be avoided if signs of nerve root involvement are present.
- The sudden onset of 'saddle' paraesthesia and/or anaesthesia (that is, perineal) is suggestive of spinal cord compression.

SUMMARY

Spinal pain is a complex phenomenon and it is not always possible to determine its source reliably. For example, if a patient presents with low back pain and sciatica to the knee, it may be impossible for the clinician to diagnose whether the pain originates from the intervertebral disc, the apophyseal joint or other spondylogenic structures. However, it is possible to recognise basic patterns of pain and this certainly helps facilitate a provisional diagnosis.

Manual procedures on the spine, including injection therapy, require the therapist to have an appropriate working knowledge of the anatomical structures and basic pathophysiology. Increased knowledge implies a better diagnostic acumen – firstly, for distinguishing visceral, vascular and psychogenic causes from the commoner spinal causes and, secondly, for attempting a working diagnostic hypothesis for the dysfunctional (mechanical) causes of spondylogenic pain originating from the moving parts of the spine.

While it is not always possible to differentiate discogenic from apophyseal disorders, a clearer understanding of the pathogenesis leads to a more perceptive and logical clinical methodology, including the selection of appropriate investigations.

Spinal diagnostic tests such as nerve and joint blockade, MRI and CT scanning may be necessary to help establish the origin of the problem.

An important clinical dimension is that of specificity, because many of the treatment modalities presented in this book require specific clinical localisation of the lesion to the affected mobile segment.

2
A diagnostic approach to spinal pain

Contents

A well planned and perceptive diagnostic approach to spinal pain is obviously essential. It behoves the practitioner with a special interest in musculoskeletal disorders of the spine (as, indeed, it behoves any practitioner) to avoid that complacency which might lead to the overlooking of one of the less common causes of spinal pain, especially the life-threatening ones such as dissecting aneurysm, osteomyelitis, malignant disease and pulmonary infarction.

For those practitioners who perform spinal manipulation it is imperative not to manipulate a diseased spine. They have a particular responsibility to be watchful and make a correct diagnosis, which should be achieved by adopting a knowledgeable systematic approach to the history of the pain and to the physical examination.

This does not imply that it is essential to clinically pinpoint the precise cause of musculoskeletal pain, be it apophyseal joints, interspinous ligament or the annulus fibrosus or nucleus pulposus of the intervertebral disc. Accuracy to this level is often impossible, but what is important is to localise the causes and consider carefully non-mechanical causes. Typical examples of important diseases that are often missed include polymyalgia rheumatica, ankylosing spondylitis, metastatic disease, multiple myeloma, multiple sclerosis and peripheral vascular disease.

KEY CHECKPOINTS

- Back pain accounts for at least 5 per cent of all presenting problems in general practice in Australia and 6.5 per cent in Great Britain.
- Approximately 85 per cent of the population will experience back pain at some stage of their life.
- At least 70 per cent of these people will recover completely within one month but recurrences are frequent and have been reported in 40 to 70 per cent of patients.
- The most common age groups are the 30s and 40s, the average age being 42 years.
- The most common cause of back pain is a minor strain to muscles and/or ligaments, but people suffering from this type of back pain usually do not seek medical treatment as most of these soft tissue problems resolve rapidly.
- The main cause of back pain presenting to the doctor is dysfunction of the intervertebral joints of the spine due to injury, also referred to as mechanical back pain (at least 70 per cent).
- The apophyseal (facet) joint has been shown to be a major site of back pain. It is a synovial joint which can cause severe pain if injured, and many modern therapies rely on directing treatment to this joint.
- The second most common cause of back pain is spondylosis (synonymous with osteoarthritis and degenerative back disease). It accounts for about 8 per cent of cases of low back pain and can be alleviated by mobilisation techniques.
- Back pain has to be considered in the three regions – cervical, thoracic and lumbar – because the causes and clinical presentations do show significant regional variations.
- The most common cause of cervical (neck) pain presenting in general practice appears to be dysfunction of the apophyseal joints.
- The most common causes of thoracic (dorsal) back pain are dysfunction of the costo-vertebral joints and dysfunction of the apophyseal joints, with the former considered to be more significant.
- The most common causes of lumbar pain are dysfunction of the apophyseal joint and dysfunction of the intervertebral disc – the exact balance being uncertain.

CAUSES OF BACK PAIN

Knowledge of the causes of back pain is essential in order to build a framework for a diagnostic strategy. The same applies to any painful problem such as headaches, chest pain or abdominal pain: if the practitioner does not understand what is common and what is rare, and what is life-threatening and what is not, then he or she will flounder. So, in addition to a knowledge of the causes of back pain, it is important to know the anatomical function and to have a systematic clinical plan.

Obvious trauma to the back causing deep-seated injuries such as fractures and haematomas will not be discussed in detail but injuries to the soft tissue and the intervertebral joints caused by lifting and twisting, by postural alterations, and following falls or other accidents, will constitute the basis of this book.

There can be a significant difference in aetiology between acute and chronic back pain (pain lasting longer than six weeks). Figure 2.1 outlines important causes of acute back pain, while Figure 2.2 summarises the usual causes of chronic back pain. The acute onset of pain can have sinister implications, especially in the thoracic spine, where various life-threatening cardiopulmonary and vascular events have to be kept in mind. The pulmonary causes of acute pain include spontaneous pneumothorax, pleurisy and pulmonary infarction. Tho-

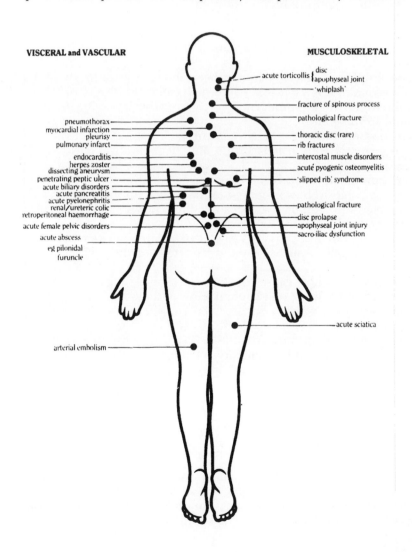

VISCERAL and VASCULAR

MUSCULOSKELETAL

acute torticollis {disc / apophyseal joint
'whiplash'
fracture of spinous process
pathological fracture
thoracic disc (rare)
rib fractures
intercostal muscle disorders
acute pyogenic osteomyelitis
'slipped rib' syndrome
pathological fracture
disc prolapse
apophyseal joint injury
sacro-iliac dysfunction

pneumothorax
myocardial infarction
pleurisy
pulmonary infarct
endocarditis
herpes zoster
dissecting aneurysm
penetrating peptic ulcer
acute biliary disorders
acute pancreatitis
acute pyelonephritis
renal/ureteric colic
retroperitoneal haemorrhage
acute female pelvic disorders
acute abscess
eg pilonidal
furuncle

acute sciatica

arterial embolism

Figure 2.1 Causes of acute back pain (direct trauma excluded).

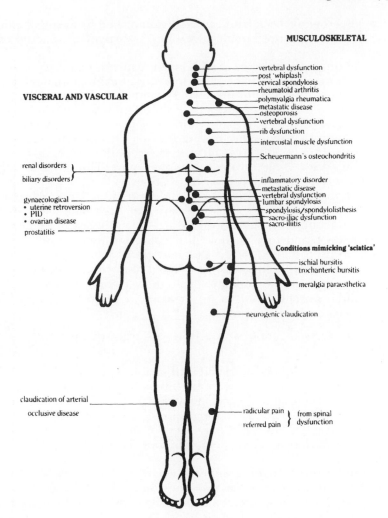

MUSCULOSKELETAL

- vertebral dysfunction
- post 'whiplash'
- cervical spondylosis
- rheumatoid arthritis
- polymyalgia rheumatica
- metastatic disease
- osteoporosis
- vertebral dysfunction
- rib dysfunction
- intercostal muscle dysfunction
- Scheuermann's osteochondritis

- inflammatory disorder
- metastatic disease
- vertebral dysfunction
- lumbar spondylosis
- spondylosis/spondylolisthesis
- sacro-iliac dysfunction
- sacro-iliitis

VISCERAL AND VASCULAR

- renal disorders
- biliary disorders

- gynaecological
  - uterine retroversion
  - PID
  - ovarian disease
- prostatitis

Conditions mimicking 'sciatica'

- ischial bursitis
- trochanteric bursitis
- meralgia paraesthetica
- neurogenic claudication

- claudication of arterial occlusive disease

- radicular pain } from spinal
- referred pain } dysfunction

Figure 2.2 Causes of chronic back pain.

racic back pain may be associated with subacute bacterial endocarditis due to embolic phenomena. The ubiquitous myocardial infarction or acute coronary occlusion may, uncommonly, cause interscapular back pain, while the very painful dissecting or ruptured aortic aneurysm may cause back pain with hypotension. Hepato-biliary and pancreatic disorders – notably biliary colic, acute cholecystitis and acute pancreatitis – can cause acute upper lumbar pain. Similarly, acute renal infection and renal colic can cause pain in this region.

Gynaecological abnormalities, including retroversion and prolapse of the uterus, are not as commonly a cause of back pain as some authorities hold, but nevertheless should be considered in women presenting with chronic low back pain, especially if it radiates to the front of the thighs and is associated with a menstrual abnormality.

Other visceral causes of referred pain to the back include prostatitis, diverticulitis, visceroptosis and malignancy of the oesophagus.

● Viscerogenic back pain can be distinguished from spinal pain by the fact that it is not usually aggravated by activity or relieved by rest.

Various inflammatory disorders can cause spinal pain and thus the practitioner should know how to recognise inflammatory pain. The significant disorders are ankylosing spondylitis and rheumatoid arthritis. Rheumatoid arthritis involves the cervical spine and can be assumed not to involve the thoracic and lumbar spines, although asymptomatic radiological changes in these areas may be present. Uncommonly, Reiter's disease, psoriasis, and the enteropathies ulcerative colitis and Crohn's disease, can involve the lumbar spine. This group is referred to as the seronegative spondyloarthropathies.

Although metabolic causes, including osteomalacia, ochronosis and chondrocalcinosis, are listed as causes of back pain, such causes are most uncommon. The disorders are generally asymptomatic, except when they lead to a pathological compression fracture – typically a fracture in the osteoporotic thoracic spine.

Pathological fractures are associated also with a focus of malignant disease and chronic osteomyelitis in the vertebrae. Malignant disease is usually metastatic but can be primary in origin – notably, multiple myeloma and osteosarcoma.

● The thoracic spine is a significant target of metastatic malignant disease.

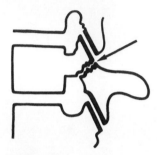

Figure 2.3
Spondylolysis: showing a stress fracture of the pars interarticularis.

Back pain may be associated with various structural anomalies of the lumbosacral spine, such as spina bifida, hemivertebrae, lumbarisation of S1, sacralisation of L5 and spondylolysis. It must be remembered that these conditions are a radiological diagnosis and may not cause pain themselves, but indirectly, because of associated mechanical problems; or they may be a coincidental finding in the presence of another problem.

Spondylolysis is the condition where a defect exists between the upper and lower articular processes on each side of the neural arch (Figure 2.3). If a spontaneous displacement or shift occurs here, the problem is termed spondylolisthesis (Figure 2.4), which can cause pain by the stretching of intervertebral ligaments and nerve roots. Not all cases of spondylolisthesis cause back pain.

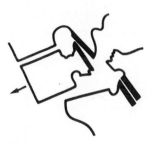

Figure 2.4
Spondylolisthesis: showing a shift of one vertebra on another.

● Think of herpes zoster for the unusual presentation of radicular pain, especially of the thorax, in an older person.

A common pitfall for the practitioner is herpes zoster (shingles) which causes radicular pain for some days before the vesicular eruption appears. This is more likely to be present in the thoracic area of an older person.

Psychogenic or non-organic causes of back pain can present a complex dilemma in diagnosis and management. The causes may be apparent from the incongruous behaviour and personality of the patient, but often the diagnosis is reached by a process of exclusion. There is obviously some functional overlay to everyone with acute or chronic pain – hence the importance of appropriate reassurance to these patients that their problem invariably subsides with time and that they do not have cancer.

Back pain in children

The common mechanical disorders of the intervertebral joints, especially acute torticollis and thoracic dysfunction, cause back pain in children, which must always be taken seriously. Like abdominal pain and leg pain, it can be related to psychogenic factors, so this possibility should be considered by diplomatically evaluating problems at home, at school or with sport.

Especially in children under the age of ten, it is very important to exclude organic disease. Infections such as osteomyelitis and tuberculosis are rare possibilities, and 'discitis' has to be considered. This painful condition can be idiopathic, but can also be caused by the spread of infection from a vertebral body. It has characteristic radiological changes.

Tumours causing back pain include the benign osteoid osteoma and the malignant osteogenic sarcoma. Osteoid osteoma is a very small tumour with a radiolucent nucleus that is sharply demarcated from the surrounding area of sclerotic bone. Although more common in the long bones of the leg, it can occur in the spine.

In older children and adolescents the organic causes of back pain are more likely to be inflammatory, congenital, or from developmental anomalies and trauma.

Inflammatory disorders to consider are juvenile ankylosing spondylitis and spinal osteochondritis (Scheuermann's disease), which may affect adolescent males in the lower thoracic and upper lumbar spines. The latter condition may be asymptomatic, but can be associated with back pain, especially as the patient grows older.

It is important to screen adolescent children for idiopathic scoliosis, which may be without associated backache. A prolapsed intervertebral disc, which can occur (uncommonly) in adolescents, can be very unusual in its presentation. There is often marked spasm, with a stiff spine and lateral deviation which may be out of proportion to the relatively lower degree of pain.

Back pain in the elderly

Traumatic spinal dysfunction is still the most common cause of back pain in the elderly and may represent a recurrence of earlier dysfunction. It is amazing how commonly disc prolapse and apophyseal joint injury can present in the aged. However, degenerative joint disease is very common and, if advanced, can present as spinal stenosis with claudication and nerve root irritation due to narrowed intervertebral foraminae.

Special problems to consider in the older person are:

- malignant disease, e.g. multiple myeloma
- occlusive disease, presenting as leg pain
- osteoporosis
- vertebral pathological fractures
- degenerative spondylolisthesis
- Paget's disease (may be asymptomatic).

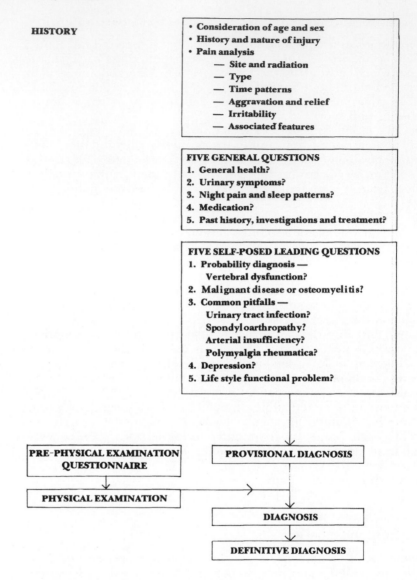

HISTORY

- Consideration of age and sex
- History and nature of injury
- Pain analysis
    — Site and radiation
    — Type
    — Time patterns
    — Aggravation and relief
    — Irritability
    — Associated features

FIVE GENERAL QUESTIONS
1. General health?
2. Urinary symptoms?
3. Night pain and sleep patterns?
4. Medication?
5. Past history, investigations and treatment?

FIVE SELF-POSED LEADING QUESTIONS
1. Probability diagnosis —
    Vertebral dysfunction?
2. Malignant disease or osteomyelitis?
3. Common pitfalls —
    Urinary tract infection?
    Spondyloarthropathy?
    Arterial insufficiency?
    Polymyalgia rheumatica?
4. Depression?
5. Life style functional problem?

PRE-PHYSICAL EXAMINATION QUESTIONNAIRE

PROVISIONAL DIAGNOSIS

PHYSICAL EXAMINATION

DIAGNOSIS

DEFINITIVE DIAGNOSIS

Figure 2.5 The diagnostic process for back pain.

THE DIAGNOSTIC APPROACH

A working background knowledge of the preceding causes of back pain and their clinical patterns permits the practitioner to develop a logical and confident approach to the history and examination for the individual patient. Careful attention to detail will help alert one to those nuances that indicate a different picture to the norm and thus point the way to the diagnosis of an uncommon disorder.

Diagnosis usually depends on the patient's description of the pain, which may not be altogether accurate, and on observation of the patient's behaviour during certain manoeuvres. This includes watching the patient proceed from the waiting room into the consulting room, noting his or her movements and demeanour during the consultation, and observing the manner of leaving.

It is important to appreciate that there are significant differences from the normal medical examination. In addition to the routine medical history, special attention must be focused on the behaviour of the symptoms and the mechanical factors involved.

As well as providing a diagnosis, the assessment should cover the diagnosis of exclusion – for example, of malignant disease. While the history informs us what area to examine, the aim of the physical examination is to determine the specific level of provocation which reproduces the patient's symptoms. The key element to achieve this is digital palpation whereby the examiner is feeling for altered joint play, which presents as pain and stiffness. This is often referred to as the zone of irritation and there are accompanying soft tissue changes, in the form of skin and subcutaneous tenderness, as well as myotendinitis.

THE HISTORY

Initially the overall patient assessment is most important, because assessment of his or her back pain, be it acute or chronic, demands a full understanding of the patient. This includes such features as age, sex, occupation, height:weight ratio, reactions to stress and pain, and his or her social, family and work status. One must relate this information to the amount of incapacity attributed to the back pain.

We must bear in mind that back pain is a symptom of an underlying functional, organic or psychological disease. Preoccupation with organic causation of symptoms may lead to serious errors in the assessment of patients with back pain. The possibility of depressive illness, masquerading as back pain, should always be kept in mind.

Many patients presenting with acute back pain are in such agony that making them comfortable and affording symptomatic relief should be the first consideration, before subjecting them to a thorough examination. Similarly, patients with chronic back pain may be silently anxious (occasionally, distraught with fear) that they have cancer, and this fact should be considered in their management.

The pain should be analysed in the traditional way of the diagnostic evaluation of pain: namely, site and radiation, onset and offset, type (quality and intensity), frequency and duration, precipitating factors, aggravating and relieving factors and associated features.

It is important to focus on the main presenting complaint. So often patients presenting with back pain complain of multifocal sites of musculoskeletal pain. To establish the prime problem, ask the patient to point to the exact areas of the pain with one finger and then to indicate areas to which the pain spreads.

Consideration of age

The age of the patient may provide a pointer to the aetiology of their back pain. Acute vertebral dysfunction, including a disc prolapse, can affect anyone from the age of 16 to 80, especially in the middle years. Similarly, psychogenic causes can straddle all age groups.

Children under the age of 13 may suffer from discitis, a febrile illness (e.g. tonsillitis), urinary tract infections, congenital abnormalities and postural problems.

In the teenage group consider Scheuermann's disease, ankylosing spondylitis (especially in males), structural defects (such as spondylolisthesis), drug addiction, malingering, and dysmenorrhoea, urinary and pelvic infection (especially in females).

The older the patient, the more likely one is to encounter malignant disease, degenerative disease (spondylosis) and arterial vascular disease leading to claudication.

If any patient over the age of 50 presents with back pain, always consider the possibility of malignant disease. For women over 65, consider the possibility of a stress fracture secondary to osteoporosis and, for men over that age, consider prostatic disease.

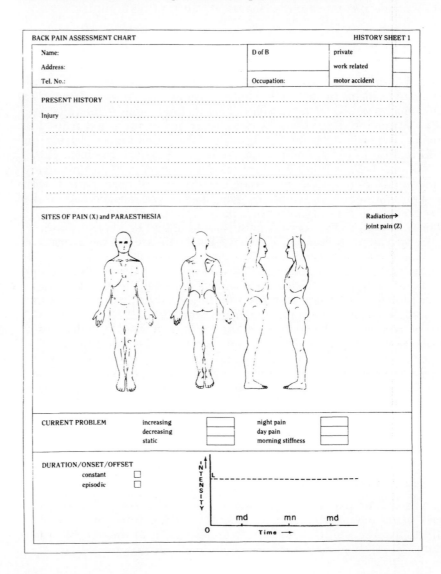

Figure 2.6 Back pain assessment chart – history sheets.

All patients over 60 (especially women) presenting with neck and shoulder girdle pain should be considered as possibly suffering from polymyalgia rheumatica until proven otherwise.

History and nature of injury

Where there is a history of injury, the mode of onset and history of injury is significant. It is important to consider any past history of back injury, and especially the immediate trauma (if any) that preceded the onset of this pain. A dramatically sudden onset is always suggestive of a

---

BACK PAIN ASSESSMENT CHART   HISTORY SHEET 2

AGGRAVATING AND RELIEVING FACTORS

    Agg by .... Eas by ....
    ....
    ....

EFFECT OF LIFESTYLE FACTORS

standing		cough/sneeze	
walking		straining	
sitting		tension/stress	
lying		rest	
bending		warmth	
exercise		relaxation	

ASSOCIATED SYMPTOMS

malaise		abdominal pain		urinary	
weight loss		joint pain		headache	
fever		diarrhoea		dizziness	
fatigue		rash		numbness	

PAST HISTORY ....
....
....
....

Specific:	childhood arthritis		TB		Treatment:	MUGA	
	rheumatic fever		colitis			epidural	
	psoriasis		R arthritis			operation	
	diabetes mellitus		carcinoma			manual	

DRUG HISTORY

| | analgesics | | steroids | |
| | anti-coagulants | | NSAIDs | |

PSYCHO SOCIAL CHECK LIST

| Problems at: | work | | attitude | | stress | | depression | |
| | home | | motivation | | anxiety | | abnormal behaviour | |

INVESTIGATION RESULTS

mechanical disruption such as a disc prolapse or subluxation of an apophyseal joint (especially the latter). This event is unlikely to have a serious cause, with the exception of a spontaneous vertebral collapse in an elderly woman with osteoporosis.

Many back problems, notably a disc prolapse which is due to a slow nucleus pulposus protrusion, have a delayed onset of pain from the time of injury. This may vary from a few to many hours. The classic example is the patient who woke with severe back pain after lifting a heavy object the day before when, although he felt something give in his back, he carried on without any discomfort.

These pain relationships are especially significant in the neck following a motor vehicle accident. Consider, for example, the patient seen on day five who is getting worse (with neck and arm pain following mild neck pain on day one) compared with the reverse situation in another patient who is rapidly improving.

Subacute pain, increasing relentlessly without relief, suggests a progressive lesion, usually inflammatory or neoplastic (benign or malignant). If the pain is not affected by activity a neoplasm is most likely.

Table 2.1 *Injury and back pain: possible correlations between the nature of the injury and the likely effect of such an injury.*

NATURE OF INJURY	LIKELY EFFECT
Twisting force, if violent	Muscular tear ± apophyseal joint injury Fractured transverse or spinous process

Lifting strain	Ligamentous injury including
	  (a) posterior longitudinal ligament
	  (b) interspinous ligament (sprung back)
	Disc injury

Lifting and twisting strain with spine flexed	Apophyseal joint injury Intervertebral disc prolapse
Crushing force	Bone injury – compression fracture
Direct force	Soft tissue injury Bone injury including fracture
Heavy fall while seated	Coccygeal injury

The nature of the preceding injury may provide a clue to the possible diagnosis (Table 2.1). Don't forget, when dealing with the very young or the very old, that trauma may be unreported.

Site and radiation of pain

With back pain it must be realised that the actual localisation of pain may differ from its anatomical site, so that finding the source of the pain is difficult. Sacro-iliac strain and coccydynia, for example, have been favoured diagnoses mainly because pain and tenderness is experienced over the sacro-iliac joint and the coccyx respectively. However, the pain is usually referred from other sites, perhaps from an upper or lower disc prolapse exerting pressure on the posterior longitudinal ligament or dura mater (Figure 1.7), or from dysfunction of an apophyseal joint (Figure 1.3).

Confusion in diagnosis arises when lesions at various levels can refer pain distally and anteriorly – for example, a lesion of the mobile segment at the thoraco-lumbar junction can cause referred pain to the abdomen or groin and can mimic appendicitis and testicular pain. Similarly, lesions of T8, T9 or T10 can mimic biliary pain and lead to unnecessary cholecystectomies.

Nerve root compression leading to radicular pain can be easier to recognise, especially in the cervical and lumbar spines.

Type of pain

The nature of the pain may reveal its likely origin. Ask such questions as 'is the pain intense or is it a dull ache?' Establish where the pain is worst – whether it is central (proximal) or peripheral.

Aching throbbing pain suggests inflammation, including spondylosis, whereas a deep aching diffuse pain is characteristic of referred pain (for example, dysmenorrhoea) or a disc prolapse against adjacent painful tissues. A superficial steady diffuse pain is typical of local pain – for example, muscular strain – while boring deep pain arises from bone disorders like neoplasia and Paget's disease.

Table 2.2 *Comparison of the patterns of pain for inflammatory and mechanical causes of low back pain.*

FEATURE	INFLAMMATION	MECHANICAL
History	Insidious onset	Precipitating injury/previous episodes
Nature	Aching, throbbing	Deep dull ache, sharp if root compression
Stiffness	Severe, prolonged morning stiffness	Moderate, transient
Effect of rest	Exacerbates	Relieves
Effect of activity	Relieves	Exacerbates
Radiation	More localised, bilateral or alternating	Tends to be diffuse, unilateral
Intensity	Night, early morning	End of day, following activity
Effect of NSAIDs	Effective	Variable effect – usually minimal

Root compression pain – for example, sciatica – is a more intense sharp or stabbing pain, often superimposed on the dull ache of referred pain.

A comparison of the significant features of the two common most types of pain – mechanical and inflammatory – is presented in Table 2.2.

Time patterns and present state

The time pattern, including the onset, duration and offset of the pain should be established. Specific questions include:

- What is the relationship of the pain to the time of day? (This can be charted on a small daily graph and include an indication of pain intensity.)
- Is night pain present? If so, how long does the pain continue into the day? Is it associated with morning stiffness and how long does the stiffness last?
- Is the pain continuous or episodic? If episodic, is it on/off or more intense on a constant background of a dull ache, and what is its frequency, duration and regularity? Are the episodes related to specific activities?
- Is the patient presently improving, or is the situation static or getting worse? This question is important since it foreshadows the management plan. For example, if the pain is getting worse and the patient is receiving treatment the problem could reflect an incorrect diagnosis or inappropriate treatment.

Aggravating and relieving factors

Factors influencing pain are vital features to elicit in the history because it may be possible to identify patterns that lead to the diagnosis. The patient should be directly asked 'What makes the pain worse?' and 'What makes the pain better?' Following the general open-ended question, direct questions about specific factors should be asked. These factors include stress, movement, activity, bending and twisting (for example making the beds, vacuuming, gardening), sitting, walking, standing, sleeping, turning over in bed, coughing, sneezing and straining at the toilet.

Coughing, sneezing and straining often aggravate pain due to space-occupying lesions, including disc protrusion. Pain provoked by walking suggests claudication (vertebral stenosis or ischaemia) or instability, such as spondylolisthesis. Some of the aggravating and relieving factors for chronic back pain are summarised in Table 2.3.

The question of *irritability* must be addressed (see Chapter 3). This is achieved by estimating how easily the pain is triggered by various activities.

Back pain referred from visceral disease which is usually experienced in the abdomen and flanks may be modified by the state of activity of the viscera. Posture and movements of the back have relatively little effect on the pain. For example, back pain affected by eating habits is suggestive of a penetrating peptic ulcer.

Table 2.3 *Back pain: aggravating and relieving factors and some conclusions.*

AGGRAVATING FACTORS	RELIEVING FACTORS	THINK OF ...
Coughing Sneezing Straining	Lying flat	Disc prolapse Intrathecal tumour (rare)
Sitting forward position	Assuming upright position	Disc prolapse Ligamentous strain
Standing Walking	Sitting	Spondylolisthesis
Activity – Walking (especially uphill)	Remaining stationary (including standing)	Claudication (a) gluteal (ischaemia) (b) cauda equina (spinal canal stenosis)
Turning over in bed in morning	Flexed hips and knees over pillow	Disc prolapse
Movement in any direction	Immobility	Malignant disease Fracture Osteomyelitis

Associated features

Relevant symptoms that are often associated with causes of back pain should be elicited during history taking and correlated with the nature of the pain.

Fever, for example, might be associated with urinary tract infection, osteomyelitis, malignant disease (such as renal carcinoma, myeloma and lymphoma), acute tonsillitis and, indeed, any systemic febrile illness which may cause back pain as part of its symptom complex.

The presence of obvious serious constitutional symptoms such as debility, malaise and weight loss should point to malignant disease, but other diagnoses to consider include osteomyelitis (pyogenic, tuberculosis, brucellosis), endogenous depression, pelvic abscess and (rarely) ankylosing spondylitis.

Urinary symptoms such as frequency and dysuria indicate urinary tract infection, prostatic carcinoma or acute prostatitis.

Respiratory symptoms such as cough and dyspnoea might be associated with pulmonary carcinoma, pleurisy with pneumonia, pulmonary infarction and a dissecting aneurysm.

Sensory disturbances of the lower limb are suggestive of a disc prolapse with nerve compression, a subtle neurological disease such as multiple sclerosis and, if acute, embolic arterial obstruction.

For neck pain, relevant associated symptoms such as headache, vertigo and visual disturbances may be significant. Vertigo is of special concern if manipulative treatment of the cervical spine is contemplated.

Evidence of the rash of herpes zoster should be sought, particularly where suspected in an older person.

THE DIAGNOSTIC PROCESS – A USEFUL STRATEGY

Five self-posed leading questions

Whenever a patient presents for the first time with back pain, the practitioner should ask himself, or herself, five leading questions. These form the basis of a 'fail-safe strategy'.

Question 1: What is the probability diagnosis?

Traumatic musculoskeletal disorders leading to vertebral dysfunction are the most common cause of back pain. Muscle or ligament tears are uncommon causes of acute or chronic pain presenting to the doctor. Most problems involve the joints of the spine, either the apophyseal joint or the intervertebral joint where disc prolapse applies pressure to adjacent pain-sensitive structures or the costo-vertebral joint of the thoracic spine.

Question 2: What serious disorder must not be missed?

It is imperative not to overlook malignant disease, especially if physical therapy is contemplated. The usual clue is unremitting back pain at night as well as during the day, especially if the patient is elderly. Malignancies include myeloma and secondary metastases from primary tumours in the prostate, breast, lung, kidney or thyroid or from a melanoma. It is of special significance with pain in the thoracic spine. Similarly it is vital not to overlook infection such as spinal tuberculosis or osteomyelitis.

Question 3: What conditions are often missed? (The pitfalls of diagnosis)

Inflammatory disorders must be kept in mind, especially the spondyloarthropathies which include psoriatic arthropathy, ankylosing spondylitis, Reiter's disease, inflammatory bowel disorders such as ulcerative colitis and Crohn's disease, and reactive arthritis. The spondyloarthropathies are more common than appreciated and must be considered in the younger person presenting with features of inflammatory back pain, i.e. pain at rest, relieved by activity. The old trap of confusing claudication in the buttocks and legs due to a high arterial obstruction with sciatica must be avoided.

The possibility of a urinary tract infection must be considered in upper lumbar pain, especially if the patient is a young woman and pregnant. Dysuria and frequent micturition are not always present with a urinary infection.

Polymyalgia rheumatica should be considered in the older person presenting with pain around the neck and shoulder girdle.

General pitfalls:

● Being unaware of the characteristic symptoms of inflammation and thus misdiagnosing one of the spondyloarthropathies.

- Overlooking the early development of malignant disease or osteomyelitis. If suspected and an X-ray is normal a radionuclide scan should detect the problem.
- Failing to realise that mechanical dysfunction and osteoarthritis can develop simultaneously, producing a combined pattern of pain.
- Overlooking anticoagulants as a cause of a severe bleed around the nerve roots, and corticosteroids leading to osteoporosis.
- Not recognising back pain as a presenting feature of the drug addict.

Question 4: Is the patient depressed?

Depression often masquerades as back pain. Does this patient have a past history or family history of depression or other psychological disorders?

Question 5: Is the patient trying to tell me something?

The patient might be unduly stressed, not coping with life or malingering. It may be necessary to probe beneath the surface of the presenting problem. Does the patient have financial or emotional problems causing stress?

General considerations

Bearing the five self-posed leading questions in mind, the practitioner should ask many questions of the patient during the history taking but there are five matters which should always be taken into consideration for patients presenting with back pain.

General health

The patient's general state of well-being should be considered: this includes symptoms such as malaise, fever, loss of weight and reduced energy.

Urinary symptoms

This consideration applies especially to women and to older patients of both sexes. The symptoms to note are dysuria, frequency, and incontinence.

Night pain and sleep patterns

This important question provides considerable information about the patient's problem and might be a pointer to neoplasia or non-organic causes such as anxiety and depression. The presence of stiffness and the effect of turning over in bed is significant for inflammatory disorders and more severe mechanical disorders such as a disc prolapse.

Medication

This is an essential question. The specific drugs to consider are analgesics, corticosteroids, other anti-inflammatory agents, anti-coagulants and self-medication with opiates and alcohol. It must be remembered that acute back pain may be the mode of presentation of a drug addict. Corticosteroid therapy predisposes to osteoporosis which in turn predisposes to a pathological fracture of a vertebrae. Rarely, an analgesic nephropathy has been known to cause renal papillary necrosis with ureteric colic presenting as acute back and loin pain.

Past history

The past history, including investigations and treatment, should be carefully evaluated. This applies particularly to similar previous episodes and includes past behaviour, outcome, treatment, investigations and whether full or partial recovery took place. The behaviour of the previous symptoms will provide an indication for the management of the current episode.

It is important to establish the outcome of any previous injection therapy, surgery and manual procedures. The presence of a previous inflammatory episode would be relevant and evidence of childhood arthritis, possible rheumatoid arthritis (for example, monoarticular arthritis, carpal tunnel syndrome), psoriasis, manifestations of Reiter's disease and inflammatory bowel disease should be sought.

A past history of rheumatic fever, tuberculosis and diabetes mellitus should be considered.

It is appropriate to consider the *family history*, since some arthropathies have a genetic or familial factor. Such diseases include rheumatoid arthritis, Crohn's disease and ulcerative colitis, ankylosing spondylitis and psoriasis.

THE PRE-PHYSICAL EXAMINATION QUESTIONNAIRE

The practitioner's completion of the pre-physical examination questionnaire is a very useful procedure which reinforces the accuracy of the diagnostic process and sets an appropriate course for the physical examination. It incorporates the essential components of the five self-posed leading questions and has an inbuilt safety mechanism which keeps the therapist from overlooking important causes less usually encountered.

It directs the therapist towards the importance of both the organic and the non-organic (functional) components of the patient's problem – that is, consideration of the whole person and what the problem means to that patient.

It helps one take into account the question of irritability (see Chapter 3) and thus assists in establishing the degree of vigour with which the physical examination can be performed.

It addresses the question of possible visceral causes or metastatic disease and, hence, the additional responsibility of extending the physical examination to sites other than the spine and the limbs. This

---

PRE-PHYSICAL EXAMINATION QUESTIONNAIRE

1. What musculoskeletal (MS) structures lie under the painful area?

   Joints

   Muscles

   Ligaments

   Bursa

2. What other musculoskeletal structures are capable of referring symptoms to this area?

3. Possible other non-musculoskeletal causes

   under the area of pain?

   distal but capable of referring?

4. What is the probability diagnosis?

5. Other possible diagnoses

   Checklist (not to be missed)

   Malignant disease

   Ankylosing spondylitis

   Arterial insufficiency

   Rheumatoid arthritis

   Polymyalgia rheumatica

   Depression

6. Is the history consistent with the severity of the symptoms?   Yes [   ]   No [   ]

7. Do you consider there is a functional element involved?   Yes [   ]   No [   ]

   If yes, to what degree?   Mild [   ]   Moderate [   ]   Severe [   ]   Total [   ]

8. Are non-organic (functional) tests likely in this patient?   Yes [   ]   No [   ]

9. What is the *irritability* of the pain?   Low [   ]   Moderate [   ]   High [   ]

10. Will you be able to:

    Reproduce the patient's complaint?   Yes [   ]   No [   ]

    Find a comparable sign?   Yes [   ]   No [   ]

    Find an appropriate level?   Yes [   ]   No [   ]

11. The examination: will it need to be: Gentle [   ]   Moderate [   ]   Rigorous [   ]

12. Is there more than one area of pain?

    If so, are they related or separate?

13. Is there any radicular or nerve root pain?   Yes [   ]   No [   ]

14. Will a neurological examination of the limb be necessary?   Yes [   ]   No [   ]

15. Will a vascular examination of the lower limb be necessary?   Yes [   ]   No [   ]

Figure 2.7 Pre-physical examination questionnaire.

---

may include a rectal examination and a vascular examination of the abdomen and lower limbs.

The authors recommend that a few minutes be set aside for the therapist to complete this questionnaire for every new patient. The questionnaire is presented in Figure 2.7.

THE PHYSICAL EXAMINATION

The all-important physical examination which will be presented as a brief overview in this chapter will be described in detail for each section of the spine in later chapters, namely the cervical spine (Chapter 9), the thoracic spine (Chapter 16), and the lumbo-sacral spine (Chapter 23).

The basic aims of the physical examination are

● to reproduce the patient's symptoms and
● to detect the level of the dysfunction

by provocation of the affected joints or tissues, and are obviously most applicable for back pain of mechanical origin.

The main components of the physical examination are:

1. Inspection
2. Active movements
   forward flexion
   extension   } to reproduce the patient's
   lateral flexion (R and L)   symptoms
   rotation (R and L)
3. Provocative tests
4. Palpation   } to detect level of dysfunction
5. Passive movement
6. Neurological testing of limbs (if appropriate)
7. Testing of related joints (shoulder, hip, sacro-iliac)
8. General medical examination.

See Figure 2.8 (Back pain assessment chart – the physical examination).

1.   Inspection

Every clue is useful in this aspect of the examination. Is there an observable abnormality that could explain (or contribute to) the patient's problem?

Some information about the patient can be obtained by observation in the waiting room. If the patient is found standing rather than sitting, then a disc prolapse is a significant possibility. As the patient arises from the chair in the waiting room and walks to the consulting room much information can be gained about the severity of the back complaint. It is often possible to diagnose an acute disc lesion by the movement which is usually guarded, slow and deliberate, so that jarring is avoided.

If the movements are bizarre and exaggerated, hysteria, depression or malingering should be suspected. Careful note should be taken of the manner of getting on and off the couch. Some patients can be caught unguarded, getting off the couch with an ease incompatible with their supposed degree of disability.

The patient should be stripped to a minimum of clothing so that a careful examination of the back can be made. This essentially involves the basic procedure of *look*, *feel* and *move*. Examination of other relevant parts of the body should not be neglected.

2.   Active movements

These are movements performed by the patient with the aims of reproducing the symptoms and of assessing the general degree of

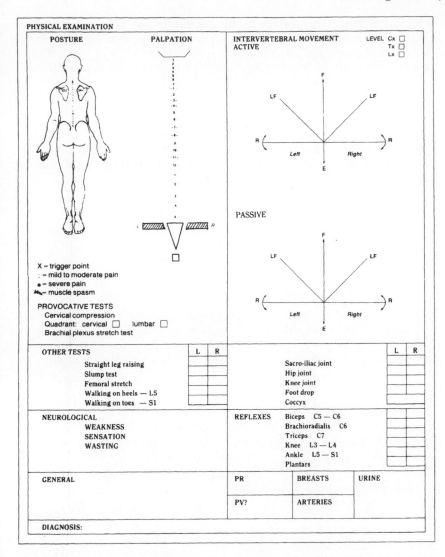

PHYSICAL EXAMINATION

POSTURE   PALPATION

X = trigger point
: = mild to moderate pain
● = severe pain
〰 = muscle spasm

PROVOCATIVE TESTS
  Cervical compression
  Quadrant: cervical ☐   lumbar ☐
  Brachial plexus stretch test

INTERVERTEBRAL MOVEMENT   LEVEL Cx ☐
ACTIVE   Tx ☐
                                 Lx ☐

PASSIVE

OTHER TESTS	L	R			L	R
Straight leg raising			Sacro-iliac joint			
Slump test			Hip joint			
Femoral stretch			Knee joint			
Walking on heels — L5			Foot drop			
Walking on toes — S1			Coccyx			

NEUROLOGICAL			REFLEXES	Biceps C5 — C6		
WEAKNESS				Brachioradialis C6		
SENSATION				Triceps C7		
WASTING				Knee L3 — L4		
				Ankle L5 — S1		
				Plantars		

GENERAL	PR	BREASTS	URINE
	PV?	ARTERIES	

DIAGNOSIS:

Figure 2.8 Back pain assessment chart – the physical examination.

restriction of pain on biomechanical movements. There are some differences in these movements between the three general areas of the spine.

3. Provocation tests

These are employed only when no symptoms have been produced by full active movements and additional strategies are required to reproduce the symptoms.

The provocation can initially be undertaken with gentle overpressure by applying a moderate yet firm passive force at the end range of the movement. Sometimes the symptoms are present only at the end range which the patient tends to avoid by a movement falling short of this point.

Should gentle overpressure fail to reproduce the pain, greater stress on the structure can be achieved by coupling movements in two or three directions – for example, the quadrant test. This much firmer provocation test, which has considerable capacity to reproduce the patient's pain, is described in Chapters 9 and 23.

4.   Palpation

This essential and sensitive component of the examination helps to locate the correct level of segmental dysfunction by examining the components of the dysfunction, namely pain, stiffness and muscle spasm. No other part of the examination can achieve this.

5.   Passive movement

Following palpation, passive movement (that is, movement initiated by the examiner) assists in assessing the degree of segmental stiffness or hypomobility.

6.   Neurological examination

The neurological examination of limbs is performed if the symptoms and signs point to neurological dysfunction. Such indications include pain below the elbow or knee, paraesthesia, anaesthesia or weakness in the limbs. An important aspect is to determine contra-indications to manual therapy.

7.   Testing of related joints

To determine if pain arises from related joints such as the shoulder joint, sacro-iliac or hip joints instead of, or in addition to, the spine, it is necessary in some instances to test these joints.

8.   General medical examination

The general examination is necessary for a complete assessment, in some patients, to obtain a total picture of their health and exclude other possible diagnoses.

Whether a general examination is required can depend on which part of the back is affected – for example, a patient presenting with thoracic back pain may need a thorough examination of the chest.

Likely sources of metastases should be carefully checked. It is good practice to perform a routine urine examination (protein, sugar and blood) on all patients presenting with low back pain.

INVESTIGATIONS

Investigations for back pain can be classified into three broad groups:

● front line screening tests
● specific disease investigation
● procedural and pre-procedural diagnostic tests.

Screening tests

These important tests are ordered to exclude serious disease and to obtain an overall picture of the patient's condition.

They include:

- plain X-ray   } for *ACUTE* pain
- urine examination
- erythrocyte sedimentation rate (ESR)   } for *CHRONIC* pain
- serum alkaline phosphatase
- prostatic specific antigen (in males)

Table 2.4 *Typical radiological and laboratory findings for important causes of back pain.*

	PLAIN X-RAY	WCC	Hb	ESR	SERUM CALCIUM	SERUM PHOSPHATE	ALKALINE PHOSPHATASE
Mechanical	Normal or degeneration	N	N	N	N	N	N
Neoplastic Myeloma	Rounded, punched or mottled ± osteoporosis	N	↓	↑↑↑	N rarely ↑	N	N or ↑
Metastases	Sclerotic or porotic lesions	N or ↑	N or ↓	↑	N rarely ↑	N	↑
Inflammatory Ankylosing spondylitis	Sacro-iliitis (sclerosis SIJ) bamboo spine (late)	N	N rarely ↓	↑	N	N	N
Reiter's disease	Sacro-iliitis	N	N	↑	N	N	N
Infective Pyogenic osteomyelitis	Localised decalcification, subperiosteal calcification	↑	N or ↓	↑	N	N	N
Polymyalgia rheumatica	Normal	N	N rarely ↓	↑↑↑	N	N	N
Osteoporosis	Normal (up to 30%) or demineralisation ? Vertebral collapse	N	N	N	N	N	N
Osteomalacia	Demineralisation, osteoid seams	N	N	N	N or ↓	↓	↑
Paget's disease	Sclerotic (dense) expanded bone	N	N	N	N rarely ↑	N	↑↑↑

WCC, white cell count; ESR, erythrocyte sedimentation rate.

The urine examination can simply be an office dipstick urinalysis for albumin, glucose, blood and nitrite. The purpose is to screen for urinary infection, while albuminuria may provide a clue to multiple myeloma.

The plain X-rays should be taken in the erect and supine positions. The erect position is important to detect an early spondylolisthesis.

A summary of the typical results of investigations for various diseases causing back pain is presented in Table 2.4. An examination of this table indicates why the above tests are the most informative and economical screening tests and why some that are often ordered (such as full blood tests and serum calcium and phosphate) are not so relevant. The chest X-ray would be an important screening test for some causes of thoracic back pain.

Specific disease investigation

Such tests include:

- peripheral arterial studies
- HLA-B27 antigen test for spondyloarthropathies
- rheumatoid factor for rheumatoid arthritis
- serum electrophoresis for multiple myeloma
- brucella agglutination test
- blood culture for pyogenic infection and infective endocarditis
- bone scanning to demonstrate inflammatory or neoplastic disease and infections (e.g. osteomyelitis) before changes are apparent on plain X-ray
- tuberculosis studies
- X-rays of shoulder and hip joint
- electromyographic (EMG) studies to screen leg pain and differentiate neurological diseases from nerve compression syndromes.

Procedural and pre-procedural diagnostic tests

These tests should be kept in reserve for chronic disorders, especially mechanical disorders, that remain undiagnosed and unabated, and where surgical intervention is planned for a disc prolapse requiring removal.

Depending on availability and merit, such tests include:

- computerised tomography (CT scan)
- myelography or radiculography
- discography
- magnetic resonance imaging (MRI)
- radio-isotope scanning
- technetium pyrophosphate scan of sacro-iliac joint (SIJ) for ankylosing spondylitis
- selective anaesthetic block of apophyseal joint under image intensification
- selective anaesthetic block of medial branches of posterior primary rami and other nerve roots.

SUMMARY

The practitioner needs to have a perceptive diagnostic strategy for managing the patient presenting with back pain because it represents one of the most complex areas of medicine and one with a weight of responsibility. It is complex because the mechanical causes are hard to differentiate in many patients, and the responsibility springs from the fact that a diseased spine must on no account be subjected to manual therapy, or to other perhaps questionable therapies used by many practitioners.

It is, however, the moving parts of the back which are the most common origin of back pain at the primary care level, following dysfunction due to acute trauma or simply chronic wear and tear. In order to recognise other causes which may be life-threatening or cause long-term suffering if the diagnosis is delayed, the practitioner must have a diagnostic plan based on a knowledge of the causes and patterns of disease. Diagnosis by exclusion of these causes is good practice.

The main objectives of the physical examination are to reproduce the patient's symptoms and determine the level of the affected vertebral segment.

The most useful screening tests for the patient presenting with, PSA chronic back pain are the plain X-ray, the ESR, the serum phosphatases, PSA and urine analysis. It is very unlikely that serious spinal disease can exist in the presence of an ESR under 30 mm/h and a normal X-ray.

The use of questionnaires and assessment charts to assist in the recording of information is recommended. Although initially time-consuming, it saves time in the long term and permits a safer diagnostic approach and better monitoring of progress and treatment. The first consultation with a patient should occupy 30 to 45 minutes and this is the time to carefully record information on these assessment charts.

SUMMARY OF DIAGNOSTIC GUIDELINES FOR SPINAL PAIN

- Continuous pain (day and night) indicates neoplasia especially malignancy or infection.
- The big primary malignancy is multiple myeloma.
- The big three metastases are from lung, breast and prostate.
- The other three metastases are from thyroid, kidney/adrenal and melanoma.
- Pain with standing/walking – relief with sitting – indicates spondylolisthesis.
- Pain (and stiffness) at rest – relief with activity – indicates inflammation.
- In a young person with inflammation, think of spondyloarthropathy – for example, ankylosing spondylitis, Reiter's disease, reactive arthritis.
- Stiffness at rest, pain with or after activity – relief with rest – indicates osteoarthritis.

- Pain provoked by activity – relief with rest – indicates mechanical dysfunction.
- Pain in bed at early morning indicates inflammation, depression or malignancy/infection.
- Pain in periphery of limb: discogenic → radicular
  or vascular → claudication
  or spinal canal stenosis → claudication.
- Pain in calf (ascending) with walking indicates vascular claudication.
- Pain in buttock (descending) with walking indicates neurogenic claudication.
- One disc lesion indicates one nerve root (exception is L5–S1 disc).
- One nerve root indicates one disc (usually).
- Two or more nerve roots – consider neoplasm.
- The rule of thumb for the lumbar nerve root lesions is L3 from L2–L3 disc, L4 from L3–L4, L5 from L4–L5 and S1 from L5–S1.
- A large disc protrusion can cause bladder symptoms, either incontinence or retention.
- A retroperitoneal bleed from anti-coagulation therapy can give intense nerve root symptoms and signs.

3
The concept of irritability

Contents
- [ ] Key checkpoints
- [ ] Implications
- [ ] Assessment factors
- [ ] Levels of irritability
- [ ] Diagnostic clues
- [ ] The physical examination
- [ ] Practice tips
- [ ] Summary

One of the definite characteristics of the pain experienced by each patient is that of irritability.

It is an important concept because an understanding of the level of irritability for a particular patient's problem will provide the therapist with a general management plan for that patient. The reason for the aggravation of the condition of some patients by spinal manipulation is that the therapist failed to recognise the correct level of irritability.

Definition

Irritability is the degree to which the patient's spinal condition can be aggravated by various provoking factors. This is a combination of the intensity of the pain provoked and the subsequent time required for resolution once the provoking factor has ceased.

Irritability is classified simply as *low, moderate* and *high*. A high irritability exists when the patient's problem is provoked to an intense level by relatively simple activities and subsequently takes a long time (longer than 24 hours) to slowly subside.

A low irritability exists, for example, when a person may notice a dull back pain some hours after commencing heavy work such as digging or housework, but can continue working with the pain, which subsides rapidly once the activity is ceased.

Questions to ask the patient

Specific questions can quickly aid evaluation of the degree of irritability:

- What activity brings on or aggravates your pain?
- How long can you perform this activity before the onset of pain?
- After the onset of pain, can you keep on working and, if so, for how long?
- After you cease the activity, how long does the pain take to settle?

KEY CHECKPOINTS

- The level of irritability of the spine is important for assessing the manner of the conduct of the physical examination and for the selection of manual therapy.
- Irritability is classified as low, moderate or high.
- Most patients with back pain exhibit low irritability.
- A patient's limit of tolerance is an important guideline to assess the level of irritability.

IMPLICATIONS

Although patients experience the same area of distribution of pain they will have different levels of irritability and will therefore need to be treated differently.

Failure to consider this factor could result in the selection of the wrong manual technique, resulting in:

- prolonged post treatment pain
- aggravation of the patient's condition or even deterioration, causing alteration of management
- adverse psychological reaction by the patient, with a very negative reaction to manipulative therapy which, in fact, could be beneficial in the longer term.

ASSESSMENT FACTORS

The three factors that should be determined are:

1. The nature of the activity to provoke symptoms. This may range from a simple movement, such as rotating the neck, to heavy manual work.
2. The intensity of the pain provoked. The key factor to consider is whether the patient can tolerate the pain and continue the activity or whether he or she has to stop.
3. The time span between the onset and offset of the pain.

These concepts are outlined in general terms in Figure 3.1.

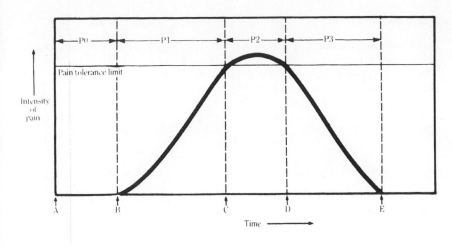

Figure 3.1 Graphic illustration of (moderate) irritability.

A: start of activity
B: onset of back pain
C: cessation of provoking activity (because of pain intolerance)
D: point at which pain starts subsiding below tolerance limit
E: offset of back pain
P0 = AB: pain-free time span
P1 = BC: time between onset of pain and cessation of activity (because of pain)
P2 = CD: severe pain, above limit of tolerance
P3 = DE: time for pain subsidence

LEVELS OF IRRITABILITY

1. High irritability

Fortunately only a relatively small number of patients have high irritability, but it is important to identify these patients, since the problem requires cautious management. Their history is characterised by severe pain (often incapacitating) which is provoked or aggravated relatively easily by light, even innocuous activities.

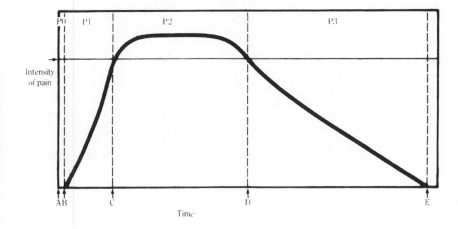

Figure 3.2 Graph of high irritability: This shows a very short P0 and P1 with a rapid ascent, a relatively long P2 and a prolonged P3.

After the rapid onset of pain the patient soon stops the provoking activity. The pain then lasts for hours despite the cessation. In addition, there is a tendency to develop referred or radicular pain.

The typical pattern for high irritability is illustrated in Figure 3.2, and a typical case history follows.

Case history

A 33-year-old woman has an eight week history of recurrent episodes of severe neck pain often provoked by simple neck rotation to the left. The pain rapidly deteriorates despite the application of a collar and then radiates into the left shoulder and arm with paraesthesia of the middle three fingers of the left hand.

The pain, which is unrelieved by medication, is intense for four to six hours, after which it slowly subsides over 24 hours or longer.

2.   Moderate irritability

Moderate irritability is found in a large group of patients. It is categorised into two types, depending on whether the pain tolerance level is reached, with the offending activity therefore having to be ceased.

Figure 3.1 represents a case of more severe moderate irritability. The two types are illustrated in Figure 3.3: M1 is the more severe while M2 is less severe, does not reach the limit of tolerance and hence the person can usually continue the pain-producing activity.

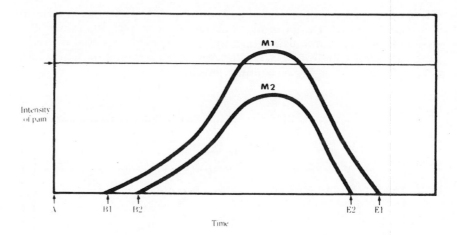

Figure 3.3 Graphs for moderate irritability: M1 represents a more severe degree, M2 a lesser degree; P2 is not present in M2.

The patient with a history of moderate irritability has a definite pain-free period, then a gradual onset of pain, usually slow, initially, but then building up to the level at which he or she is forced to cease the activity, or finds it uncomfortable to continue. The pain usually ceases within one or two hours but may persist for up to four hours.

3.   Low irritability

The majority of patients with back pain fall into the low irritability category. A typical case is illustrated in Figure 3.4, with a long delay in the onset of pain, which may require strenuous activity to initiate it. The pain level rises slowly, keeps within the pain tolerance limit so that the

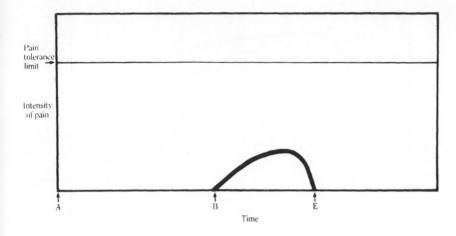

Figure 3.4 Graph for low irritability: Long P0, P1 has gentle incline, P2 absent, short P3.

patient can usually continue the activity, although some patients may cease the activity because of the discomfort. Upon cessation of the activity the pain settles quite rapidly, usually within 15 to 30 minutes.

Case history

A 50-year-old woman who, after gardening for two hours, notices the gradual onset of low back pain, continues this activity until she stops for morning tea. By the time she has rested for 15 minutes the pain has disappeared and she returns to her gardening.

DIAGNOSTIC CLUES

Scrutiny of the pain irritability patterns can provide clues to the diagnosis. Any condition, if severe enough, can reach the limit of tolerance, but certain conditions reach this level more easily. For highly irritable conditions the important factor is not so much the intensity of the pain but its behaviour.

Case history A

Take, for example, the case of a 42-year-old carpenter (patient A: Figure 3.5) who experiences the sudden onset of right-sided neck pain after carrying a bag of tools. The pain rapidly gets worse, despite cessation of this provoking activity, and exceeds the tolerance limit. The pain then starts to radiate into the region of the right shoulder and supraclavicular area, with paraesthesia developing in the middle fingers. After 30 minutes the neck pain subsides but the peripheral pain and paraesthesia persist, to subside only some hours later.

The significant feature of this problem is the importance of radicular pain or nerve root irritation. This aspect has to be evaluated carefully during the physical examination, and appropriate care taken to handle the examination and subsequent treatment cautiously.

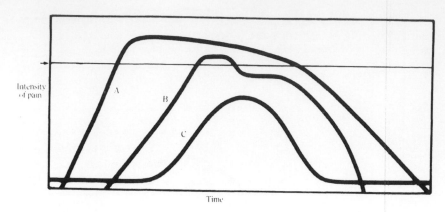

Figure 3.5 Pain patterns for various clinical conditions. A: High irritability neck pain with nerve root irritation. B: Moderate irritability with acute dysfunction of the apophyseal joint. C: Moderate irritability with typical apophyseal joint dysfunction.

Case history B

A 28-year-old plumber, after working for one hour, starts to experience left-sided low back pain (patient B: Figure 3.5). As he continues to work the pain intensity steadily increases, until he is forced to stop after approximately one hour. The pain remains quite severe for approximately 30 minutes then starts to slowly decrease for a while until it reaches a constant level at which it remains for approximately two hours, then subsiding quite rapidly over the next two hours. This pattern of moderate irritability is typical of an acute dysfunction of the apophyseal joint.

Case history C

The graph depicted for patient C (Figure 3.5) represents the most common pattern for apophyseal joint dysfunction and is usually an acute pattern on a chronic background. It is a pattern of moderate irritability and, like most apophyseal joint problems, keeps within the patient's tolerance limit.

However, there is a variability between these patterns and the next episode of pain in the patient could exhibit a different pattern.

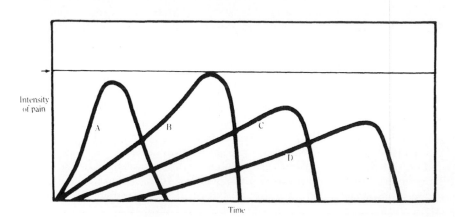

Figure 3.6 Typical pain pattern for soft tissue injuries such as muscle and tendons.

Figure 3.6. shows typical pain patterns for soft tissue injuries such as strained ligaments and muscles. The main characteristic is a rapid P4 time but there is considerable variability with P0 and P1.

THE PHYSICAL EXAMINATION

The assessment of the patient's degree of irritability will inevitably modify the approach to the examination and management of the patient.

1. High irritability

The examination will have to be as gentle and as brief as possible. Only a brief examination will be required to reproduce the patient's symptoms and signs. The examination has to proceed with considerable caution. With treatment there is less margin for error and the

Table 3.1 *Levels of irritability – typical history patterns.*

	IRRITABILITY LEVEL		
	LOW	MODERATE	HIGH
P0 time	● Prolonged ● Very slow onset	● Long ● Variable but slow onset	● Short ● Rapid onset, within minutes
Typical time span	2 or more hours	30 mins–2 hours	1–30 minutes
P1 time	● Prolonged ● Slow build-up	● Long ● Variable but gradual build-up	● Short ● Almost immediate ● Rapid cessation of activity
Typical time span	Hours	30–60 mins	1–30 mins
P2 time	● Usually not reached	● Variable	● Cannot continue
Tolerance level	● Can continue activity ● Sometimes ceases	● May continue ● Often ceases	● Pain may get worse
Typical time span		10–60 mins	24–48 hours
P3 time	● Very short ● Subsides within a few minutes	● Variable	● Very long
Typical time span	1–20 mins	2–8 hours	24–48 hours
Type of provoking activity	● Heavy e.g. heavy lifting digging making beds	● Variable but usually moderate physical activity e.g. vacuuming making beds gardening	● Minimal e.g. simple movements intercourse sitting light lifting

therapist has to be as conservative as possible – for example, mobilisation may have to be used instead of manipulation, or perhaps no manual therapy should be used at all. On the other hand, manipulation is not necessarily contra-indicated in all cases with high irritability. It may be necessary to prescribe rest and analgesics for two or three days or longer to decrease the level of irritability to the stage where other methods can be used.

2.   Moderate irritability

It is relatively easy to reproduce the symptoms and find the relevant signs during the examination. Obviously, caution has to be used with the more sensitive cases. A wider selection of techniques for treatment is available.

3.   Low irritability

It may be necessary to use special provocative tests to reproduce the symptoms in patients with back pain of low irritability. There is a very wide range of treatment options to choose from.

PRACTICE TIPS

- A gentle and brief examination is necessary for patients with high irritability back pain.
- It is usually possible to subject a patient with low irritability to a rigorous examination.
- Asking questions to determine the level of irritability for a patient gives a subjective idea of that patient's level of pain tolerance.
- A highly irritable pain problem must be treated with utmost care: spinal manipulation is usually contra-indicated.

SUMMARY

Back pain can be assessed for the important characteristic of irritability, which can be classified as low, moderate or high. It is usually determined by asking specific questions related to the patient's pain, such as: What actually brings on your pain? Does the activity make you stop because of the pain? How long is this period before you are forced to stop? How long does the pain take to settle once you stop?

The division of pain into the three categories assists in establishing the extent of the physical examination and subsequent treatment.

4
Mobilisation and manipulation

Contents
- [ ] Key checkpoints
- [ ] Mobilisation
- [ ] Manipulation
- [ ] Aspects of manipulation
- [ ] Why bother with manual therapy for the spine?
- [ ] Practice tips
- [ ] Summary

The term 'manipulation', as applied to the spine, is so widely used and misrepresented that it will be necessary to provide a clear definition of its meaning in this text.

Used in a general sense, manipulation refers to the skilful use of hands for therapeutic techniques. Hence it can refer to any manual technique involving a passive movement, be it specific manipulation, mobilisation, traction, soft tissue techniques or massage. In this text, however, manipulation is used only to refer to those manual techniques that apply a high velocity thrust at the end range of the joint.

KEY CHECKPOINTS

- Manipulation is a high velocity thrust at the end range.
- Mobilisation is a gentle, coaxing, repetitive rhythmic movement.
- Mobilisation can be given over three stages of the range of movement of the joint, according to the level of pain and stiffness.
- Mobilisation and manipulation diminish muscle spasm, stiffness and pain.
- Maigne's MID (minor intervertebral derangement) concept explains how manipulation can break the pain cycle.
- Follow Maigne's 'direction of manipulation' rule – 'opposite movement and no pain'.

MOBILISATION

Definition

Mobilisation is a passive movement directed at the apophyseal joint without any high velocity thrust and within the range of the joint.

Description

It is a gentle, coaxing, repetitive rhythmic movement of a joint that can be resisted by the patient. Unlike manipulation, it can be performed over a wide range and can thus involve a series of movements referred to as stages.

Manipulation, on the other hand, being a very rapid, passive movement at the end range of a joint, is far more forceful than mobilisation and cannot be controlled by the patient.

The differences are compared in Figures 4.1 and 4.2. In Figure 4.1, consider the movement as rotation of the head to the right from the neutral position A to reach the normal active limit B, a range of about 80 degrees. If the person now rotates the head further by tightening the neck muscles the head will move to the elastic limit C. This range from A to C is known as the mobilisation range.

It is not possible for the person to actively rotate the head any further but movement past this elastic limit C or end or range can be achieved by the forceful thrust of manipulation which produces a very small arc of movement from C to the anatomical limit of the joint D. This range from C to D is known as the manipulation range.

Mobilisation can be performed in a *physiological direction* (namely rotation, extension, lateral flexion or flexion) or in a *non-physiological*

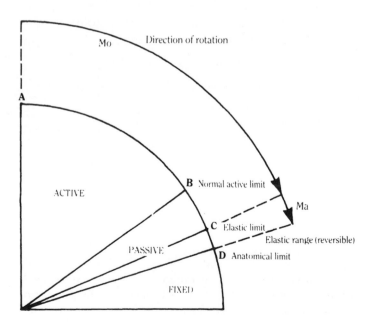

Figure 4.1 Schematic representation of movement (by rotation) of a joint.

Mobilisation (Mo)   A → C
Manipulation (Ma)   C → D

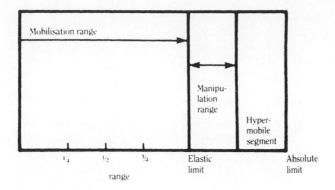

Figure 4.2 Schematic range of movement.

direction (for example, longitudinal traction or anterior directed (posterior–anterior) gliding). In practice it is mainly employed in rotation, posterior–anterior gliding and traction.

Mobilisation can be a surprisingly effective technique, with many therapists claiming it to be almost as, if not as, effective as manipulation. The great hallmark of mobilisation is its relative safety. Although there are many mobilisation techniques, it is necessary to become proficient with a few only.

It is often used to prepare the joint for manipulation; however, if there are relative contra-indications for manipulation, mobilisation provides an alternative treatment strategy. The authors prefer the use of mobilisation over manipulation for the cervical spine, especially the upper cervical spine, and for very painful conditions of the spine.

Some therapists tend to use either manipulation alone or, where contra-indications for its use are present, nothing at all. The patient is consequently disadvantaged by not having the benefit of a useful technique to initiate treatment.

Stages of mobilisation

Mobilisation procedures or techniques are considered in three stages over the relatively wide range of movement of the joint (Figure 4.3). It will be appreciated that manipulation can only produce a very small range of movement which is almost imperceptible at times.

Stage 1 refers to the small amplitude movement at or near the commencement of the movement from the neutral or central position A.

Stage 2 refers to a large amplitude of movement spanning the mid range and can virtually occupy most of the range A to C.

Stage 3 represents a small amplitude movement at or near the end range C.

Stage 1 or 2 mobilisation is usually employed for more painful conditions, while stage 3 mobilisation is very useful where less pain and greater mobility are present (Table 4.1).

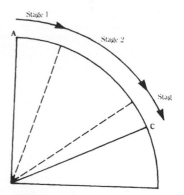

Figure 4.3 Illustrating the three stages of mobilisation on the rotation model.

Table 4.1 *Stages of mobilisation.*

	STAGE 1	STAGE 2	STAGE 3
Range	Start of range	Mid range	End of range
Amplitude	Small	Large	Small
Indication	Acute painful hypomobile joints	Pain and stiffness	Stiffness and pain

Guidelines for the technique selection

- Keep just short of reproduction of the symptoms, or just 'nip' the pain.
- Staying too short with a small amplitude means that the technique is less effective.
- Going too far into the painful area will aggravate the symptoms.

Once the stage has been determined the oscillations should be kept steady and rhythmic.

The aim with all mobilisation is to decrease the pain and increase the mobility at the appropriate level.

MANIPULATION

Definition

Manipulation is a high velocity thrust of small amplitude performed in rotation, in lateral flexion, in flexion or in extension, either separately or as a combination of these directions.

The effect of manipulation

Although there are many theories as to the manner in which manipulation achieves its effect the general consensus is that the effect of manipulation at the appropriate level is to:

- diminish pain
- decrease stiffness
- diminish muscle spasm.

Practitioners of manipulation who assess their patients after the procedure are aware of an improved range of movement with concomitant decrease in pain and muscle spasm.

Manipulation addresses the problem of hypomobility or stiffness. On examination, it is important to establish not only the level of hypomobility but also the degree of pain-related loss of movement. When a joint becomes painful there is associated loss of movement – not only of physiological movement (such as active flexion or extension) but also non-physiological or accessory movement. This explains why direct palpation over the spinous process of the affected vertebral level, or transverse pressure on the side of that spinous process, can be so painful – the accessory movements at that level are diminished. This is known as 'joint play'. Following manipulation, re-examination will often show improved movement and less pain on palpation.

The net result is that when mobility is improved with manipulation there is restoration of physiological and accessory movement with accompanying decrease of pain.

Contrary to the views of some other groups of practitioners, loss of mobility (stiffness) without accompanying pain is, the authors consider, not significant. Clinically, pain is more important than stiffness. To subject patients to a prolonged course of manual therapy for stiffness in the absence of pain is considered inappropriate.

Other theories on the effect of manipulation

The apophyseal joint syndrome

It has been postulated that the painful hypomobility is caused by a subluxation or an internal derangement of small meniscoid-like bodies, nipped synovial fringes or a 'joint lock' of the apophyseal joint. Manipulation applies a distracting force to one or more of these joints, thus correcting the mechanical problem.

The intervertebral disc lesion

A prolapsed disc bulging into the spinal canal can cause either local or referred pain. Manipulation moves or relocates the position of the bulge – for example, it can shift a fragment of disc to a lateral recess away from unrelated or entrapped painful structures. It is inconceivable that manipulation could return a prolapsed or extruded fragment of disc back to the confines of the disc. However, manipulation may reposition the nucleus pulposus, thus relieving pressure on the weakened outer pain-sensitive layers of the annulus fibrosus.

Reflex inhibition of muscle spasm

A logical theory about the mechanism of manipulation and other manual techniques such as mobilisation and muscle energy therapy is that, whatever else the technique may do, it provides reflex inhibition of acute or chronic muscle spasm which has become self-perpetuating.

Painful muscle spasm can be produced by nociceptive (painful) activity from the joints, and the action of passive stretching can reduce this nociceptor activity, in accordance with the 'gate' theory of Melzack and Wall. A relatively common example of this concept is seen in the treatment of a painful wry neck in considerable spasm, when an immediate increase in relaxation, and thus in range of movement, follows the application of a manual technique.

The effect on the minor intervertebral derangement (MID)

The MID theory of Maigne has been outlined in Chapter 1. Maigne points out that MID exists when the painful segmental area is the consequence of a mechanical, postural or traumatic disturbance and is reversible when manipulation makes it disappear. The MID will thus not improve until manipulation re-establishes normal function by producing a reflex inhibition of the spasm.

The direction of manipulation

The direction of manipulation is determined by the examination findings and then following the basic rule of *'opposite movement and no pain'*.

This generally means that manipulation achieves *a gapping or opening up of the painful side* – for example, if rotation of the neck is painful to the left but not painful to the right, manipulation needs to be in rotation to the right (see Figure 4.5).

This gapping achieves two biomechanical effects:

● opening up the intervertebral foramen
● maximally stretching the posterior wall of the synovial capsule of the apophyseal joint.

It follows that the physical examination must determine the pain-free direction or directions of movement as well as the painful directions. Consider the direction of movement (DOM) diagram (Figure 4.4)

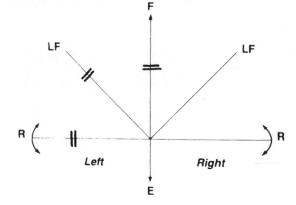

Figure 4.4 DOM diagram illustrating restricted and painful movements (blocked indicated by //) in flexion, left lateral flexion and left rotation but pain-free extension, right lateral flexion and right rotation (free movements).

which indicates that the patient's movements are restricted and painful in flexion, lateral flexion and L rotation but pain-free in extension, R lateral flexion and R rotation. The direction of manipulation is therefore towards the right and can be either R lateral flexion or R rotation (Figure 4.5) or a combination of these two directions (Figure 4.6) – that is, either unidirectional or multi-directional.

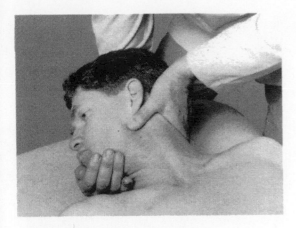

Figure 4.5 Uni-directional manipulation of the neck by rotation to the right in the patient with pain on the left side but with painless movement to the right. The painful joint or joints on the left are gapped open.

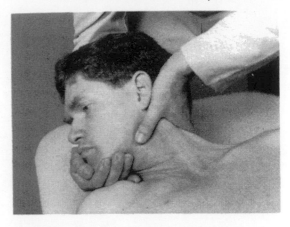

Figure 4.6 Multi-directional manipulation of the neck in the same patient including lateral flexion to the right.

ASPECTS OF MANIPULATION

Direct and indirect

Spinal manipulation techniques can be considered in their general types which are basically *direct* and *indirect*.

A direct manipulation is one where direct pressure is exerted on the affected vertebral segment as illustrated in Figure 4.7, while indirect manipulation is achieved by the use of the lever principle and mainly applies to rotational methods (Figure 4.8).

Indirect techniques are generally more appropriate, both from the viewpoint of effectiveness and for greater patient comfort.

Degree of specificity

In the rules of procedure it is emphasised that it is important to localise the treatment as much as possible. The more specific (or localised) the manipulative thrust to the affected region, the less chance there is of other non-affected or asymptomatic areas being involved and the more effective the treatment is likely to be. The specificity is classified as non-specific (or general), semi-specific and specific.

A non-specific technique is shown in Figure 4.8, where the entire lumbar region is subjected to the manipulative force.

A specific technique requires a very precise thrust at a specific level to achieve gapping of the joints at that level. This means that no other level is brought to the end range. The principle of the lever cannot be used and thus considerable skill is required to achieve precise specificity by the indirect rotational technique. Thus a specific technique is often a direct thrust performed exactly in the right direction at the specific level (Figure 4.7).

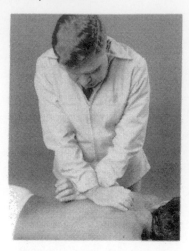

Figure 4.7 Direct manipulation. This manipulation of the thoracic spine demonstrates a direct thrust on the affected vertebral segment. The manipulation is also specific for that level.

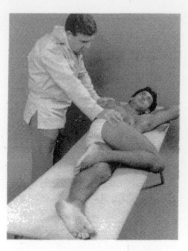

Figure 4.8 Indirect manipulation. This rotation of the lumbar spine which gaps the painful joint uses a lever principle and is obviously a general or non-specific method.

A semi-specific technique is a combination of non-specific and specific techniques, and is usually performed with a hand located at the specific level to guide the thrust during a non-specific rotational technique (Figure 4.9). This also involves a combination of direct and indirect methods.

It should be obvious that, the more specific the technique, the greater is the required degree of skill and dexterity, not only in applying the technique but also during the physical examination, where establishment of the precise affected level is imperative. This represents one of the constant challenges of manipulation: each day produces new tests of skill, as not only is each patient different,

Figure 4.9 Semi-specific manipulation of the neck. Note how a general indirect rotation is applied to the head while the reinforcing thrusting hand is placed directly over the painful level.

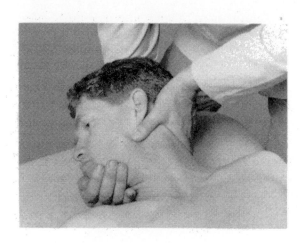

requiring a variation of a technique, but the same patient, depending on the condition, can vary from consultation to consultation, necessitating a different technique or approach.

Degree of limitation

The spine has variable directions or degrees of movement, generally up to six directions – namely flexion, extension, lateral flexion (R and L [right and left]) and rotation (also R and L).

The practical working rule is that for manipulation to be effective there must be three degrees (directions) of freedom (Maigne, 1986). In Figure 4.4 there are three blocked movements and three free movements. Thus manipulation in one or a combination of these movements should be effective.

For the patient with a painful neck (illustrated in Figure 4.10) there is freedom in only one direction, namely R lateral flexion, and although manipulation in this direction is possible it should not be

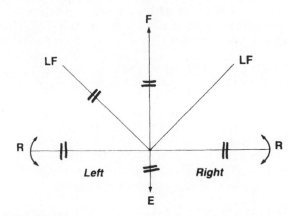

Figure 4.10 DOM diagram illustrating blockage of five movements in a patient with a painful neck. Manipulation is possible in one direction only (right lateral flexion) and is not only likely to fail but will aggravate the problem.

attempted. This is because, since five other directions are blocked, the manipulation will either be ineffective or cause post-treatment pain. The pain arises because the end range has been exceeded and the limited degrees of freedom tend to cause a flare-up of the problem.

Mobilisation, however, is not excluded in this situation, because it does not exceed the end range.

Taking up the slack

One of the mandatory rules of procedure for manipulation is 'the joint(s) must be at absolute full stretch prior to manipulation'. Achieving full stretch is referred to as 'taking up the slack', and is not necessarily as easy at it appears, being particularly difficult for beginners to master.

The set routine is to approach the end of range carefully but not quickly. As one approaches this end range it is important to be sensitive to the joint at the elastic limit (Figure 4.11). This is termed the 'end feel' and can be described as either HARD or SOFT.

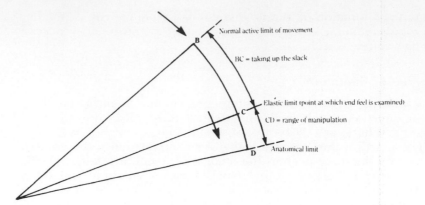

Normal active limit of movement

B

BC = taking up the slack

Elastic limit (point at which end feel is examined)

C

CD = range of manipulation

D   Anatomical limit

Figure 4.11 Illustration of the end feel during rotatory movement of the joint (small angle exaggerated for illustration purposes). At the elastic limit C the examiner determines if the end feel is 'hard' or 'soft'.

A hard end feel indicates that the joint is abnormal or pathological for this direction and that manipulation should not proceed. If the hard end is associated with pain and reproduction of the patient's symptoms it is referred to as a HARD STOP. This indicates that it is not a pain-free direction.

HARD END FEEL ⎫ No elasticity = Pathological = Manipulation
HARD STOP ⎭ at end range   joint movement   contra-indicated

This concept is important as it represents a biomechanical contra-indication for manipulation which will not be evident prior to examining the end range and planning the procedure.

A soft end feel or SOFT STOP indicates a definite elastic movement and thus the particular direction is not pathological, and manipulation can proceed in this pain-free direction.

SOFT END FEEL   Elastic end = Normal joint = Manipulation
feel   movement   can proceed

The cracking sound of manipulation

The 'cracking' sound is caused by the rapid formation of a gas bubble (considered to be carbon dioxide) which forms in the joint from synovial fluid. It must be emphasised that an audible 'crack' is not essential to signify a successful manipulation.

Management plan

Once it has been decided to perform a manipulative thrust there is a set routine through which to proceed. This consists of:

● gentle handling, and providing the patient with explanation and reassurance
● correct comfortable physical positioning of both patient and therapist

- correct positioning of the joint at the end range
- correct direction, velocity and amplitude of the thrust.

The manipulative thrust, which must never be lax, violent or forceful, should be skilfully controlled at the end range. At the position of end range, when all the slack in the joint is taken up by stretching, the patient should notice that the appropriate area is tight but not painful. This is an important nuance because what may appear to be a pain-free or active movement may not be so when passive over-pressure is applied at the end range. If it is painful, then proceeding with the thrust would result in aggravation of the patient's symptoms. Therefore until one carefully feels the end range and evaluates the patient's response to this position it is not known if the manipulation is possible. An appropriate plan is presented in Figure 4.12.

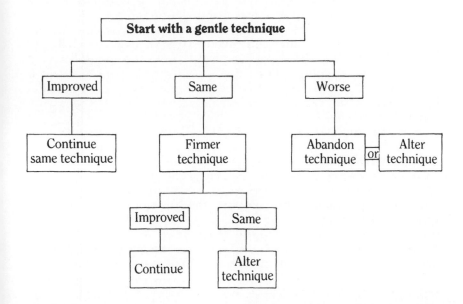

Figure 4.12 Management plan for spinal manipulation.

It is wise to commence with a gentle technique and, upon review (whether immediately or at a later consultation), to continue or alter the technique depending on the patient's response to treatment. If the patient is the same then there is a choice of repeating a technique (especially if mobilisation is used initially) more firmly, or changing to a different technique, or retaining the initial technique and adding another.

However, if the patient is worse the technique should be stopped, the reason established, the patient reassessed and another technique added if appropriate.

The authors recommend that after performing a manipulation or mobilisation the patient should always be reassessed immediately. This will determine the next technique to be selected.

No more than three manipulations to one region should be performed in any treatment session.

WHY BOTHER WITH MANUAL THERAPY FOR THE SPINE?

The issue of the efficacy of spinal manipulation and mobilisation has always been a subject of controversy within the medical profession, some practitioners associating it with quackery while others, especially rural general practitioners, claim that it is an essential component of their daily practice. A highly significant observation is that so many back pain sufferers gravitate to practitioners of the art, seeking relief with varying success.

One of the problems as perceived by the medical profession is that the therapy is often treated as a business rather than a science. In addition, its reputation has been blurred by some of its advocates claiming far too much for its effectiveness and using it as a panacea.

Another observation is that many patients have been subjected to a prolonged and failed trial of spinal manipulation.

The conduct of credible scientific trials in this area is difficult and the ideal of the double-blind controlled trial is virtually impossible to achieve. Many trials to date have been handicapped by design flaws but the better trials generally indicate that manipulation or mobilisation is better than rest in bringing about an earlier return to normal function – see Farrell and Twomey (1982) and Sims-Williams and Jayson (1978).

Parker, Tupling and Pryor (1978) showed that, in the treatment of migraine by manual therapy, both mobilisation and manipulation achieved significantly better results than controls and, interestingly, that mobilisation was as effective as manipulation.

All the above mentioned trials have considerable clinical and economic implications and support the opinion and claims of exponents of manual therapy.

Of course we do have empirical evidence of the excellent results achieved by manual therapy and anecdotal accounts of individual dramatic results in many patients who were in despair about their spinal problem. Empirical methodology certainly has an important place in medicine.

However, it is the authors' contention that the results and reputation of manual therapy would be considerably enhanced if its practitioners were generally more skilled, more clinical and scientific in their approach. The ability to screen patients to obtain appropriate indications and contra-indications for this therapy, and to employ proper safety guidelines, would inevitably lead to better results.

PRACTICE TIPS

- If in doubt use mobilisation in preference to manipulation.
- Always mobilise or manipulate in the direction of no pain.
- Always assess the patient immediately after the treatment.
- Don't give more than three treatments to one level in one treatment session.

Table 4.2 *Comparison of the essential features of mobilisation and manipulation.*

	MOBILISATION	MANIPULATION
Techniques	Passive Gentle rhythmic oscillatory Within range of joint Better patient control	Passive High velocity thrust At limit of joint range Greater force
Advantages	Safer if doubtful Greater patient comfort Wide variety of techniques	Quicker response Fewer treatments required
Disadvantages	Slower response More treatments required Not as effective as manipulation	Higher level of skill required Diagnosis must be accurate Can aggravate some spinal problems

- Aim to provide a specific treatment wherever possible.
- Dysfunction of the disc can indirectly cause dysfunction of the apophyseal joint.
- It is never known if manipulation is possible until the slack is taken up and the end range examined to determine whether it is a hard or a soft stop.

SUMMARY

A comparison of mobilisation and manipulation is presented in Table 4.2. Basically, mobilisation is performed inside the range of the joint while manipulation is performed at the end range at high velocity. If the therapist has any doubt about the selection technique, mobilisation should be chosen because it is safer and there is a chance that manipulation can aggravate the patient's condition. It is important to test the 'end feel' of that joint at the elastic limit and determine whether it is 'hard' or 'soft'. If it is 'soft', manipulation can proceed, but this is contra-indicated if it is 'hard'.

However, mobilisation is generally slower to achieve results. More treatments are usually required and it is normally not as effective as manipulation, especially in the thoracic spine. Used in combination, where mobilisation prepares a stiff painful joint for manipulation, the techniques can be very effective.

Manipulation is a safe procedure provided that the appropriate indications and safety guidelines are followed carefully. Although manipulation is more forceful than mobilisation the therapist does not necessarily have to use great force: the force can be restricted and controlled.

The basic effect of these manual techniques is to increase mobility of the joint and achieve pain relief. There is an inseparable relationship between the two.

5
Muscle energy therapy

'No muscle uses its power in pushing but always in drawing to itself
the parts that are joined to it.'

Leonardo da Vinci (1452–1519)

Contents
- ☐ Key checkpoints
- ☐ Physiological principles
- ☐ Clinical applications
- ☐ Clinical principles of muscle energy therapy

Spinal manipulation is the most effective technique in manual therapy
for treatment of spinal disorders that produce pain and stiffness. It
certainly produces a more effective and rapid return to normal
function of the vertebral segment or segments. However, some spinal
problems, especially acute syndromes of the cervical spine, are not
suitable for manipulation.

One of the alternative techniques to using forceful thrusting
techniques in the cervical spine is the muscle energy or neuromuscular
technique: it is basically simple in concept and execution, is safe and
involves no thrusting.

Its theory is based on an old and basic neurophysiological principle
known as Sherrington's second law: 'When a muscle gets stimulation
for contraction, the antagonist receives an impulse for relaxation'.

Use of muscle energy therapy is indicated where there is increased or
altered muscle tone in the presence of cervical dysfunction (for the
cervical spine).

In practice, therapists use the ability to achieve muscle relaxation
following not only contraction but also stretching of muscles. Painful
tight muscles can be safely mobilised in the post-contraction and post-
stretching phases.

KEY CHECKPOINTS

- The synonyms for muscle energy therapy include 'neuromuscular therapy', and 'proprioceptive neuromuscular facilitation'.
- Muscle energy is essentially a mobilisation technique using
  muscular facilitation and inhibition.
- It is effective for acute musculoskeletal disorders of the neck –
  for example, acute torticollis.

- Muscle energy treats segmental vertebral dysfunction by addressing faults in muscle activity which, through abnormal motor neurone discharge, cause an imbalance of forces acting on joints.
- Abnormalities in posture and movement can be caused through abnormal shortening or lengthening of muscles in response to injury and pain. Muscle energy therapy will restore the muscle range to normality.

PHYSIOLOGICAL PRINCIPLES

Muscle contraction

When a muscle is subjected to very strong contraction, especially if the tension becomes excessive, contraction suddenly ceases and the muscle relaxes (Ganong, 1981). This relaxation in response to strong tension is called the inverse stretch reflex or autogenic inhibition and conforms with Sherrington's second law. All this process is happening in the same muscle – it is an inbuilt safety mechanism for a particular skeletal muscle.

An important receptor for the inverse stretch reflex is the Golgi tendon organ, which consists of a netlike collection of knobby nerve endings among the fascicles of a tendon. The fibres from the Golgi tendon organs comprise the Ib group of myelinated, rapidly conducting sensory nerve fibres that terminate in the spinal cord onto inhibitory neurones. Strong contractions of muscles stimulate the Golgi tendon organs, which are in series with the muscle fibres and thus cause reflex inhibition of the muscle. The pathway is illustrated in Figure 5.1.

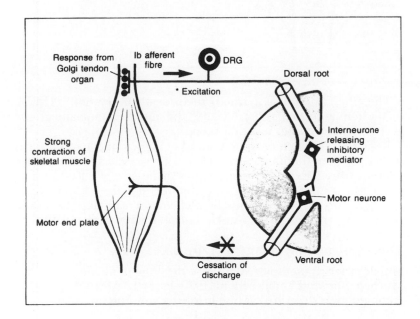

Figure 5.1 Diagram illustrating the pathway for the autogenic inhibition reflex following strong muscular contraction (after Ganong).

Muscle stretching

When a muscle is stretched, muscle spindles or stretch receptors in the skeletal muscles are stimulated and impulses pass up the Ia group afferent nerve fibres to excite motor neurones supplying the muscle from which the impulses arise (the agonist muscle). At the same time an inhibitory pathway, via interneurones of the spinal cord, inhibits the motor neurones that supply the antagonists of that muscle acting on the same joint or joints. This pathway is illustrated in Figure 5.2.

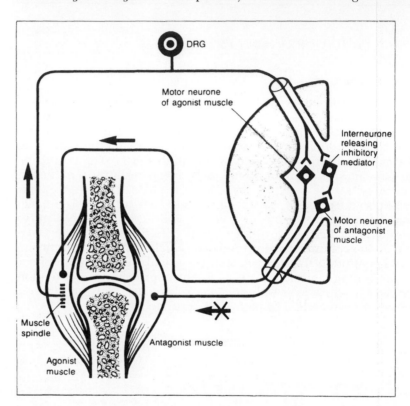

Figure 5.2 Diagram illustrating the pathway for the inhibition of antagonists to a muscle contraction in response to stretching (after Ganong).

The phenomenon is termed 'reciprocal innervation'. This means that when a stretch reflex occurs, the muscles that antagonise the action of the muscles involved relax.

Research has demonstrated another reflex mechanism involving stretch or lengthening receptors in the muscle fascia via group II afferent fibres. Excessive lengthening of muscle will lead in a similar way to autogenic inhibition giving an effect like the 'clasp knife' reflex, which occurs in spastic muscle. Relaxation can also be evoked by stimulating (rubbing) the muscle fascia (Rymer et al., 1979).

Theory of muscle energy therapy

Muscle energy therapy (MET) was developed in the 1940s by F. L. Mitchell Snr and published in 1979 by F. L. Mitchell Jr et al. The technique was described as one involving voluntary muscle contraction in a controlled manner at clearly determined localised segments opposed by an appropriate counterforce.

The muscle energy method employs the method of muscle contraction by the patient followed by relaxation and stretching of antagonist and agonist muscles. It is an indirect form of mobilisation of a joint that involves no thrusting.

The mobilisation of the joint is necessary because it is stiff and perhaps 'locked', with the responsible muscles acting on the joint being abnormally contracted (maybe in spasm). Such a contracted muscle is painful and creates a 'motion barrier' across the affected joint.

The objective of therapy is to relax that abnormal muscle at the affected level, increase its length and movement and thus increase the range of movement of the joint.

In practice, this objective cannot be achieved rapidly by one or two 'contraction–relaxation–stretching' manoeuvres because only a small degree of muscle relaxation and mobilisation of the joint or joints can be achieved by one manoeuvre. Treatment requires the summation of a successive series of manoeuvres which then produces a significant increase in range of movement, reduction of the motion barrier and a decrease in pain.

The contraction of the muscle or muscle tone can be synergised or reinforced by two important although simple functions: inspiration and ocular movements (Lewit, 1985) (upwards and towards the direction of activity of the contracting muscle).

Alternatively, the relaxation of the muscle is facilitated by expiration and by looking downwards in the direction in which relaxation is desired. These facilitatory factors are summarised in Table 5.1

Table 5.1 *Role of respiration and ocular movement in muscle energy.*

	FACILITATION OF MUSCULAR CONTRACTION	FACILITATION OF MUSCULAR RELAXATION
Respiration	Inspiration	Expiration
Ocular movement	Towards contraction Superior	Towards relaxation Inferior

The application of visual impulses on the contraction and relaxation of agonist–antagonist muscles of the neck can be determined locally when reflecting on the situation of a person hearing a wild animal or similar threatening danger from one side. The sudden rotation of the neck towards that side is accompanied by reciprocal relaxation of the side away from the darting eyes.

CLINICAL APPLICATIONS

Muscular energy therapy is most effective for relatively acute musculoskeletal disorders of the neck, especially acute torticollis.

The neck is particularly prone to develop painful musculoskeletal problems in response to trauma. Abrahams (1979) considers that in comparison with other musculature the neck has an abundance of muscle spindles. In addition, nociceptors in the cervical articulations are very active and produce reactive muscle guarding similar to the intense nociceptor activity that causes muscle rigidity over an inflamed appendix. The ability to reduce this nociceptor activity from cervical joints may be one of the important mechanisms behind the effectiveness of the therapy described in this chapter.

Muscular energy therapy can be and is used to treat a variety of disorders of the thoracic and lumbar spine (Lee, 1986) but has limited application compared with spinal manipulation. It can be very effective in treating pelvic dysfunction, where large muscles influence the function of joints in this region – namely, the sacro-iliac, hip and lumbo-sacral joints. Specific muscular energy therapy can be directed to iliopsoas, quadratus lumborum, hamstrings, piriformis and extensors of the lumbar spine (Guymer, 1986).

Another important clinical dimension is the ability to produce specific self-administered exercise programmes for patients, based on muscle energy. This is most obviously applicable to the neck and pelvic area, and the stretching exercise programmes developed by athletes are based on these principles.

CLINICAL PRINCIPLES OF MUSCLE ENERGY THERAPY

Although specific ME techniques vary for the various muscles and joints involved, they do share eight common steps that *must* be repeated for all ME techniques. The outline of specific techniques that follows does not always mention each of these steps, but they are nevertheless implied with each of the techniques.

The eight essential tips for ALL muscle energy techniques are:

1. Accurate structural *diagnosis*.
2. Engage the restrictive *barrier* in all three planes (flexion/extension, sidebending left/right, rotation left/right).
3. Underlying *counterforce* (Operator Force = Patient Force).
4. Appropriate patient *muscle effort* (isometric).
   (a) Correct amount of force.
   (b) Correct direction of effort – away from the restrictive barrier.
   (c) Correct duration of effort (5 to 7 seconds).
5. *Complete relaxation* after the muscle effort (both operator and patient relax their counterforces simultaneously).
6. *Repositioning* to the new restrictive barrier in all three planes – monitor motions with palpation.
7. *Repeat* steps 3 through 6, three to five times.
8. *Retest* (repeat structural diagnosis).

The most common errors that are made include the following:

1. Not monitoring motion with palpation of involved joint.
2. Too forceful a muscle contraction by the patient.
3. Too short a duration of muscle contraction by the patient.
4. Not allowing the patient to totally relax before repositioning to new restrictive barrier (forcing the new motion barrier).
5. Forgetting to retest.

6
Safety guidelines

'I will keep my patients from harm and injustice.'

Hippocrates

Contents
- ☐ Rules of procedure for manual therapy
- ☐ Key checkpoints
- ☐ Contra-indications to mobilisation and manipulation
- ☐ Practice tips
- ☐ Summary

One of the basic tenets of the Hippocratic Oath is to 'do no harm'. This must be a guiding principle in the application of manual therapy, particularly spinal manipulation. Deaths and severe injuries have followed inappropriate cervical manipulation when safety guidelines were not followed. Forceful manipulation of the cervical spine presents the biggest problem, and some teachers counsel that this technique should not be used except in the most experienced hands.

Similarly in the lumbar spine, a massive sequestration of lumbar disc can follow an inappropriate manipulation, with dangerous compromisation of the lumbosacral nerve roots or cauda equina.

Another particular concern is the number of patients on anticoagulant therapy who have developed permanent damage to nerve roots following a spontaneous retroperitoneal haemorrhage. The likelihood of precipitating such an event with a manipulative thrust is very real and represents a contra-indication to manipulation.

RULES OF PROCEDURE FOR MANUAL THERAPY

1. **Do no harm**: consider contra-indications and those conditions requiring care or gentleness.
2. Carefully assess symptoms and signs prior to treatment.
3. Localise the problem and, consequently, localise the treatment wherever possible.
4. Use economy of vigour of the technique.
5. Let treatment be guided by assessment and reassessment throughout its course.
6. Stop any treatment that causes deterioration of symptoms or signs.
7. Continue treatment if the patient is improving.
8. Be careful and very conservative in your approach to people aged 65 and over.

```
┌─────────────────────────────────────────────────────────────┐
│ KEY CHECKPOINTS                                               │
│                                                               │
│ ● Cerebrovascular accidents (CVAs), quadriplegia or sudden    │
│   death can follow inappropriate manipulation in rotation of  │
│   the cervical spine.                                         │
│ ● Provocative tests for vertebro-basilar insufficiency are    │
│   important.                                                  │
│ ● Rheumatoid arthritis can cause instability of the cervical  │
│   spine.                                                      │
│ ● Large disc protrusions can be aggravated by manipulation.   │
│ ● Unrelenting pain, day and night, suggests severe spinal     │
│   disease.                                                    │
│ ● Bilateral 'sciatica' or more than two nerve root lesions in │
│   the upper limb suggest sinister pathology.                  │
│ ● Avoid giving patients with non-organic pain a course of     │
│   manual therapy.                                             │
└─────────────────────────────────────────────────────────────┘
```

CONTRA-INDICATIONS TO MOBILISATION AND MANIPULATION

Contra-indications to mobilisation and manipulation can be considered under the following categories:

1. Absolute (no mobilisation; no manipulation)
2. Relative (mobilisation with care; no manipulation)
3. Care.

The specific conditions are summarised in Table 6.1.

Table 6.1 *Contra-indications to mobilisation and manipulation.*

ABSOLUTE	RELATIVE	CARE
Neoplasia: benign or malignant	Vertebro-basilar insufficiency	Pregnancy
Active infection or inflammation, including rheumatoid arthritis	Spondylolisthesis	Dizziness
	Anticoagulation (warfarin) therapy	Elderly patient
		Trivial back pain
Neurological changes such as: spinal cord compression cauda equina compression	History of stroke	Psychogenic pain
	Drop attacks	Undiagnosed pain
	Osteoporosis	Severe pain
Instability following trauma	Maldevelopment of bone	Hypermobility
	Inability of patient to relax	Post laminectomy
	Marked foraminal encorachment (oblique X-ray)	Post spinal fusion
	Evidence of severe disc protrusion or acute nerve root irritation/compression	

Absolute contra-indications

1. Neoplasia

Fortunately, tumours of the spine are uncommon. Nevertheless, they occur frequently enough for the full-time practitioner in back disorders to encounter some each year, especially metastatic disease.

The three common primary malignancies that metastasise to the spine are those originating in the lung, the breast and the prostate (all paired structures). The less common primaries to consider are the thyroid, the kidney and adrenals, and malignant melanoma.

Malignancies arising from the gastrointestinal tract – for example, from the stomach, large bowel and pancreas – and from the female genital organs can reach the spine by direct spread and thus are well advanced.

Reticuloses such as Hodgkin's disease can involve the spine. Primary malignancies that arise in the vertebrae include multiple myeloma and sarcoma.

Benign tumours to consider are often neurological in origin. An interesting tumour is the osteoid osteoma, which is aggravated by consuming alcohol.

The tumours affecting the spine are summarised in Table 6.2.

The symptoms and signs that should alert the clinician to malignant disease are:

● back pain occurring in an older person
● unrelenting back pain, unrelieved by rest (this includes night pain)

Table 6.2 *Significant tumours affecting the spine.*

	BENIGN	MALIGNANT

Of bone:	Osteoid osteoma
	Haemangioma
	Osteoblastoma
	Aneurysmal bone cyst
	Eosinophilic granuloma
		Primary
		    Multiple myeloma
		    Lymphomas e.g. Hodgkin's
		    Sarcoma

Spinal:	**Extradural**
	    Lipoma
	    Neuroma
	    Fibroma
	
	Intradural
	    Neuroma
	    Ependymoma
	    Chordoma
	    Meningioma
		Secondary
		    Breast
		    Lung
		    Prostate
		    Adrenals/kidney
		    Thyroid
		    Melanoma
		
		Direct spread
		    Stomach
		    Large bowel
		    Pancreas
		    Uterus/cervix/ovary

- rapidly increasing back pain
- constitutional symptoms – for example, weight loss, fever, malaise
- a history of treatment for cancer – for example, excision of skin melanoma
- major neurological signs without severe nerve root pain
- bilateral 'sciatica'
- the involvement of more than one nerve root
- muscular spasm, especially with lateral flexion.

2. Active infection or inflammation

Infective conditions that can involve the spine include osteomyelitis, tuberculosis, brucellosis, syphilis and salmonella infections.

Such conditions should be suspected in young patients (osteomyelitis), farm workers (brucellosis) and migrants from South East Asia and third world countries (tuberculosis). The presence of poor general health and fever necessitates investigations for these infections.

Inflammatory disorders can involve the spine and are often overlooked if the associations are not kept in mind by the clinician. In particular, rheumatoid arthritis is important, because it can involve the cervical spine, affecting the transverse ligament and allowing the odontoid process of the axis to sublux. This atlanto-axial subluxation may be asymptomatic and is diagnosed by special X-rays in flexion (lateral view) and by oral views. This subluxation is clinically significant since it may result in severe cord compression, causing quadriplegia and even death.

Rheumatoid arthritis may also erode the odontoid, causing a fracture, with subsequent impingement on the foramen magnum.

It is dangerous to manipulate the spine in the presence of disorders such as ankylosing spondylitis, Reiter's disease, psoriasis (which can involve sacro-iliac joints), ulcerative colitis and Crohn's disease. The inflammatory bowel disorders cause an apophyseal joint arthropathy.

The distribution of the target joints in the spine is shown in Figure 6.1. The distribution of osteoarthritis is shown for comparison but it does not represent an absolute contra-indication to therapy.

3. Severe neurological changes

It is mandatory that the therapist recognises the early clinical features of spinal cord and cauda equina compression, because urgent referral for surgical correction (if appropriate) is essential. Unfortunately this emergency can follow manipulation of the lumbar spine. The commonest cause is a large central disc protrusion.

The symptoms and signs are outlined in Chapter 21.

4. Instability of the spine

It is important to diagnose instability since the performance of a procedure that increases mobility will further weaken the unstable area. The area of concern is the cervical spine with rheumatoid arthritis (already mentioned), but the other problem is post trauma, especially the common problem of whiplash, which can produce instability in any region of the cervical spine, especially the upper and mid regions.

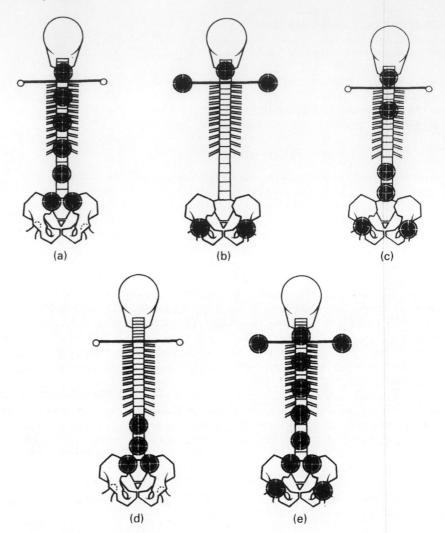

Figure 6.1 (a) Target areas of Crohn's disease and ulcerative colitis. (b) Target areas of rheumatoid arthritis. (c) Target areas of osteoarthritis. (d) Target areas of Reiter's disease. (e) Target areas of ankylosing spondylitis and psoriatic arthropathy.

Symptoms and signs indicating instability are:

- chronic persistent pain
- persistence of symptoms beyond the expected time of improvement
- bilateral pain, and paraesthesia and abnormal signs, especially in the upper limbs
- bilateral symptoms present in both limbs simultaneously or fluctuating between limbs
- symptoms crossing the midline
- symptoms relieved by immobilisation, for example, a proper cervical collar.

The diagnosis is made radiologically by plain radiographs or CT scans of the upper cervical region. The plain radiographs should include lateral views in flexion and extension and an anteroposterior view in lateral flexion.

Relative contra-indications

Not all the conditions included in the list will be discussed but the important condition of vertebro-basilar insufficiency will be covered in some detail.

1. Vertebro-basilar insufficiency (VBI)

Although this problem is likely to increase with age it can occur in younger patients, some of whom have vascular abnormalities. However, in others there may be no demonstrable abnormality.

It is the single most important condition to be on the alert for before manipulating the cervical spine. Any patient diagnosed as having VBI should only receive gentle mobilisation or soft tissue treatment.

End range techniques must not be used because of the devastating complication of a complete cerebrovascular accident due to vertebro-basilar infarction; sudden death can occur as a result of using end range techniques with patients in this category.

The clinical features of vertebro-basilar ischaemia and carotid artery ischaemia (for comparison) are shown in Figure 6.2. They can be summarised thus:

● any age of onset, but especially likely in the elderly
● symptoms include: vertigo or dizziness, blurred vision, diplopia, headache, nausea, tinnitus, drop attacks and dysarthria
● symptoms precipitated or aggravated by rotation of the neck in extension, for example, looking up into a high cupboard.

A clinically provocative test which tests for these symptoms, especially vertigo and the sign of nystagmus, should be conducted prior to any cervical manipulation.

Figure 6.2 Cerebral arterial circulation with some important clinical features of carotid and vertebro-basilar ischaemia.

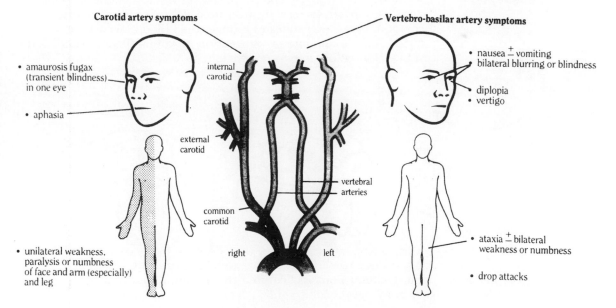

Carotid artery symptoms

Vertebro-basilar artery symptoms

• amaurosis fugax (transient blindness) in one eye

• aphasia

internal carotid

external carotid

common carotid

vertebral arteries

right   left

• unilateral weakness, paralysis or numbness of face and arm (especially) and leg

• nausea ± vomiting
bilateral blurring or blindness

• diplopia
• vertigo

• ataxia ± bilateral weakness or numbness

• drop attacks

The problem arises because of the anatomical course of the vertebral artery which enters the costo-transverse foramina of C6 and runs to the axis through the costo-transverse foramina. It then enters the costo-transverse foramina of the atlas and exits to form a posterosuperiorly directed loop before entering the skull.

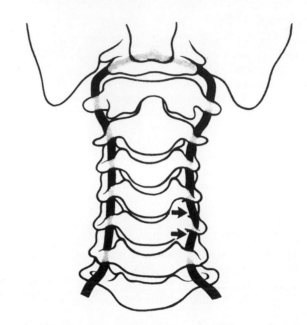

Figure 6.3 Schematic representation of the vertebral arteries which join to form the basilar artery. The osteophytes (arrowed) are generally not a significant problem and unlikely to produce symptoms but can compromise arterial flow with sharp rotations of the neck (after Dvorak, 1984).

When the head is rotated the contralateral vertebral artery is angulated at the level of the atlanto-axial junction (Figures 6.3, 6.4). The blood flow may be compromised, especially in the presence of disease within the artery or narrowed foramen due to osteophyte formation. However, extension reduces the blood flow further (in both arteries) and, if combined with rotation or lateral flexion, renders the cerebral flow vulnerable to insufficiency.

Figure 6.4 Movements of the left vertebral artery in three positions of the head (after Fielding, 1957).

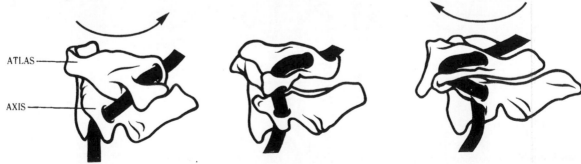

A. *atlas rotation to the left*   B. *mid position*   C. *atlas rotation to the right (note the angulation)*

The clinical provocation tests for VBI will be outlined in Chapter 12 on cervical manipulation.

2. *Spondylolisthesis*

Spondylolisthesis is a reasonably common condition of forward subluxation of the body of one vertebra on the vertebra below, especially of L5 over the body of the sacrum (Figure 6.5). The term is derived from the Greek word *listhesis* which means a falling or slipping. The clinical features are presented in Chapter 21.

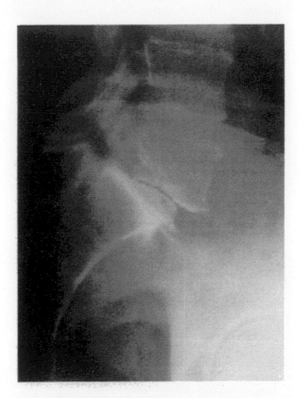

Figure 6.5 Lateral X-ray of the lumbo-sacral spine showing spondylolisthesis of L5 on the body of the sacrum: manipulation is contra-indicated in this patient at this level.

Manipulation of patients with this condition should be avoided, because not only will it fail to improve the problem, but any manipulative thrust into extension may cause aggravation.

Management consists essentially of a strict flexion exercise programme to be maintained for a minimum period of three months.

3. *Anti-coagulant therapy*

With the increase in the number of people having heart surgery, the number of those taking anti-coagulant medication is increasing, thus highlighting the need to consider this as a routine question in the history. Patients tend to forget to remind the therapist about this fact as it is such a normal routine for them.

Bleeding around nerve roots can occur spontaneously in those with a low prothrombin level, with the high probability of permanent damage. Hence forceful techniques must be avoided. The presence of unusual bruising should alert the therapist to this possibility. Some therapists do not consider giving even mobilisation to these patients, and favour an exercise programme and other very conservative techniques.

4.   Osteoporosis

Osteoporosis is a special problem in the post-menopausal woman complaining of back pain, because a mainpulative technique runs a significant risk of causing a compression fracture of a vertebra or a rib fracture.

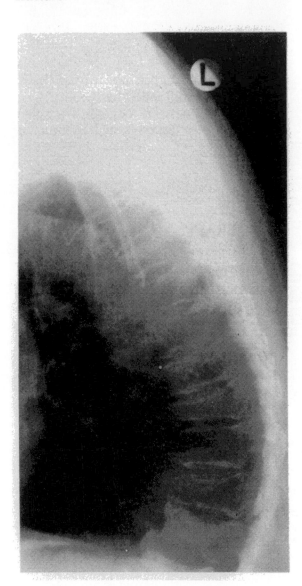

Figure 6.6 Plain X-ray showing osteoporosis in the spine in a 65-year-old woman: note the presence of compression fractures of the vertebrae. (It takes about 10 years and a loss of at least one-third of bone mass to diagnose osteoporosis on a plain X-ray.)

The diagnosis of osteoporosis is usually made on a plain X-ray (Figure 6.6) but it takes approximately 10 years and a loss of one-third of bone mass before it is apparent on such X-rays. An early diagnosis prior to this stage can be made only with more sophisticated techniques including densitometry, dual photonspectrometry and CT scans.

The golden rule is to exercise extreme caution with the elderly, and with the post-menopausal female presenting with thoracic back pain: if in doubt, don't manipulate.

5.   Inability of the patient to relax

If a patient cannot relax then it is difficult to perform a satisfactory manipulation.

Some patients are anxious and cannot relax because of their predisposition and because they do not feel relaxed or confident with the therapist. Similarly, they may have heard unfavourable reports about manual therapy. If it is not possible to reassure and relax the patient, manipulation should not be attempted. It should never be attempted in a patient who states that he or she does not want to be treated with a forceful technique. Such a patient can be given mobilisation or a muscle energy technique as an alternative and this may be both psychologically and physically therapeutic.

6.   Marked foraminal encroachment

An X-ray showing foraminal encroachment (Figure 6.7) in a patient with neck pain or low back pain may not be responsible for the patient's

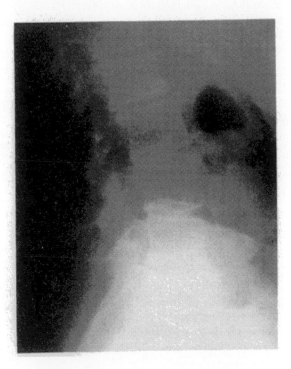

Figure 6.7 Lateral X-ray of a lumbar spine with degenerative disease showing significant narrowing of the intervertebral foramen.

presenting problem, but such a finding may be very significant, especially in the presence of intervertebral disc degeneration. Manipulation in the wrong direction may precipitate radicular pain which was not present previously. It must be remembered that narrowed intervertebral foramina may be present bilaterally, so the opening up of the foramen on one side will compress the foramen on the opposite side, with corresponding compression of the nerve root. This situation applies to moderate to severe narrowing but not to mild narrowing.

The appropriate physical treatment for these patients is mobilisation, especially traction, but no post end range technique should be attempted.

7.   Evidence of a severe disc protrusion or acute nerve root involvement

The therapist must be continually on guard for clinical evidence of a severe disc protrusion which must not be subjected to a manipulative thrust. This runs the risk of sequestration of the disc into the juxtaposed neurological structures including the spinal cord and cauda equina.

The following symptoms and signs are pointers to a large disc protrusion:

- delayed onset of pain (hours after injury)
- radicular pain – sciatica below knee
  – arm pain below the elbow
- paraesthesia and anaesthesia in the limbs
- a feeling of a floppy foot and weakness in the leg
- marked scoliosis/lateral deviation of the spine
- an 'irritable' spine
- sensitive slump test
- straight leg raising < 30 degrees.

Interpreting radicular pain

It should be recognised that patients presenting with radicular pain in the leg can have two nerve roots involved – for example, an L5–S1 disc protrusion can compress both the L5 and S1 nerve roots – but this is not the case at the cervical level, where a disc lesion will affect one nerve root only. If a patient presents with involvement of two or more roots in the arm then often diagnosis such as a tumour should be considered.

Care with manual therapy

1.   Pregnancy

Back pain, especially low back pain, is common during pregnancy and special care has to be taken, as the joints are being 'softened' and tend to be hypermobile due to the release of prolactin in preparation for parturition. Particular attention must be paid to the sacro-iliac joints. However, manual therapy can be extremely effective for pregnant patients but certain safety rules should be followed.

First trimester   use normal manual therapy
Second trimester   use supine side lying rotation and sitting
techniques only
Third trimester   avoid manual therapy if possible

The guidelines for treatment are:

- keep mobilisation and manipulation to a minimum
- use mobilisation in preference to manipulation
- use specific manipulation techniques rather than general
- safeguard the sacro-iliac joints in the last trimester
- encourage exercise as much as possible
- avoid medications wherever possible.

In the post partum phase back pain is common, especially thoracic back pain due to lifting and lumbar pain following a difficult birth (especially in the lithotomy position). Manual therapy is not contra-indicated; indeed it is advisable, but should be administered carefully especially in the first two weeks. Poor muscle tone is a common predisposing factor and an exercise programme is to be encouraged.

2.   Trivial and psychogenic back pain

There is a tendency for a therapist trained in a particular method, be it spinal manipulation, acupuncture, hypnotherapy or some other method, to become a zealot for their beloved therapy which is perceived as a cure for most problems. This enthusiasm can be counterproductive in some patients, especially those with a psychoneurosis, including anxiety, depression, conversion disorder (hysteria), hypochondriasis, malingering and compensation neurosis.

The treatment does not help on a long-term (even short-term) basis and often aggravates the problem because it reinforces the sick role. The cause has to be treated, not the effect. A reliable sign that such a patient has a psychoneurotic disorder is the fact they often claim that the treatment felt marvellous as they leave the consulting room but call later in the day to say that their pain is worse.

Similarly those with trivial pain should be managed with caution and it may be appropriate to advise them about self care rather than to administer manual therapy.

Prevention is an important goal in medicine and it is good therapy to recognise or foreshadow the problem patient who will become a victim of the chronic pain cycle (Figure 6.8). The merry-go-round of multiple treatment and referrals must be avoided initially or subsequently ceased with wise counselling and appropriate referral with consideration being given to referral to a pain clinic.

3.   Hypermobility

Hypermobility, or segmental instability, is generally due to a specific group of causes. These include post-traumatic 'whiplash', inflammation (notably, rheumatoid arthritis in the cervical region), spondylolisthesis in the lumbar spine and severe disc degeneration (cervical and lumbar).

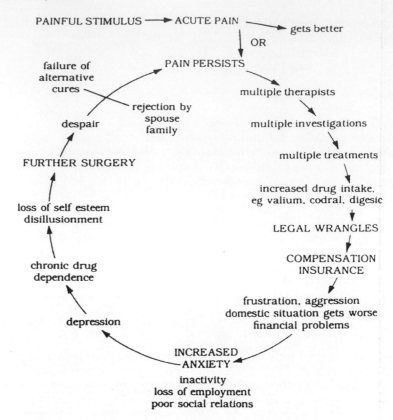

Figure 6.8 The chronic pain cycle (courtesy Dr Terry Little): Appropriate early treatment and counselling should prevent your patient becoming a victim of this complex 'nightmare'.

The low back pain in patients with hypermobility is aggravated by both activity and inactivity. Prolonged sitting and standing causes aching; stiffness in the morning is common, and minor injury can cause acute pain with diffuse radiation into the buttocks. The classic sign is that of lumbar insufficiency, evidenced by movement which is the opposite of the normal movement when extending from the flexed position. Instead of extending the upper trunk over the buttocks, the patient brings the buttocks and legs forward beneath the upper trunk in a ducking, irregular movement.

Most of these disorders are in the absolute or relative contra-indications category. Hypermobile conditions can be dangerous to handle and, in some instances, surgical stabilisation is needed, not manual therapy.

PRACTICE TIPS

- Don't manipulate the patient who is on anti-coagulant therapy.
- 'One disc lesion – one nerve root' is the rule for the cervical spine.
- An L5–S1 disc lesion can involve both the L5 and S1 nerve roots.

- Vertigo is the key symptom and nystagmus the key sign of vertebro-basilar insufficiency.
- As a rule, manipulation should be avoided in most patients over the age of 65.
- Narrowing of the intervertebral foramen is usually bilateral.
- Manual therapy is usually safe in the first six months of pregnancy.

SUMMARY

It is vital that practitioners of manual therapy be aware of safety guidelines. Irrespective of the current medico-legal climate, the guiding rule should be 'do no harm'.

A good practitioner is one who is trained in and acquainted with the global medical picture of organic and non-organic causes of pain in the back and who is clinically perceptive in quickly diagnosing disease and recognising danger signs.

Patients need and appreciate early referral where appropriate.

Important areas that demand special surveillance and caution are:

Cervical spine:	rheumatoid arthritis
	instability due to 'whiplash' and disc degeneration
	vertebro-basilar insufficiency
	nerve root compression with radicular pain
Thoracic spine:	osteoporosis
	metastatic disease
Lumbar spine:	spondylolisthesis
	large disc protrusion
	nerve root compression with radicular pain
	spinal cord and cauda equina pressure
	metastatic disease

General factors such as infection, tumours and anti-coagulant therapy should be kept in mind.

Section 2
The Cervical Spine and Upper Limb

7
Neck pain and related clinical features

'We have all heard of the courtiers who mimicked the wry neck of Alexander the Great.'

William Heberden (1710–1801)

Contents
- ☐ Key checkpoints
- ☐ Functional anatomy
- ☐ Dermatome patterns
- ☐ Causes of neck pain
- ☐ A diagnostic approach to neck pain
- ☐ Clinical syndromes
- ☐ Practice tips
- ☐ Summary

Disorders of cervical origin are very common in both sexes at most ages. Pain of cervical origin may be experienced as neck pain or referred to the head, shoulders and chest. There are 35 cervical joints, and, as is the case with the lumbar spine, pain may arise from any of these (especially the apophyseal joints), the intervertebral disc and the muscles. The other major symptom, apart from neck pain, is limited movement or stiffness.

KEY CHECKPOINTS

- Headache can be caused by abnormalities in any structure innervated by the upper cervical nerves (C2 and C3).
- Common sources of neck pain are the apophyseal joints, the intervertebral discs, the pre-vertebral and post-vertebral muscles.
- Disorders of any of these cervical structures can refer pain to the head, shoulder, upper limb, the posterior and anterior chest wall; depending on the site of the lesion.
- Strains and fractures of the apophyseal joints, especially after a 'whiplash' injury, are difficult to detect, and are often over-looked causes of neck and referred pain.

- Cervical nerve root compression can be caused by a disc protrusion or osteophytic encroachment on the transverse foramen.
- The commonest cause of neck pain is dysfunction of the facet joints with or without a history of injury.
- Cervical spondylosis is a disorder of ageing: radiological signs occur in 50 per cent of people over the age of 50 and in 75 per cent over the age of 65.
- In cervical spondylosis, osteophytic projections may produce nerve root and spinal cord compression, resulting in radiculopathy and myelopathy respectively.
- Radiculopathy can be caused by a soft disc protrusion (usually unilateral), a hard calcified lump and osteophytes (may be bilateral).
- Cervical disorders are aggravated by vibration – for example, riding in a motor vehicle.

FUNCTIONAL ANATOMY

The cervical spine is a complex of 35 joints which permits exceptional mobility. This mobility is enhanced by the anatomical arrangement of the atlas and axis, by the relative smallness of the antero-posterior diameter of the vertebral body relative to the height and by the sagittal apophyseal angle of 45 degrees which permits movement in every direction.

The apophyseal joints, which are very important for mobility, are absent between the atlas and skull (the atlanto-occipital joints: C0–C1) and between the atlas and the axis (the atlanto-axial joints: C1–C2). These weight-bearing joints lie in a firm column called the articular pillar. On palpation they feel like rather small domes and lie deep beneath the trapezius muscle. They are prone to osteoarthritis, with the C2–C3 joints being referred to as the 'headache joints' and the C5–C6, C6–C7 joints as the 'osteoarthritic joints', an important cause of pain in the upper limb. Figure 7.1 shows an illustration of a transverse section

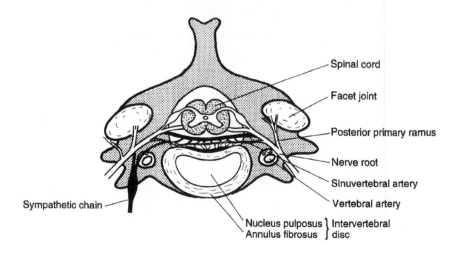

Figure 7.1 Transverse section illustrating the functional unit and nervous network of the cervical spine.

Spinal cord

Facet joint

Posterior primary ramus

Nerve root

Sinuvertebral artery

Vertebral artery

Sympathetic chain

Nucleus pulposus ⎱ Intervertebral
Annulus fibrosus ⎰ disc

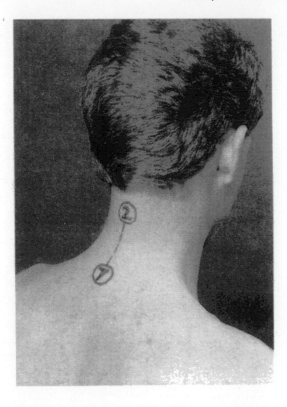

Figure 7.2 Surface anatomy of the neck highlighting the positions of the spinous processes of the cervical spine.

through the cervical spine. The relationship of nerves and blood vessels is quite unique.

The main muscles are the extensors, trapezius, splenius and the smaller rotators. These muscles, which have an exceptionally high innervation ratio, are capable of very rapid and delicate movements.

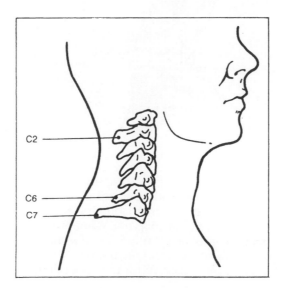

Figure 7.3 Relative sizes of spinous processes of the cervical spine.

The surface anatomy of the spinous processes is of paramount clinical importance in establishing the exact level of pain originating in the cervical spine. The first large projection beneath the occiput is the spinous process of C2. The spinous processes of C3, C4 and C5 are difficult to palpate because of the cervical lordosis. C6 is easily palpable but disappears under the palpating finger on extension of the neck. The largest 'fixed' prominence is the spinous process of C7 (Figures 7.2 and 7.3).

The palpable tip of the transverse process of the atlas (C1) lies between the angle of the jaw and the mastoid process. The apophyseal pillar (two to three centimetres from the midline) is felt as a series of small ridges, especially when the neck is flexed.

DERMATOME PATTERNS

The cervical spine is a prolific source of referred pain patterns. Generally, this can arise from one of two mechanisms, nerve root pain (radicular) or segmental dysfunction (spondylogenic). Nerve root pain can arise from nerve root compression caused by a prolapsed disc or by narrowing of an intervertebral foramen. Segmental dysfunction, which is by far the commonest cause, results in irritation of the posterior primary rami causing referred pain in the dermatomal pattern (refer to Chapter 1). Practitioners should be familiar with the dermatomal

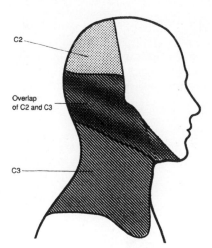

Figure 7.4 Dermatomes of the head: typical patterns (note the overlap of C2 and C3).

patterns for all cervical nerves and should be aware of overlapping patterns and individual variations in patterns. The dermatomes of the head (Figure 7.4) highlight those for the second and third cervical nerves with the overlap in distribution. Roots of these nerves can refer pain in the distribution of the fifth cranial (trigeminal) nerve, especially the ophthalmic branch.

The typical patterns for the upper limb are presented in Figure 7.5.

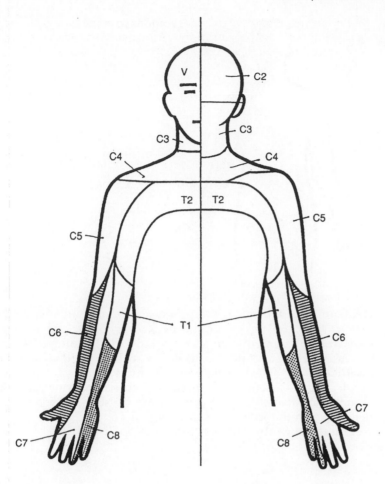

Figure 7.5 Dermatomes of the upper limb.

CAUSES OF NECK PAIN

Vertebral dysfunction, especially of the apophyseal joints, and spondylosis, known also as degenerative osteoarthrosis or osteoarthritis, are the main causes of neck pain.

In children and adolescents neck pain, often with stiffness, may be a manifestation of infection or inflammation of cervical lymph nodes, usually secondary to an infected throat – for example, tonsillitis or pharyngitis. However, it is vital to consider the possibility of meningitis. Sometimes a high fever associated with a systemic infection or pneumonia can cause meningism. In the presence of fever the rare possibility of poliomyelitis should be kept in mind. In both children and adults the presence of cerebral pathology such as haemorrhage, abscess or tumour are uncommon possibilities.

In adults the outstanding causes are dysfunction of the joints and spondylosis, with the acute febrile causes encountered in children being rare. However, cerebral and meningeal disorders may cause pain and stiffness in the neck.

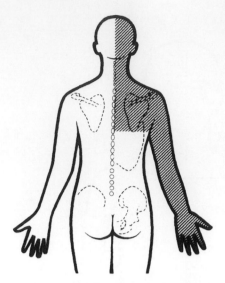

Figure 7.6 Zone of possible pain distribution (radicular or referred) caused by cervical disc lesions on the right side.

Rheumatoid arthritis is the prime severe inflammatory arthropathy that involves the neck, but the neck can be affected in ankylosing spondylitis, Reiter's disease and psoriasis. The painful acute wry neck can affect all ages and is considered to be caused mainly by acute disorders of the apophyseal joints rather than a disc prolapse. However, disc lesions do occur and can cause referred pain or radicular pain (Figure 7.6). Radicular pain can be caused also by impingement of the nerve root in the intervertebral foramen.

A summary of the causes is presented in Table 7.1.

Table 7.1 *Causes of neck pain.*

Musculoskeletal	**Infective**	**Neoplasia****
Joint dysfunction	Spinal	benign
apophyseal	osteomyelitis	malignant
intervertebral disc	tuberculosis	
	herpes zoster	**Psychogenic**
Muscular/ligamentous		
	Extraspinal	**Referred visceral**
Trauma	cervical adenitis	heart
'whiplash'	poliomyelitis	oesophagus
fracture	tetanus	carcinoma lung
other disorders		
	Extracervical	
	meningitis	**Referred cranial**
Inflammation	febrile states –	haemorrhage, e.g.
osteoarthritis*	meningism	subarachnoid
rheumatoid arthritis	malaria	tumour
ankylosing spondylitis		abscess
psoriasis	**Degenerative**	
Reiter's disease	spondylosis*	
polymyalgia rheumatica		
thyroiditis		

*   Osteoarthritis or spondylosis is inflammatory and degenerative.
** Neoplasia of the cervical spine is rare.

A DIAGNOSTIC APPROACH TO NECK PAIN

A summary of the Murtagh safety diagnostic model is presented in Table 7.2.

Probability diagnosis

The main causes of neck pain are vertebral dysfunction, especially of the facet joints, and traumatic strains or sprains affecting the

Table 7.2 *Neck pain: diagnostic strategy model.*

Q.	*Probability diagnosis*
A.	Vertebral dysfunction
	Traumatic 'strain' or 'sprain'
	Cervical spondylosis
Q.	*Serious disorders not to be missed*
A.	Cardiovascular
	angina
	subarachnoid haemorrhage
	Neoplasia
	primary
	metastasis
	Pancoast's tumour
	Severe infections
	osteomyelitis
	meningitis
	Vertebral fractures or dislocation
Q.	*Pitfalls (often missed)*
A.	Disc prolapse
	Myelopathy
	Cervical lymphadenitis
	Fibromyalgia syndrome
	Outlet compression syndrome, e.g. cervical rib
	Polymyalgia rheumatica
	Ankylosing spondylitis
	Rheumatoid arthritis
	Oesophageal foreign bodies and tumours
	Paget's disease
Q.	*Seven masquerades checklist*
A.	Depression ✓
	Diabetes –
	Drugs –
	Anaemia –
	Thyroid disease ✓
	Spinal dysfunction ✓✓
	UTI –
Q.	*Is the patient trying to tell me something?*
A.	Highly probable. Stress and adverse occupational factors relevant.

musculoligamentous structures of the neck. Spondylosis, known also as degenerative osteoarthrosis and osteoarthritis, is also a common cause, especially in the elderly patient.

Serious disorders not to be missed

Conditions causing neck pain and stiffness may be a sign of meningitis or of cerebral haemorrhage, particularly subarachnoid haemorrhage, or of a cerebral tumour or retropharyngeal abscess. Angina and myocardial infarction should be considered in anterior neck pain. Tumours are relatively rare in the cervical spine but metastases do occur and should be kept in mind, especially with persistent neck pain present day and night.

Pitfalls

There are many pitfalls in the clinical assessment of causes of neck pain and many of them are inflammatory.

Rheumatoid arthritis is the prime severe inflammatory arthropathy that involves the neck but the neck can be affected by the seronegative spondyloarthropathies, particularly ankylosing spondylitis, psoriasis and the inflammatory bowel disorders.

While polymyalgia rheumatica affects mainly the shoulder girdle, pain in the lower neck, which is part of the symptom complex, is often overlooked. Diffuse neck pain in myofascial soft tissue with tender trigger areas is part of the uncommon but refractory fibromyalgia syndrome.

Seven masquerades checklist

Cervical spinal dysfunction is the obvious outstanding cause. Thyroiditis may cause neck pain, as in the extremely rare cases of acute specific infection in the thyroid (e.g. syphilis, pyogenic infections) which cause severe pain; non-specific thyroiditis (de Quervain's thyroiditis) produces painful swelling with dysphagia. The association between depression and neck pain is well documented.

Psychogenic considerations

The neck is one of the commonest areas for psychological fixation following injury. This may involve perpetuation or exaggeration of pain because of factors such as anxiety and depression, conversion reaction and secondary gain.

CLINICAL SYNDROMES

Pain originating from the cervical spine is commonly, but not always, experienced in the neck. The patient may complain of headache, or pain around the ear, face, shoulder, arm, scapulae or upper anterior chest.

If the cervical spine is overlooked as a source of pain the cause of symptoms will remain masked and mismanagement will follow.

Clinical problems of cervical origin

- neck pain
- neck stiffness
- headache
- 'migraine' like headache
- arm pain (referred or radicular)
- facial pain
- ear pain (periauricular)
- scapular pain
- anterior chest pain
- torticollis
- dizziness/vertigo
- visual dysfunction

Figure 7.7 indicates typical directions of referred pain according to the patterns described in Chapter 1.

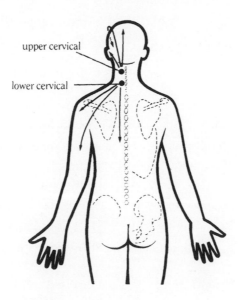

upper cervical

lower cervical

Figure 7.7 Possible common directions of referred pain from the cervical spine.

Pain in the arm (brachialgia) is common and tends to cover the shoulder and upper arm area indicated in Figure 7.7. This is the zone of referred pain which is not caused by nerve root compression. It can be a difficult diagnostic dilemma because pain reference from the fifth cervical nerve segment (C5) involves musculoskeletal, neurological and visceral structures. Virtually all shoulder structures are innervated by C5.

The practitioner must first determine whether the pain originates from the cervical spine or the shoulder joints, or from both simultaneously, or whether it originates from some other structure.

The often missed diagnosis of polymyalgia rheumatica should be considered in the elderly patient presenting with pain in the zone indicated, especially if bilateral.

Cervical dysfunction

Dysfunction of the 35 intervertebral joints that comprise the cervical spine complex is responsible for most cases of neck pain. The problem can occur at all ages and appears to be caused by disorder (including malalignment) of the many facet joints, which are pain-sensitive. Dysfunction of these joints, which may also be secondary to intervertebral disc disruption, initiates a reflex response of adjacent muscle spasm and myofascial tenderness. Dysfunction can follow obvious trauma such as a blow to the head or a sharp jerk to the neck, but can be caused by repeated trivial trauma or activity such as painting a ceiling or gentle wrestling. People often wake up with severe neck pain and blame it on a 'chill' from a draught on the neck during the night. This is incorrect because it is usually caused by an unusual twist on the flexed neck for a long period during sleep.

A typical profile

Age:	Typical range 12–50 years.
Radiation:	● To occiput, ear, face and temporal area (upper cervical). ● To shoulder region especially suprascapular area (lower cervical). Rarely refers pain below the level of the shoulder.
Site:	Usually localised to neck.
Occality:	A dull ache (may be sharp).
Precipitating factors:	Follows trauma or unaccustomed activity such as painting a ceiling.
Aggravating factors:	Above activities, reversing car, lying in bed.
Relieving factors:	Heat and massage, exercises.
Associations:	Stiffness of varying degrees. Neck tends to lock with certain specific movements.
Examination:	Localised unilateral tenderness over affected joints. Variable restriction of movement (may be normal).

Cervical disc disruption

Disruption of a cervical disc can result in several different syndromes.

1. Referred pain over a widespread area due to pressure on adjacent dura mater.
   Note: A disc disruption is capable of referring pain over such a diffuse area (Figure 7.6) that the patient is sometimes diagnosed as functional, e.g. hysterical.

2. Nerve root or radicular pain (radiculopathy). The pain follows the dermatomal distribution of the nerve root in the arm.
3. Spinal cord compression (myelopathy).

Radiculopathy

Apart from protrusion from an intervertebral disc, nerve root pressure causing arm pain can be caused by osteophytes associated with cervical spondylosis. The pain follows neurological patterns down the arm, being easier to localise with lower cervical roots especially C6, C7 and C8.

Note: 1. The cervical roots exit above their respective vertebral bodies. For example, the C6 root exits between C5 and C6 so that a prolapse of C5–C6 intervertebral disc or spondylosis of the C5–C6 junction affects primarily the C6 root (Figure 7.8).

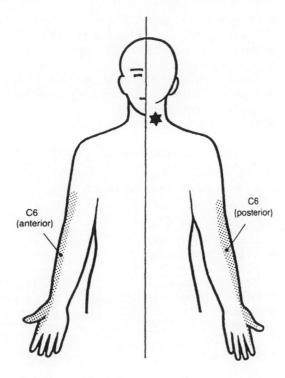

Figure 7.8 Typical C6 nerve root (radicular pain).

2. One disc–one nerve root is the rule.
3. Spondylosis and tumours tend to cause bilateral pain, i.e. more than one nerve root.

Clinical presentation

● A sharp aching pain in the neck, radiating down one or both arms.
● Onset of pain may be abrupt, often precipitated by a sudden neck movement on awakening.

- Stiffness of neck with limitation of movement.
- Nocturnal pain, waking patient during night.
- Pain localised to upper trapezius and possible muscle spasm.

Investigations

- Plain X-ray (A-P, lateral E and F, oblique views to visualise foramina); good for diagnosis, not for surgery.
- Plain CT scan.
- CT scan and myelogram – excellent visualisation of structures but invasive.
- MRI – excellent but expensive, sometimes difficult to distinguish soft disc from osteophytes.

Myelopathy

Clinical features:

- Older patients, typically men over 50.
- Insidious onset: symptoms over 1–2 years.
- Numbness and tingling in fingers.
- Leg stiffness.
- Numb clumsy hands, especially with a high cervical lesion.
- Signs of UMN: spastic weakness, increased tone and hyper-reflexia (arms > legs).
- Neurological deficit which predicts the level with reasonable accuracy.
- Bowel and bladder function usually spared.

Note: LMN signs occur at the level of the lesion and UMN signs and sensory changes below this level.

Causes

- Cervical spondylosis.
- Atlanto-axial subluxation
     rheumatoid arthritis
     Down's syndrome.
- Primary spinal cord tumours, e.g. meningiomas.
- Metastasis to cervical spine leading to epidural spinal cord compression.

Investigations

- CT scan with myelogram (very accurate).
- MRI (also accurate).

Cervical headache

Cervical headache is usually suboccipital and unilateral but can be bilateral. Although commonly misdiagnosed as migraine, a careful history will differentiate between headaches of cervical origin and classic migraine. Routine investigation of headache should involve examination of the cervical spine. The neck may be responsible also for so-called 'tension' headache but clinical differentiation can be more difficult.

A typical profile

Site:	Suboccipital.
Radiation:	Parietal region and vertex of skull. May spread to behind one or both eyes, or sometimes is frontal.
Quality:	Nagging aching pain of mild to moderate severity.
Frequency:	Often every day.
Duration:	Usually one to six hours but can last two to three days.
Onset:	Patient usually wakes up with it.
Offset:	Variable but settles usually around mid-day.
Precipitating factors:	Often a history of preceding trauma such as motor vehicle accident or hitting head on overhead obstacle.
Aggravating factors:	Neck movements, reversing car, extending neck for long periods such as painting ceiling, 'faulty' pillows.
Relieving factors:	Heat and neck massage, cervical mobilisation or manipulation.
Associated features (possible):	Stiffness and grating in the neck, paraesthesia of scalp, vision blurred or dull, lassitude, irritability.
Examination:	Neck movements reproduce the head pain. Spasm and tenderness of suboccipital muscles. Painful restriction C1–C2, C2–C3 (especially) on palpation.

The explanation for referral of pain from disorders of the upper cervical spine to the head and eye is that some afferent fibres from the upper cervical nerve roots converge upon cells in the posterior horn of the spinal cord (which can also be excited by trigeminal afferent fibres) thus conveying to the patient the impression of head pain through this shared pathway. It has been demonstrated that stimulation of the first cervical posterior root provokes pain in the frontal and orbital regions. Furthermore, cervical headaches have been abolished by selective anaesthetic blockage of the lateral atlanto-axial joints (C1–C2) or the C2–C3 apophyseal joints.

Cervical spondylosis

Cervical spondylosis following disc degeneration and apophyseal joint degeneration is far more common than lumbar spondylosis and mainly involves the C5–C6 and C6–C7 segments. The consequence is narrowing of the intervertebral foramen with the nerve roots of C6 and C7 being at risk of compression.

Cervical spondylosis is generally a chronic problem but it may be asymptomatic. In some patients the pain may lessen with age, while stiffness increases.

Clinical features

- Dull aching suboccipital neck pain.
- Stiffness.
- Worse in morning on arising and lifting head.
- Improves with gentle activity.
- Deteriorates with heavy activity – for example, painting.
- Usually unilateral pain – may be bilateral.
- Pain may be referred to head, arms and scapulae.
- May wake patient at night with paraesthesia in arms.
- C6 nerve root most commonly involved.
- Acute attacks on chronic background.
- Aggravated by flexion (reading) and extension.
- Associated vertigo or unsteadiness.
- Restricted tender movements, especially rotation/lateral flexion.
- Joints tender to palpation.
- X-ray changes invariable.

Acute torticollis

Torticollis (acute wry neck) means a lateral deformity of the neck and is usually a transient self-limiting acutely painful joint disorder with associated muscle spasm of variable intensity.

Clinical features (typical)

- Age of patient between 13 and 30 years.
- Patient usually awakes with the problem.
- Pain usually confined to neck but may radiate.
- Deformity of lateral flexion and slight flexion/rotation.
- Deformity usually away from the painful side.
- Restricted lateral flexion and rotation towards painful side.
- Loss of extension.
- Mid cervical spine (C2–C3, C3–C4, C4–C5).
- Any segment between C2–C7 can cause torticollis.
- Usually no neurological symptoms or signs.

The exact cause of this condition is uncertain, both an acute disc lesion and an apophyseal joint lesion being implicated, with the latter the more likely cause. Management by mobilisation and muscle energy therapy (Chapter 11) is described.

Whiplash

'Whiplash' is an emotive and overused term that probably should be confined to injuries suffered in a rear end collision between motor vehicles. Patients with the whiplash syndrome present typically with varying degrees of pain, related loss of mobility of the cervical spine, headache and emotional disturbance in the form of anxiety and depression.

The injury occurs as a consequence of hyperextension of the neck followed by recoil hyperflexion. There is reversal of sequence of these movements in a head-on collision. In addition to hyperextension, there is prolongation or anterior stretching plus longitudinal extension of the neck.

Hyperextension can be limited by a head restraint that supports the occipital region of the skull. Unfortunately, most cars have head restraints far removed from the occiput and some are set so low that they act as a fulcrum for hyperextension, thereby reinforcing the injury.

Whiplash causes injury to soft tissue structures including muscle, nerve roots, the cervical sympathetic chain, ligaments, apophyseal joints and their synovial capsules and intervertebral discs. Damage to the apophyseal joints appears to be severe, with possible microfractures (not detectable on plain X-ray) and long-term dysfunction. Table 7.3 summarises the anatomical disruption and their clinical effects.

Table 7.3 *Whiplash – summary of anatomical disruption.**

ANATOMICAL STRUCTURE INJURED	CLINICAL EFFECTS
Muscles	Stiffness
scaleni	Pain
longus colli	Headache (occipital)
sternomastoid	Dysphagia
Ligament	
anterior longitudinal	(As above)
Apophyseal joints	Stiffness
	Pain
	Headache
Intervertebral disc	Stiffness
	Nerve root pain
Sympathetic chain	Horner's syndrome
Nerve roots	Nerve root pain
(stretching)	
Oesophagus	Dysphagia

* The subsequent effects are caused by oedema, haematoma with inflammatory response and, later, by scar tissue and degenerative joint changes.

Pain and stiffness of the neck are the most common symptoms. The pain is usually experienced in the neck and upper shoulders but may radiate to the suboccipital region, the interscapular region and down the arms. The stiffness felt initially in the anterior neck muscles shifts to the posterior neck.

Headache is a common and disabling symptom that may persist for many months. It is typically occipital but can be referred to the temporal region and the eyes.

Table 7.4 *Complications of whiplash.*

Referred pain (headache, arm pain)
Visual problems
Vertigo
Dysphagia
Depression
Compensation neurosis
Disc rupture increasing to nerve root pain
Osteoarthritis becomes symptomatic

Nerve root pain can be caused by a traction injury of the cervical nerve roots or by inflammatory changes or direct pressure subsequent to herniation of a disc.

Paraesthesia of the ulnar border of the hand, nausea, dizziness, blurred vision are all relatively common symptoms.

Delayed symptoms are common. A patient may feel no pain until 24 (sometimes up to 96) hours later; most experience symptoms within six hours. Complications of whiplash are summarised in Table 7.4.

PRACTICE TIPS

- Dysfunction of the cervical spine is an underestimated cause of headache.
- Consider the cervical spine as a possible cause of shoulder pain.
- Cervical problems are aggravated by vibration, for example, riding in a motor vehicle.
- Beware of physically treating the neck in a patient with rheumatoid arthritis or Down syndrome.
- Consider dysfunction of the cervical spine as a possible cause of the tennis elbow syndrome and other so-called repetitive strain injuries of the arm.
- 'One disc – one nerve root' is a working rule for the cervical spine.
- All acutely painful conditions of the cervical spine following trauma should be investigated with a careful neurological examination of the limbs, sphincter tone and reflexes. Plain film radiology is mandatory.

SUMMARY

The cervical spine is a very mobile structure with a complex of 35 joints and all its components are capable of causing pain. Although pain and stiffness in the neck is the commonest outcome, the many referred pain patterns and associated symptoms should be kept in mind. Dysfunction of the discs and apophyseal joints are the major sources of pain, factors which become apparent with the onset of acute torticollis and the so-called 'whiplash' injury. The whiplash syndrome is particularly significant because it can cause damage to most of the musculoskeletal and neurological structures in the neck with the whole range of many clinical features including headache, brachialgia, chest pain, vertigo, sympathetic disturbance, blurred vision and stiffness.

The psychological sequelae that can follow this injury and chronic neck problems such as spondylosis convey a message to us that the state of the patient's cervical spine can profoundly affect his or her life and that we should always be aware of the whole person.

8
Pain in the shoulder and upper limb

'The patient who presents with the complaint "of pain in my shoulder" may well be referring to pain in the scapular area which could originate from the neck. Always remember that.'

James Cyriax
Lecture in London, 1976

Contents
- ☐ Key checkpoints
- ☐ Pain in the arm and hand
- ☐ Shoulder pain: neck or shoulder?

The patient who presents with pain in the region of the shoulder girdle or upper arm in particular, and into the arm in general, represents a challenging and often difficult problem. The practitioner must first determine whether the pain originates from the cervical spine or the shoulder joints, or from both simultaneously, or whether it originates from some other structure.

KEY CHECKPOINTS

- The so-called thoracic outlet syndrome is probably most often caused by 'the droopy shoulder syndrome' rather than by a cervical rib.
- Pain in the shoulder and upper arm may arise from dysfunction of the cervical spine, from disorders of the C5, C6 and C7 nerve roots, from disorders of the shoulder joints and their associated soft tissues, and from visceral causes.
- A careful history should generally indicate whether the neck or the shoulder is responsible for the patient's pain.
- Virtually all shoulder structures are innervated by the fifth cervical vertebra (C5) nerve root. Pain present in the distribution of C5 can arise from:

  - cervical spine
  - upper roots of brachial plexus
  - glenohumeral joint

- rotator cuff tendons, especially supraspinatus
- biceps tendon
- soft tissue – for example, polymyalgia rheumatica
- viscera, especially those innervated by the phrenic nerve (C3, C4, C5).

- By the age of 50 about 25 per cent of people have some wear and tear of the rotator cuff, making it more injury-prone (Bertelsen, 1969).
- Disorders of the rotator cuff are common, especially supraspinatus tendinitis. The most effective tests to diagnose these problems are the resisted movement tests (Ireland, 1986).
- The upper cervical nerve roots, comprising the brachial plexus (C5, C6, C7) with their dural investment, are capable of causing shoulder pain and arm pain which is clinically confusing. The brachial plexus tension test will help diagnose such disorders.

PAIN IN THE ARM AND HAND

Like pain in the shoulder, pain originating from the cervical spine and shoulder disorders can extend down the arm. While pain from disorders of the shoulder joint (because of its C5 innervation) does not usually extend below the elbow, radiculopathies originating in the cervical spine can transmit to distal parts of the arm (Figures 7.5 and 7.7).

Important causes are illustrated in Figure 8.1. Myocardial ischaemia must be considered, especially for pain experienced down the inner left arm.

Soft tissue disorders of the elbow are extremely common, especially tennis elbow. Two types of tennis elbow are identifiable: 'backhand' tennis elbow, or lateral epicondylitis, and 'forehand' tennis elbow, or medial epicondylitis, which is known also as golfer's or pitcher's elbow.

The various causes of the painful arm can be considered with the diagnostic model (Table 8.1).

Probability diagnosis

The commonest causes of arm pain are referred pain and radiculopathies caused by disorders of the cervical spine, the tennis elbows (lateral and, to a lesser extent, medial epicondylitis), carpal tunnel syndrome and regional pain syndromes caused by inflammation of the tendons around the wrist and thumb.

Disorders of the shoulder, particularly supraspinatus tendinitis, should be considered if the pain is present in the C5 dermatome distribution. Pain in the hand is commonly caused by osteoarthritis of the carpometacarpal joint of the thumb and the distal interphalangeal (DIP) joints and also by the carpal tunnel syndrome.

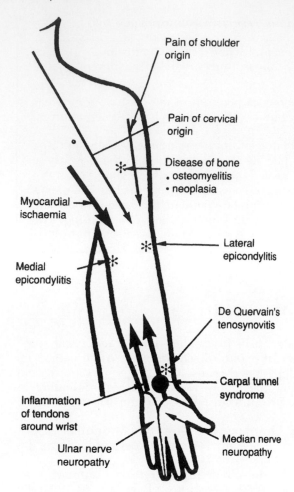

Figure 8.1 Important causes of arm pain (excluding trauma and arthritis).

Pain of shoulder origin

Pain of cervical origin

Disease of bone
• osteomyelitis
• neoplasia

Myocardial ischaemia

Lateral epicondylitis

Medial epicondylitis

De Quervain's tenosynovitis

Carpal tunnel syndrome

Inflammation of tendons around wrist

Ulnar nerve neuropathy

Median nerve neuropathy

Serious disorders not to be missed

Like any other presenting problem it is vital not to overlook malignant disease or severe infection. In the case of the arm, possible malignant disease includes tumours in bones, lymphoma involving axillary glands and Pancoast's syndrome.

In addition, myocardial ischaemia, especially infarction in the case of pain of sudden onset, should be considered for left arm pain.

Diagnostic pitfalls

Lesions of the nerve roots comprising the brachial plexus can cause arm pain, especially in the C5 and C6 distribution. These can be detected by the brachial plexus tension tests.

Other commonly missed causes include polymyalgia rheumatica, although the pain typically involves the shoulder girdle, reflex

Table 8.1 *Pain in the arm and hand: diagnostic strategy model (modified).*

Q. *Probability diagnosis*
A. Dysfunction of cervical spine (lower)
    Disorders of the shoulder
    Medial or lateral epicondylitis
    Overuse tendinitis of the wrist
    Carpal tunnel syndrome
    Osteoarthritis of thumb and DIP joints

Q. *Serious disorders not to be missed*
A. Cardiovascular
    ● angina (referred)
    ● myocardial infarction
    Neoplasia
    ● Pancoast's tumour
    ● bone tumours (rare)
    Severe infections
    ● septic arthritis (shoulder/elbow)
    ● osteomyelitis
    ● infections of tendon sheath and fascial spaces of hand

Q. *Pitfalls (often missed)*
A. Entrapment neuropathies, e.g. median nerve, ulnar nerve
    Pulled elbow – children
    Foreign body, e.g. elbow
    Rarities
    Polymyalgia rheumatica (for arm pain)
    Reflex sympathetic dystrophy
    Thoracic outlet syndrome
    Arm claudication (left arm)

sympathetic dystrophy (Sudek's atrophy) and the thoracic outlet syndromes.

The thoracic outlet syndromes include problems arising from compression or intermittent obstruction of the neurovascular bundle supplying the upper extremity – for example, cervical rib syndrome, costo-clavicular syndrome, scalenus anterior and medius syndrome, 'effort thrombosis' of axillary and subclavian veins and the subclavian steal syndrome.

The commonest cause of the thoracic outlet syndrome is sagging musculature related to ageing, obesity, and heavy breasts and arms, aptly described by Swift and Nichols as 'the droopy shoulder syndrome' (Swift and Nichols, 1984).

Cervical ribs are relatively common and may, or may not, contribute to the thoracic outlet syndrome. Often the cause is a functional change in the thoracic outlet due to the 'droopy shoulder syndrome' with no significant anatomical fault (Bertelsen, 1969).

Arm claudication is also rare. It can occur with arterial obstruction due to occlusion of the proximal left subclavian artery or the innominate artery. Exercise of the arm may be associated with central nervous system symptoms as well as claudication.

Arm pain causing sleep disturbance

Three important causes are cervical disorders, carpal tunnel syndrome and the thoracic outlet syndrome. The working rule is:

● thoracic outlet syndrome – patients cannot fall asleep
● carpal tunnel syndrome – patients wake in the middle of the night
● cervical spondylosis – the patient wakes with pain and stiffness that persists well into the day (Rathburn and MacNab, 1970).

SHOULDER PAIN: NECK OR SHOULDER?

The commonest causes of pain in the shoulder zone (Figure 8.2) are cervical disorders and periarthritis, i.e. soft tissue inflammation involving the tendons around the glenohumeral joint. The outstanding

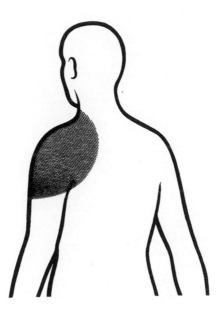

Figure 8.2 The confusion zone: pain in the shoulder and upper arms.

common disorders of the shoulder joint are the various disorders of the tendons comprising the rotator cuff and biceps tendon. Of these, supraspinatus tendon disorders are the commonest. A summary of the diagnostic model is presented in Table 8.2.

Pitfalls

The shoulder is notorious for diagnostic traps, especially for referred pain from visceral structures, but polymyalgia rheumatica is the real pitfall. A good rule is to consider it foremost in any older person (over

Table 8.2 *Shoulder pain: diagnostic strategy model (modified).*

Q.   Probability diagnosis
A.   Cervical spine dysfunction
       Supraspinatus tendinitis
       Adhesive capsulitis

Q.   Serious disorders not to be missed
A.   Cardiovascular
           angina
           myocardial infarction
       Neoplasia
           Pancoast's tumour
           primary or secondary in humerus
       Severe infections
           septic arthritis (children)
           osteomyelitis
       Rheumatoid arthritis

Q.   Pitfalls (often missed)
A.   Polymyalgia rheumatica
       Cervical dysfunction
       Osteoarthritis of acromioclavicular joint
       Winged scapula – muscular fatigue pain

---

60) presenting with bilateral shoulder girdle pain which is worse in the morning.

Specific pitfalls include:

- misdiagnosing posterior dislocation of the shoulder joint
- misdiagnosing recurrent subluxation of the shoulder joint
- overlooking an avascular humeral head (post fracture)
- misdiagnosing rotator cuff tear or degeneration.

Functional anatomy of the shoulder

A working knowledge of the anatomical features of the shoulder is essential for the understanding of the various disorders causing pain or dysfunction of the shoulder. Apart from the acromioclavicular (AC) joint there are two most significant functional joints – the glenohumeral (the primary joint) and the subacromial complex (the secondary joint) (Figure 8.3). The glenohumeral joint is a ball and socket joint enveloped by a loose capsule. It is prone to injury from traumatic forces and develops osteoarthritis more often than appreciated. Two other relevant functional joints are the scapulothoracic and stenoclavicular joints.

The clinically important subacromial space lies above the glenohumeral joint between the head of the humerus and an arch formed by the bony acromion, the thick coracoacromial ligament and the coracoid process. This relatively tight compartment houses the sub-

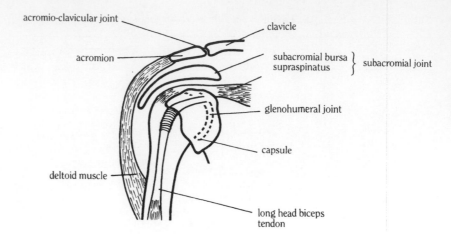

Figure 8.3. Anatomical features of the shoulder.

acromial bursa and the rotator cuff, particularly the vulnerable supraspinatus tendon. Excessive friction and pinching in this space renders these structures prone to injury.

There is a critical zone of relative ischaemia that appears to affect the rotator cuff about 1 cm medial to the attachment of the supraspinatus tendon (Rathburn and MacNab, 1970) and this area is compromised during adduction and abduction of the arm due to pressure on the rotator cuff tendons from the head of the humerus.

These factors are largely responsible for the many rotator cuff syndromes, bicipital tendinitis, subacromial bursitis and tears of supraspinatus tendon.

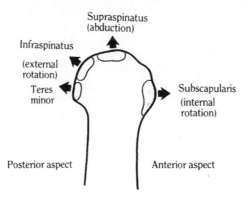

Figure 8.4 Attachment of the rotator cuff tendons.

A study of the anatomical attachments of the rotator cuff tendons to the head of the humerus (Figure 8.4) provides an understanding of the shoulder movements powered by these muscles. The muscles responsible for the various movements of the shoulder joint are summarised in Table 8.3. Several muscles can be involved in any movement of this complex joint.

Pain reference of key structures in the upper limb is presented in Table 8.4. The importance of the C5 nerve root is apparent.

Table 8.3 *Shoulder joint movements.*

MOVEMENT	NORMAL RANGE	MUSCLE(S) (main)
Flexion (anterior elevation)	180°	**Trapezius** Coracobrachialis
Extension (posterior elevation)	45°	**Teres major** Latissimus dorsi
Abduction (lateral elevation)	180°	**Supraspinatus** **Deltoid** Pectoralis major
Adduction	*30°	**Pectoralis major** Latissimus dorsi
Internal (medial) rotation	*40°	**Subscapularis** Pectoralis major
External (lateral) rotation	*90°	**Infraspinatus** Teres minor

Note. Deltoid is involved in all movements except adduction.
* American Medical Association Guidelines to Evaluation of Permanent Impairment (2nd
  Edition); movement from a neutral position.

Table 8.4 *Pain reference of key structures of the upper limb.*

STRUCTURE	MAIN NERVE ROOTS
Phrenic nerve	C3, C4, C5
Acromioclavicular joint	C4
Capsule of shoulder joint	C5
Subacromial bursa	C5
Supraspinatus	C5
Infraspinatus	C5, C6
Subscapularis	C5, C6
Biceps tendon	C5, C6
Triceps tendon	C7
Brachial plexus	C5, C6, C7, C8, T1
Radial nerve	C5, C6, C7, C8, T1
Median nerve	C6, C7, C8
Ulnar nerve	C8, T1

Examples

Supraspinatus tendinitis (typical pain profile)

Site:	The shoulder and outer border of arm. Maximal over deltoid insertion.
Radiation:	To elbow.
Quality:	Throbbing pain, can be severe.
Frequency:	Constant, day and night.
Duration:	Constant.

Onset:	Two days after straining the shoulder (e.g. dog on leash, working under car).
Offset:	Nil.
Aggravation:	Heat, putting on shirt, toilet activity, lying on shoulder.
Relief:	Analgesics only.
Associated features:	Trigger point over supraspinatus origin.

Traumatic adhesive capsulitis (typical pain profile)

Site:	Around the shoulder and outer border of arm.
Radiation:	To elbow.
Quality:	Deep throbbing pain.
Frequency:	Constant, day and night.
Duration:	Constant.
Onset:	Following minor fall onto shoulder (e.g. against wall); wakes the patient from sleep.
Offset:	Nil.
Aggravation:	Activity, dressing, combing hair, heat.
Relief:	Analgesics only (partial relief).
Associated features:	Stiffness of arm, may be frozen.

The frequently misdiagnosed condition of polymyalgia rheumatica should always be considered if an elderly patient presents with diffuse pain in the area of the shoulder girdle and if the physical examination is essentially normal. An elevated erythrocyte sedimentation rate supports the suspected diagnosis.

Referred pain to the shoulder can arise from irritation of the diaphragm due to visceral disease such as carcinoma of the lung, and can be a presentation of angina.

9
Examination of the cervical spine and shoulder

'More mistakes, many more, are made by not looking than by not knowing.'

Sir William Jenner

Contents
- ☐ Examination of the cervical spine
  - ● Key checkpoints
  - ● Inspection
  - ● Movements of the neck
  - ● Palpation
  - ● Pain provocation tests
  - ● Neurological examination
- ☐ Examination of the shoulder joint
  - ● Inspection
  - ● Palpation
  - ● Movements
- ☐ Practice tips
- ☐ Summary

EXAMINATION OF THE CERVICAL SPINE

Careful examination of the cervical spine is crucial for the correct diagnosis to be reached and for the appropriate treatment to be initiated, whether it is cervical mobilisation or manipulation.

The three objectives of the examination are to:

- ● reproduce the patient's symptoms
- ● identify the level of the lesion or lesions
- ● determine its cause (if possible).

As for other joint examinations, the examiner must follow the traditional rule of look, feel, move, test function, measure and X-ray.

A neurological examination is essential if radicular pain is present and weakness or other upper limb symptoms, including any pain or paraesthesia that extends below the elbow.

Throughout the physical examination it is important to exercise care and be aware of the degree of irritability of the spine so that unnecessary exacerbation of symptoms does not occur.

KEY CHECKPOINTS

- Examine the patient with an apparent irritable cervical spine with caution.
- Observe the length of the neck (base of skull to C7 level) during all active movements.
- If the movements are full and pain-free, apply over-pressure.
- Palpation of the neck is the cornerstone of cervical management. Palpate gently – the more one presses the less one feels.
- A neurological examination is necessary in only selected instances.

INSPECTION

Several pointers to the diagnosis may be present. It is important to observe the patient's head, neck and arm movements while he or she is undressing.

The patient should be examined sitting on a couch, rather than sitting in a chair. The body should be fully supported with the hands resting on the thighs. The following should be noted:

- willingness to move the head and neck
- position of the head
- level of the shoulders
- any lateral flexion
- contour of the neck from the side.

In the patient with torticollis the head is held laterally flexed with, perhaps, slight rotation to one side – usually away from the painful side. Patients suffering from whiplash injury and severe spondylosis tend to hold their neck stiff, their head forward and tend to turn their trunk rather than rotate their neck.

MOVEMENTS OF THE NECK

The movements are active and once again should be observed with the patient sitting on the couch.

After the patient points to where the symptoms are felt he or she is asked to follow a sequence of movements of the neck – flexion, extension, lateral flexion to both sides and rotation to both sides.

The movements should be observed from the front and side of the patient. Note the range, rhythm and degree of stiffness and pain for each movement. Note whether the arc of motion is smooth or halting, and whether combined or 'false' movements are used.

If there is a full range of pain-free movement, apply over-pressure slowly at the end range and note any pain. The range of movements

Table 9.1 *Movements of the cervical spine with normal ranges and involved joints.*

MOVEMENT	NORMAL RANGE	JOINTS INVOLVED
Flexion	45°	Atlanto-occipital Atlanto-axial Lower cervical
Extension	50°	Atlanto-occipital Atlanto-axial Lower cervical
Lateral flexion (left and right)	45°	Atlanto-occipital Lower cervical
Rotation (left and right)	75°	Atlanto-axial Lower cervical

may be recorded on the DOM diagram (Figure 2.8) or on a special grid used by some practitioners to record neck movements. The normal range of neck movements is presented in Table 9.1.

Flexion (Figure 9.1)

Stand in front of the seated patient and instruct the patient to move the chin towards the chest; normally it is possible to touch the chest. Note

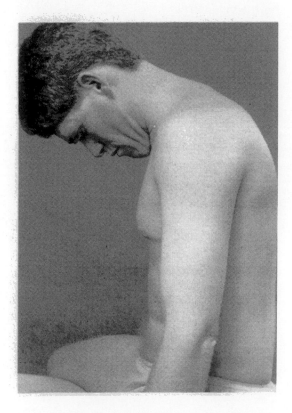

Figure 9.1 Flexion of the neck.

any asymmetry of movement. Now stand to the side and note flexion in the upper and lower cervical spine so that 'protected' non-mobile areas can be detected. Flexion is usually a most uncomfortable movement for patients with neck problems.

Extension (Figure 9.2)

Observe extension from the front and side of the patient. Instruct the patient to look up at the ceiling and extend as far as possible. Note where the movement is occurring, because 'flat spots' can occur in the upper or lower spine. Over-pressure to the head in extension can

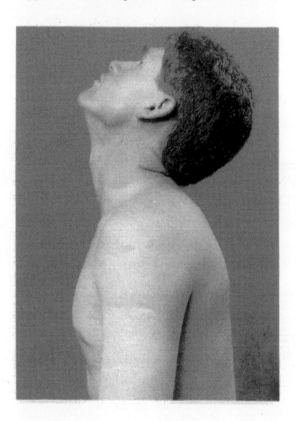

Figure 9.2 Extension of the neck.

provoke the patient's pain and can be selectively given for upper cervical or low cervical extension. Since the latter movement is often restricted it can be tested by applying over-pressure with the head in full extension (Figure 9.3).

Extension is usually restricted by disorders of the cervical spine. Normally all levels in the neck will be observed to move. Note any dizziness.

Lateral flexion (Figure 9.4)

While observing carefully from the front instruct the patient to move the ear down towards the shoulder, for left and right sides. The normal

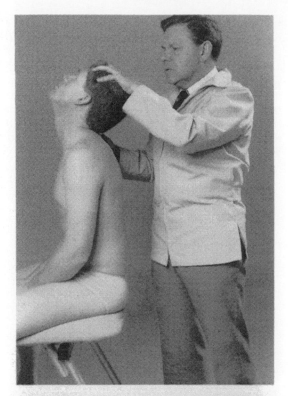

Figure 9.3 Applying over-pressure to lower cervical extension.

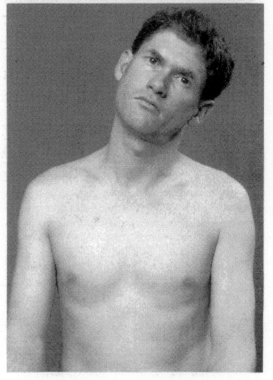

Figure 9.4 Lateral flexion of the neck.

range is about 45 degrees. The patient may compensate for limited neck movement by lifting the shoulder towards the ear. Apply over-pressure if necessary.

Rotation (Figure 9.5)

Instruct the patient to turn the head and look over the shoulder, for right and left sides. Normally the chin should almost align with the shoulder and younger people should be able to extend slightly beyond this point.

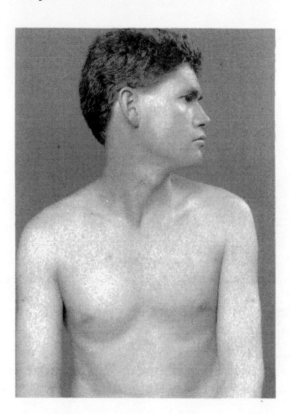

Figure 9.5 Rotation of the neck.

For each of these movements note the range, site and intensity of any pain. Correct or prevent any deviation (for example, compensation for limited rotation by using extension) and note the new range and pain response.

PALPATION

Palpation is a main component of the examination and it is essential to be familiar with the surface anatomy of the neck. The objectives are to determine the level of the lesion, the nature of the problem, and the mobility.

The patient should be prone with the forehead resting on the hands, palms up; the shoulders should be relaxed and the neck flexed forward as far as possible. The neck can also be readily palpated with the patient lying supine.

Spinous processes as reference points

Palpate the spinous processes to determine the levels of pain; palpate between them to detect thickening of the interspinous ligaments; palpate unilaterally about two to three centimetres from the midline over the apophyseal (facet) pillar.

Compare any abnormal joint with both the one above and the one opposite (at the same level). Note any increased temperature or sweating.

Central digital palpation

Stand at the patient's head. Place opposed straight thumbs on the spinous process of C2 (Figure 9.6), then methodically move down the midline on the spinous processes.

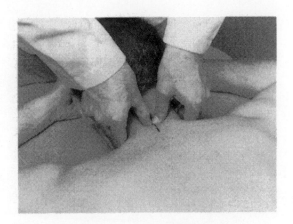

Figure 9.6 Central palpation on the spinous processes.

Press firmly two or three times over each vertebra, increasing the pressure with each oscillation to detect stiffness, pain or muscle spasm.

Unilateral digital palpation

Press with opposed straight thumbs against the articular pillar, about two to three centimetres from the midline (Figure 9.7). This will reproduce pain in the underlying apophyseal joints if they are abnormal.

Note: These palpatory procedures are not only diagnostic but also used for mobilisation therapy. Again, remember: the harder one presses, the less one feels.

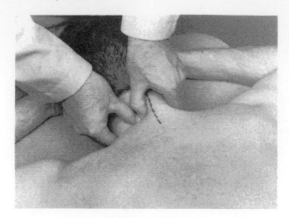

Figure 9.7 Unilateral palpation two to three centimetres from the midline over the articular pillar.

Palpation lying supine

Localised dysfunction can also be assessed with the frequently used method of palpating the neck with the patient lying in the supine position (Figure 9.8). The fingers gently palpate over each segment

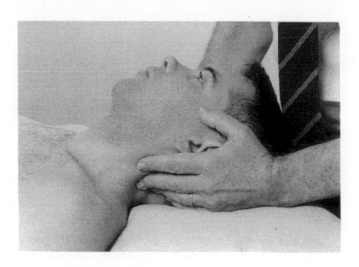

Figure 9.8 Palpation of the neck with the patient lying supine.

level feeling for tenderness and altered muscle tone. Running the fingers down each paravertebral 'gutter' helps identify localised problems.

PAIN PROVOCATION TESTS

Occasionally, palpation and movement testing will fail to reproduce the patient's pain; provocation tests, however, may achieve this essential objective. All movements are directed towards the painful side.

Compression test

The patient's head should be laterally flexed and slightly extended. Steady pressure to the head compresses the articular pillar on the painful side (Figure 9.9).

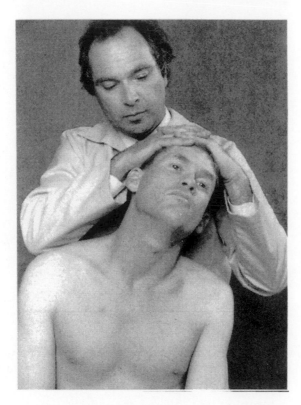

Figure 9.9 The compression test for the cervical spine.

Quadrant test

This combination of extension, lateral flexion and rotation to the painful side (Figure 9.10) narrows the intervertebral foraminae. It tests the mid and lower cervical spines if there is doubt that the pain originates from the neck.

NEUROLOGICAL EXAMINATION

Examination for nerve root lesions (between fifth cervical and first thoracic vertebrae) is indicated if neurological symptoms or signs are identified in the clinical assessment. The objective is to localise spinal segments for the origin of lower motor lesions.

Nerve root pressure is indicated by:

- pain and paraesthesia along the distribution of the dermatome
- localised sensory loss

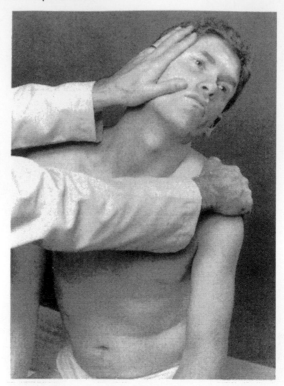

Figure 9.10 The quadrant test for the cervical spine.

- reduced muscular power (weakness or fatigue or both)
- hyporeflexia (reduced reflex amplitude or fatigue or both).

It is important to know the sensory distribution of each nerve root and the motor changes that accompany root injury. The relevant anatomical patterns are shown in Table 9.2.

Table 9.2 *Cervical nerve root syndromes.*

NERVE ROOT	SENSORY CHANGE	MUSCLE POWER	POWER LOSS	REFLEX
C5	Outer arm	Deltoid	Abduction arm	Biceps jerk
C6	Outer forearm/thumb/ index finger	Biceps	Elbow flexion Extension wrist	Biceps + brachioradialis
C7	Hand/middle and ring fingers	Triceps	Elbow extension	Triceps
C8	Inner forearm/ little finger	Long flexors finger, long extensors thumb	Grip	
T1	Inner arm	Interossei	Finger spread	

Pain distribution

Test for sensation by light touch and pin prick over the relevant dermatomes, focusing on the areas where the patient experiences paraesthesia and anaesthesia. The dermatomal patterns are outlined in Figure 7.5.

Muscle power

Muscle power in the upper limbs may be tested by a systematic approach to resisted movements.

The fifth cervical nerve root is tested by resisting abduction of the arms, which are held at an angle of about 45 degrees from the sides (Figure 9.11). This tests power in the deltoid muscle; note any weakness or fatigue.

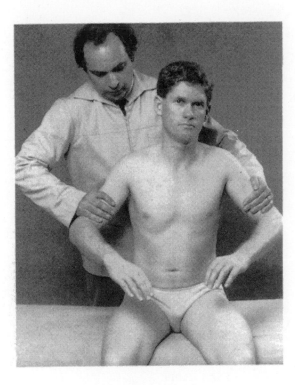

Figure 9.11 Testing deltoid power (C5).

The fifth and sixth cervical nerves innervate the biceps muscle, which is tested by resisted flexion of the elbow with the patient supine and the forearm flexed to 90 degrees (Figure 9.12).

The sixth cervical nerve is responsible for wrist extension, thus a useful test for C6 is restricted extension of the wrist (Figure 9.13).

The seventh cervical nerve innervates the triceps muscle. Test by resisted extension of the elbow as shown in Figure 9.14 (arm in same position as for the biceps muscle).

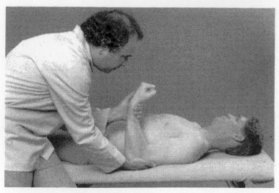

Figure 9.12 Testing biceps power (C5, C6).

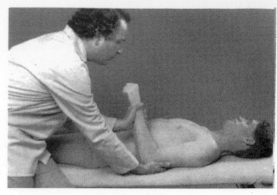

Figure 9.14 Testing triceps power (C7).

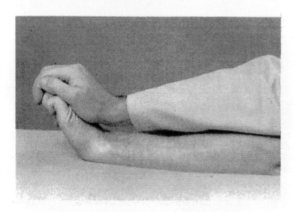

Figure 9.13 Testing wrist extension (C6).

The eighth cervical nerve is tested via two muscles: extensor pollicis longus and flexor digitorum longus. Extensor pollicis longus is assessed by resistance, against the thumb nail, to extension (Figure 9.15). The power of the long finger flexors is tested by resisting terminal phalangeal flexion (Figure 9.16).

The first thoracic nerve root is tested by assessing function of the interossei muscles (Figure 9.17). Adduction of the extended fingers is determined by the patient (with hand flat on the table) resisting removal of the paper.

Reflexes

The biceps muscle reflex (Figure 9.18) allows assessment of the function of the fifth and sixth cervical nerve roots; the brachioradialis (supinator) reflex is a function of the sixth cervical nerve root (Figure 9.19), the triceps reflex a function of the seventh (Figure 9.20).

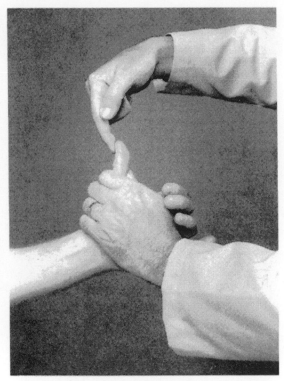

Figure 9.15 Testing extensor pollicis longus (C8).

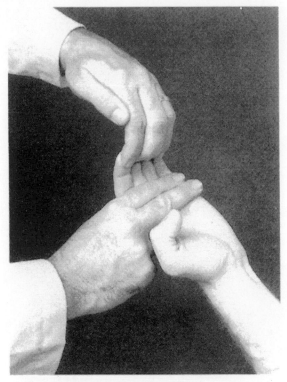

Figure 9.16 Testing flexor digitorum longus (C8).

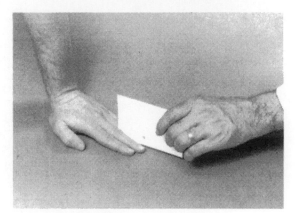

Figure 9.17 Testing the interossei (T1).

Each reflex should be tested six times to observe any fatigue, which is a pointer to nerve root dysfunction.

Measurement of muscle mass

A tape measure is used to measure the girth of the arms to detect the presence of any muscle wasting.

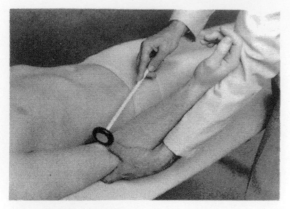

Figure 9.18 Testing biceps reflex (C5 and C6).

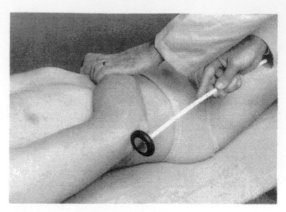

Figure 9.20 Testing triceps reflex (C7).

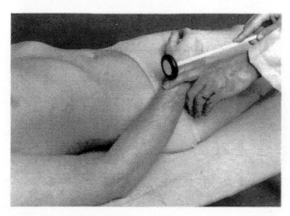

Figure 9.19 Testing brachioradialis (supinator) reflex (C6).

EXAMINATION OF THE SHOULDER JOINT

Examination of the cervical spine is followed by examination of the shoulder joint. For the examination of the shoulder it is important to understand the functional anatomy of all important tendons.

The tendon disorders are diagnosed by pain on resisted movement as shown in Table 9.3. A knowledge of the anatomical attachments of the rotator cuff tendons to the head of the humerus (Figure 8.4) provides an understanding of the shoulder movements powered by these muscles. With tendon disorders (rotator cuff tendons or biceps) there is painful restriction of movement in one direction, but with capsulitis and subacromial bursitis there is usually restriction in all directions.

Table 9.3 *Diagnosis of tendon disorders by pain on resisted movement.*

PAINFUL RESISTED MOVEMENT AT SHOULDER	AFFECTED TENDON
1. Abduction	Supraspinatus
2. Internal rotation	Subscapularis
	Teres minor*
3. External rotation	Infraspinatus
	Biceps*
4. Adduction	Pectoralis major
	Latissimus dorsi*

* Lesser role.

INSPECTION

Observe the shape and contour of the shoulder joints and compare both sides. Note the posture and the position of the neck and scapulae. The position of the scapulae provides considerable clinical information. Note any deformity, swelling or muscle wasting.

PALPATION

Stand behind the patient and palpate significant structures such as the acromioclavicular (AC) joint, the subacromial space, the supraspinatus tendon and the long head of biceps. The subacromial bursa is one area where it is possible to localise tenderness with inflammation. Feel also over the supraspinatus and infraspinatus muscles for muscle spasm and trigger points.

MOVEMENTS

The movements of the shoulder joint are complex and involve the scapulothoracic joint as well as the glenohumeral joint, with each joint accounting for about half the total range. Significant signs of a painful capsular pattern can be gained by determining the movements of flexion, abduction, external rotation and internal rotation.

For each movement, note:

● the range of movement
● any pain reproduction
● any trick movement by the patient
● scapulothoracic rotation.

Movements should be tested bilaterally and simultaneously wherever possible.

PRACTICE TIPS

- Test for supraspinatus disorders with the 'impingement test' which tests resistance of the semi-flexed and internally rotated straight arms.
- Consider the possibility of disorders of the neural tissue associated with the C5 and C6 nerve roots as a cause of unexplained pain in the shoulder and arm. Test this diagnostic hypothesis with the brachial plexus tension test.
- Consider the possibility of polymyalgia rheumatica in the older patient (over 50) who presents with shoulder pain and stiffness. Although typically bilateral, it may start as unilateral discomfort.
- Dysfunction of the cervical spine can coexist with dysfunction of the shoulder joints.

Active movements

Flexion

With palm facing medially, the patient moves the arm upwards through 180 degrees to a vertical position above the head (Figures 9.21 and 9.22).

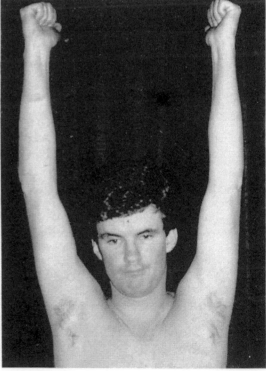

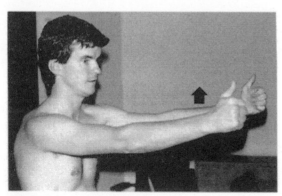

Figure 9.21 Flexion of the arms showing position of the arms.

Figure 9.22 Flexion of the arms: full range of movement.

Abduction

With the thumb pointing upwards the patient lifts the arm outwards from the sides (Figures 9.23 and 9.24). This combined glenohumeral and scapulothoracic movement should reach 180 degrees. Look for the presence of a painful arc that occurs usually between 60 and 120 degrees of abduction (Figure 9.25).

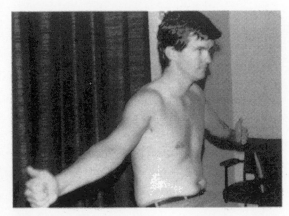

Figure 9.23 Abduction of the arms: initial movement.

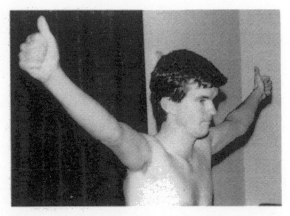

Figure 9.24 Abduction of the arms: further elevation.

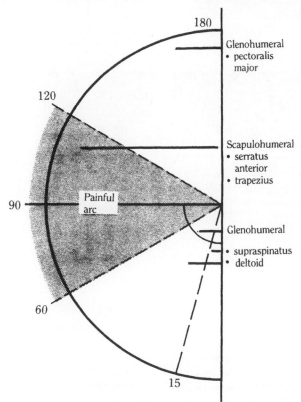

180

Glenohumeral
• pectoralis major

120

Scapulohumeral
• serratus anterior
• trapezius

90   Painful arc

Glenohumeral
• supraspinatus
• deltoid

60

15

Figure 9.25 Abduction of the arm: illustrating the responsible joints and muscles, and the painful arc.

External rotation

Following the placement of the arm by the side with the elbow flexed to 90 degrees and the palm facing medially, the patient is instructed to place the hand behind the neck (Figure 9.26). Patients with an external rotation problem caused by a lesion of infraspinatus complain of pain when brushing their hair.

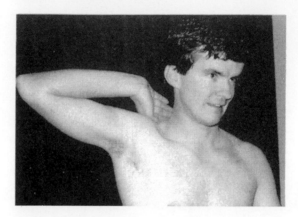

Figure 9.26 External rotation of the arm.

Internal rotation

With the same starting position as for external rotation the patient is asked to place the hand behind the back. This movement is tested bilaterally (Figure 9.27).

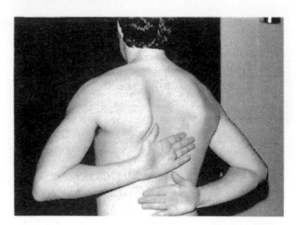

Figure 9.27 Internal rotation of the arm.

Supraspinatus/infraspinatus rapid differentiation test

A quick test that differentiates between a lesion of either of these tendons causing a painful arc syndrome is the 'thumbs up/thumbs down' abduction test.

To test supraspinatus, perform abduction with the thumbs pointing upwards (Figure 9.28). To test infraspinatus perform the same test with the thumb pointing downwards (Figure 9.29).

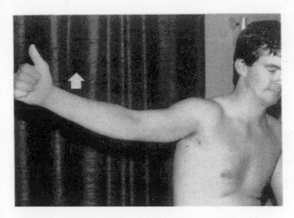

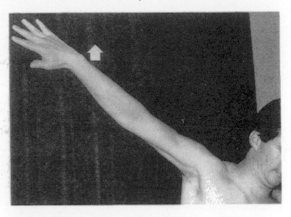

Figure 9.28 'Thumbs up' abduction test for supraspinatus.

Figure 9.29 'Thumbs down' abduction test for infraspinatus.

Resisted movements

Resisted movements (resisted isometric contractions of a muscle) are important tests for pinpointing tenderness of muscle insertions around the shoulder joint.

Abduction (supraspinatus test)

With the arm abducted no more than 15 degrees, the patient pushes the elbow away from the side while the examiner's hand resists and prevents the movement, holding for five seconds (Figure 9.30). Compare both sides and note any reproduction of the patient's pain. This is an important test for the common supraspinatus tendon lesion.

Combined movements (supraspinatus test)

The patient places the arms in the position of semiflexion (90 degrees) and internal rotation with the forearms in full pronation. The therapist

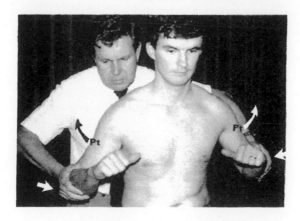

Figure 9.30 Resisted abduction: testing for supraspinatus pathology.

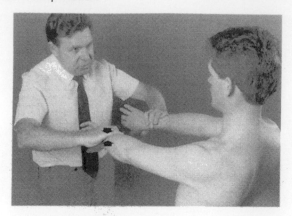

Figure 9.31 The impingement test (resisted flexion in semiflexion and internal rotation): testing for rotator cuff pathology, especially supraspinatus.

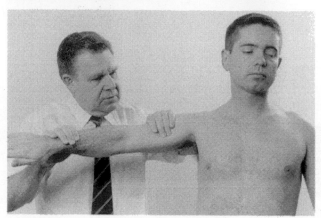

Figure 9.32 The 'emptying the can' impingement test: the arm is held at about 30 degrees of horizontal flexion.

tests resisted elevation (flexion) (Figure 9.31). If pain is reproduced, this is called a positive 'impingement sign'; it is a very sensitive test for the upper components of the rotator cuff, especially supraspinatus (Browne, 1986). Another effective test for the rotator cuff as it forces impingement of the greater tuberosity on the acromion is testing resisted elevation in the 'emptying the can' position (90 degrees of abduction, 30 degrees of horizontal flexion and full internal rotation) (Figure 9.32). This is an even more sensitive impingement test.

External rotation (infraspinatus test)

The examiner stands behind the patient and grasps the forearm near the wrist. The patient, who should keep the elbows against the trunk, presses outwards using the forearm as a lever to produce external rotation (Figure 9.33).

Internal rotation (subscapularis test)

The examiner and patient adopt a similar position as for external rotation, but the examiner grasps the palmar surface of the patient's

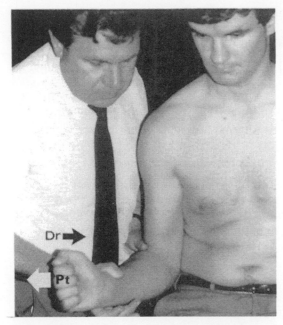

Figure 9.33 Resisted external rotation: testing for infraspinatus pathology.

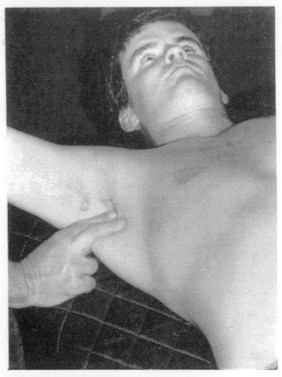

Figure 9.35 Palpation of subscapularis muscle.

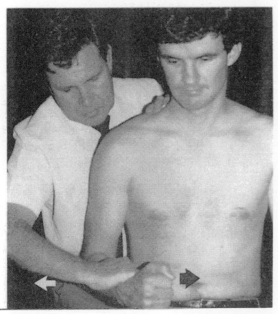

Figure 9.34 Resisted internal rotation: testing for subsapularis pathology.

wrist. The patient attempts to move the forearm medially against resistance (Figure 9.34). This tests the function of subscapularis.

Another helpful test of the subscapularis muscle is to directly palpate the muscle belly for trigger points. The anterior surface of the muscle forms a considerable part of the posterior wall of the axilla. With the patient supine and the arm abducted, the muscle is gently palpated, after it has been ensured that the palpating fingers get above the edge of latissimus dorsi (Figure 9.35). This test should be performed bilaterally to compare both muscles.

Forearm supination and flexion (long head of biceps test)

An effective test for a lesion of the long head of biceps is Yergason's test: the examiner tests resisted supination of the forearm with the elbow flexed to 90 degrees and the forearm supinated (Figure 9.36). Reproduction of pain at the antero-medial aspect of the shoulder is a positive sign.

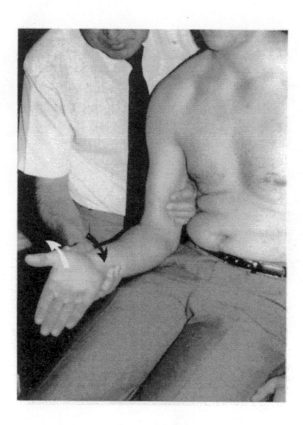

Figure 9.36 Resisted supination of flexed forearm: testing for long head of biceps.

The brachial plexus tension test

This specific stretch test for the brachial plexus (Elvey, 1983 and 1985) tests the nerve roots and sheaths of the brachial plexus without implicating the cervical spine and the glenohumeral joint.

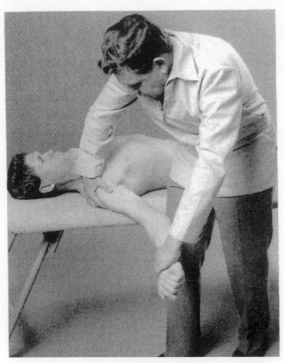

Figure 9.37 The brachial plexus tension test 1: the arm is placed into abduction and external rotation while the shoulder girdle is depressed.

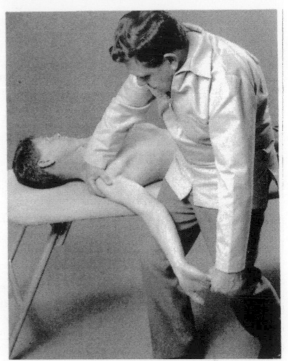

Figure 9.39 The brachial plexus tension test 3 (provocation for less sensitive conditions): the wrist is extended and the neck laterally flexed to the contralateral side.

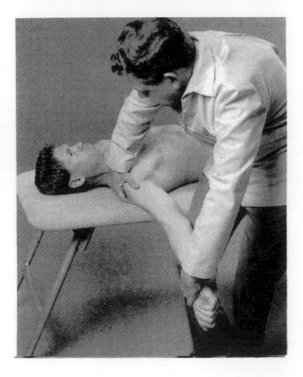

Figure 9.38 The brachial plexus tension test 2: the arm is straightened by extension of the elbow and supination of the forearm.

It tests mainly the movement of the upper cervical roots of the plexus, with their investing pain-sensitive dural sheaths and corresponding intraspinal dura. These movements occur with various movements of the arm. The test is similar in principle to the slump test, or the straight leg raising test for the lumbosacral nerve roots, but this test detects abnormalities of the C5, C6 and C7 (to a lesser extent) nerve roots with no apparent effect at C8 and T1.

According to Elvey (1986), 'The combined position of the upper quarter which places maximum tension on the cervical nerve root complexes involves glenohumeral joint abduction and external rotation with the arm behind the coronal plane, elbow extension and wrist

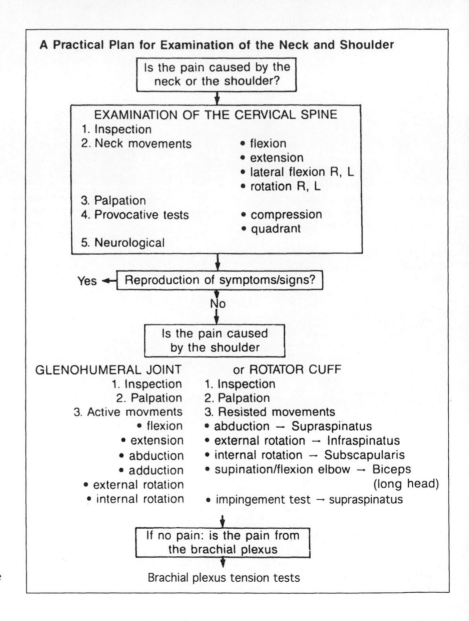

Figure 9.40 A practical plan for examination of the neck and shoulder.

extension, supination of the forearm, shoulder girdle depression and lateral flexion of the cervical spine to the contralateral side'.

Method

- The patient lies supine and the shoulder girdle is depressed.
- The arm is placed into (glenohumeral) abduction and external rotation (Figure 9.37). The arm is held to the side posterior to the coronal plane – that is, just below the level of the couch.
- The test is completed by passive extension of the elbow (Figure 9.38) and supination of the forearm.
- A positive test is one which reproduces the patient's symptoms in the limb or limbs (pain or paraesthesia).
- The sensitivity of the test can be reinforced by extension of the wrist (analogous to dorsiflexion of the foot) and lateral flexion of the cervical spine to the contralateral (non-painful) side (Figure 9.39).

SUMMARY

A summary of a practical plan for examination of the neck and shoulder is outlined in Figure 9.40.

10
Mobilisation of the cervical spine

'Doctor those gentle soothing movements you are giving to my neck feel so therapeutic and safe. I worry about heavy hands cracking my neck.'

Comment from a 66-year-old woman about mobilisation of her neck.

Contents

An outstanding advantage of cervical mobilisation is that it enables manual therapy to commence when cervical manipulation is either contra-indicated or inadvisable due to the patient's clinical condition. This is evident when acutely painful neck conditions such as a wry neck render manipulation impossible and inadvisable because of the high degree of irritability.

Cervical mobilisation permits early treatment by means of gentle oscillatory movements which have the effect of decreasing muscle spasm and pain and thus gradually improving mobility.

While there is a risk of complications with cervical manipulation, cervical mobilisation is safe as it is not a past end range technique. Furthermore, a lesser degree of skill is required for mobilisation than for manipulation.

As for the lumbar spine, mobilisation can be used as a treatment in its own right or as a pre-manipulation procedure. Six different general techniques will be presented in this chapter and they should be mastered before manipulation is attempted.

> **KEY CHECKPOINTS**
>
> - Keep in mind contra-indications and conditions that require care. 'Thou shalt do no harm.'
> - Carefully examine the cervical spine and assess signs and symptoms to determine your choice of first technique.
> - Aim to localise the problem and treat specifically at the one vertebral level wherever possible.
> - Use a mobilisation technique in preference to a manipulation technique.
> - Rotate or flex **away** from the side of the pain.
> - Discard a technique proving ineffective for that particular patient.
> - Do not overtreat the cervical spine. Cease treatment as soon as symptoms and signs subside.
> - Be careful of the irritable joint – do not push through protective muscle spasm.
> - Warn patients about soreness and temporary after-effects following treatment.

REVIEW OF MOBILISATION STAGING AND TECHNIQUES

Mobilisation techniques are generally divided into three stages for both anterior directed (postero-anterior) and rotational techniques. Stages 1 and 3 are relatively small amplitude movements while stage 2 is a larger amplitude movement that occupies the range between stages 1 and 3 (see Figures 4.3 and 10.3). The techniques may be direct or indirect, depending on whether a lever principle is used and whether it is preferable to mobilise one or several levels simultaneously. The mobilisation techniques for the cervical spine are summarised in Table 10.1.

Table 10.1 *Mobilisation techniques for the cervical spine.*

TECHNIQUE	TYPE	INDICATION
Anterior directed central gliding	Direct	Bilateral or central pain
Anterior directed unilateral gliding	Direct	Unilateral pain
Anterior directed unilateral gliding with head rotation	Direct	Unilateral pain C1/C2
Accessory rotation	Indirect	Unilateral pain Central or bilateral pain Acute pain
Lateral flexion	Indirect	Unilateral pain Acute pain
Longitudinal distraction gliding (= traction)	Indirect	Central or bilateral pain Unilateral pain
Muscle energy	Indirect	Hyperacute pain – acute torticollis usually unilateral pain

CERVICAL MOBILISATION TECHNIQUES

1. Anterior directed central gliding

This method is similar to that used for the lumbar and thoracic spine. The tips of the thumbs must be used and the technique has to be delicate.

It is suitable for the levels from C2 to C6. It can be used as an early, mid or end range technique (that is, all three grades).

Indication

Bilateral or central symptoms.

Position of the patient

- The patient lies prone.
- The head rests in a flexed position, with the forehead in the palms or on the back of the hands.
- The chin is slightly tucked in.

Position of the therapist

- The therapist stands at the patient's head, facing the patient.
- The tips of both thumbs (with nails back to back) are placed on the tip of the spinous process at the affected level.
- The other fingers are spread to each side of the patient's neck in order to stabilise the hands.

Method

- Holding the thumbs in apposition, direct the longitudinal axis of the thumbs in a direct postero-anterior direction.
- Pressure is transmitted through the therapist's thumbs by movement of the trunk and arms (Figures 10.1 and 10.2).

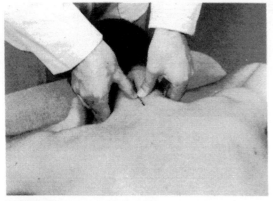

Figure 10.1 Cervical mobilisation technique 1: anterior directed central gliding using C5 as an example.

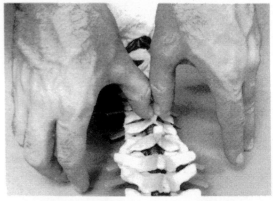

Figure 10.2 Cervical mobilisation technique 1: skeletal view showing the position of the thumbs over spinous process C6.

- Initially the oscillations are gentle and rhythmic (about one or two per second).
- Ask the patient what he or she is feeling.
- The depth and amplitude of the mobilisation can be increased according to the response. **At all times it is important to maintain constant rhythm and depth**.

Time span

- If possible, 60 seconds is ideal. The procedure can be repeated twice or three times, often increasing in range as the painful segment improves.

The various stages

It is convenient to consider this particular mobilisation in three distinct stages or ranges (Figure 10.3).

Initial range (stage 1)

This is the gentlest of all movements and is used for the initial treatment of more tender problems. A gentle oscillatory movement is imparted with the thumbs to the spinous processes and involves only a

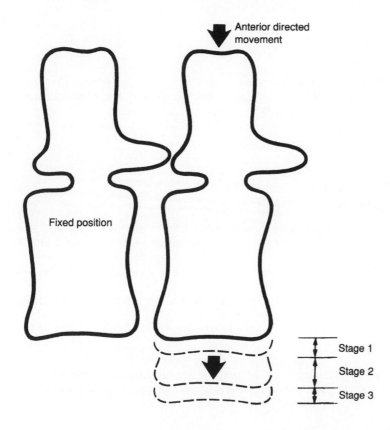

Figure 10.3 Anterior directed central gliding mobilisation, illustrating the three stages of mobilisation.

slight movement in the A-P plane. Sometimes it is too painful even to produce limited movement and so this method should be abandoned.

Mid range (stage 2)

This is a deeper movement over a wider range. The oscillations should be smooth over a constant range. This consistency is very important. The stretching pressure should not be released during this 30 to 60 seconds' treatment. The vertebral movement is surprisingly elastic but the movement should not cause pain and its depth should just stop short of any pain.

End range (stage 3)

This is the ideal range to aim for and is usually used for less painful problems or when the previous two stages have to be used to relieve pain and allow a progression to stage 3. A small amplitude to the end range is therefore permissible.

2. Anterior directed unilateral gliding

This is a very effective technique which is often used. As there is considerable movement over the apophyseal joint it can be highly effective through all three stages.

Indication

Unilateral cervical pain, especially for the common dysfunction of C2–C3 – the 'headache' joint. It is used for the lateral joints from C2–C3 to C6–C7.

Position of the patient and therapist

● As for technique 1.

Method

● The thumbs are placed over the tender level behind the articular pillar about two to three centimetres from the midline. This varies slightly from patient to patient (Figure 10.4).
● Application of pressure at the C4 level mobilises the C4–C5 joint (Figure 10.5).
● The rhythmical oscillatory movement is transmitted to the thumbs in the usual way.

Time span

● This depends on the degree of comfort, but 60 seconds is ideal. The technique can be repeated two or three times, depending on the response.

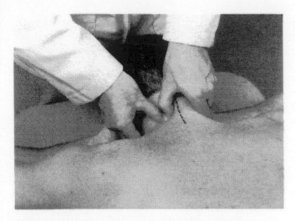

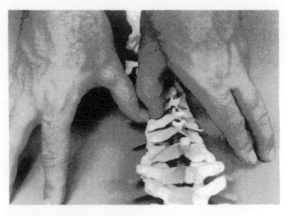

Figure 10.4 Cervical mobilisation technique 2: anterior directed unilateral gliding at the C4–C5 level.

Figure 10.5 Cervical mobilisation technique 2: skeletal view showing the position of the thumbs on the articular pillar.

3. Anterior unilateral gliding with head rotation

This is a specific method for treatment of the important C1–C2 joint which, like the C2–C3 joint, is often responsible for headache. The method is similar to technique 2 but the head is rotated towards the painful side.

Indication

Unilateral painful C1–C2 apophyseal joint.

Position of the patient and therapist

● This is similar to technique 2 except that the patient's head is rotated approximately 30 degrees towards the painful side.

Method

● The long axis of the therapist's thumbs is postero-anterior directed but tilted slightly towards the head (Figure 10.6).

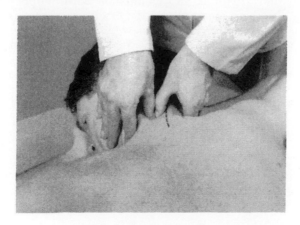

Figure 10.6 Cervical mobilisation technique 3: mobilising the left C1–C2 joint with the head rotated 30 degrees to the left.

- The oscillatory movement is transmitted through the thumbs, as with other anterior directed techniques. It is important to maintain constant rhythm and depth with this slightly different technique.

Time span

- 60 seconds or more is ideal.
- The technique can be repeated two or three times.

4. Rotation

This accessory movement is an extremely important technique for treatment of unilateral or bilateral cervical pain. For unilateral pain the head should be rotated away from the painful side.

For the demonstration of rotation techniques, rotation to the right for left-sided pain will be illustrated. The stages of rotation are illustrated in Figures 4.3 and 4.11.

Position of the patient

- The patient lies supine with the head at the edge of the couch and arms by the side.

Position of the therapist (for rotation to the right)

- The therapist crouches at the end of the couch over the patient.
- The patient's head is now gently cradled in the therapist's hands with the right forearm and hand snugly embracing the right side of the patient's head and the fingers supporting the chin without pressing against the throat.
- The therapist's left hand supports the head under the occiput with the thumb embracing the left mastoid process and the middle finger on the right mastoid process. It is essential that the patient's head be well supported at all times.

Method

- Rotation of the head and thus the cervical spine is achieved by equal and rhythmic movements of both hands working in unison to produce a smooth oscillatory movement around a constant axis of direction.
- It is important to be close to the patient and not have the arms stretched out.
- Figures 10.7 and 10.8 demonstrate a stage 1 rotation with a small amplitude of rotation.
- The amplitude can vary from small to large. The further the rotation to the right the greater the stretch and amplitude of the rotation.
- Figures 10.9 and 10.10 demonstrate stage 2 rotation with a wide arc of movement. This method is more difficult to coordinate so the therapist has to concentrate on keeping both hands oscillating evenly.
- Figures 10.11 and 10.12 illustrate stage 3 rotation, which is the ideal stage to achieve with this method.

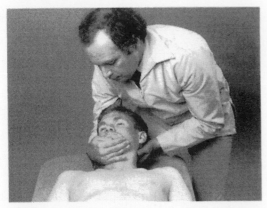

Figure 10.7 Cervical mobilisation technique 4: stage 1 rotation to the right.

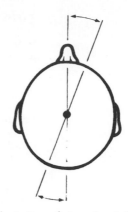

Figure 10.8 Illustration of stage 1 rotation with a relatively small arc of movement from the starting point of the range.

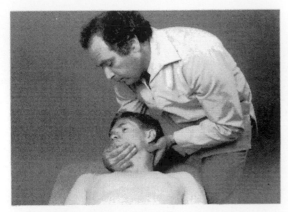

Figure 10.9 Cervical mobilisation technique 4: stage 2 rotation to the right.

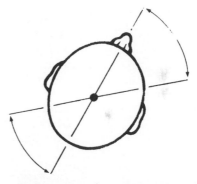

Figure 10.10 Illustration of stage 2 rotation with a wide arc of movement. The nose indicates the starting point of the range.

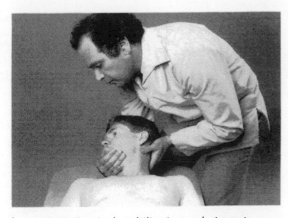

Figure 10.11 Cervical mobilisation technique 4: stage 3 rotation to the right – a small oscillation at the end of range.

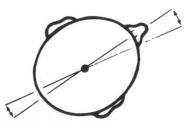

Figure 10.12 Illustration of stage 3 rotation with a small arc of movement at the end range.

Time span

- 60 seconds or more is ideal.
- This technique can be repeated two or three times.

Achieving some specificity for an indirect technique

Variations to the accessory rotation technique can be applied to give more specificity – for example, the lower the cervical area to be mobilised, the greater the degree of neck flexion.

For the upper cervical spine the patient's neck is held on the same plane as the body, as shown for Figures 10.7–10.12.

For the mid cervical spine the neck is flexed to about 30 degrees.

For the lower cervical spine the neck is flexed to about 45 degrees.

Localisation is achieved by placing the hand over the appropriate level.

5. Lateral flexion

Mobilisation in lateral flexion is often underrated, but it can be a very effective technique. It can be used effectively when rotation is painful and restricted because this means that lateral flexion is also restricted and limiting rotation. Lateral flexion mobilisation can be used as a general or as a specific technique, depending on whether the objective is to mobilise the entire cervical spine or only one or two levels. To achieve specificity at a given level, the proximal aspect of the lateral border of the index finger of the near hand applies pressure on the neck against the affected level of the articular pillar.

Indications for use

- Unilateral pain in neck and referred pain.
- Rotation decreased and/or painful.
- Lateral flexion decreased and/or painful.

Rules of procedure

- In lateral flexion it is the *opposite side* that is being handled – for example, if the left side (as shown in Figure 10.13) is the side requiring treatment, the neck is flexed to the right because this affects gapping of the stiff joints on the left.

   Lateral flexion is therefore away from the painful side.
- The head is used as a body lever.
- Lateral flexion is most effective as a stage 2 or 3 procedure.

Position of the patient

- The patient lies supine with the head resting on the couch (the head can be taken over the end of the couch for the procedure but it is not necessary).

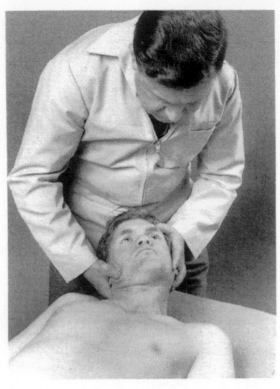

Figure 10.13 Cervical mobilisation technique 5: lateral flexion for a left-sided problem.

Position of the therapist

- The therapist stands above the patient and to the side – that is, alongside the shoulder opposite to the painful side. *Note*: this method is shown for a painful left side in Figure 10.13.
- The patient's head is cradled in a neutral position mid-way between flexion and extension (for the upper cervical spine) and slightly flexed for treating the lower cervical spine.
- One hand cradles the occiput while the other is placed at the base of the neck (or at a specific level) with the thumb resting anteriorly and to the side and the four fingers curled posteriorly around the neck with the palmar surface of the index finger wedged against the articular pillar.

Method

- The patient's head is laterally flexed away from the painful side and firmly held against the therapist's body.
- The lateral flexion mobilisation is produced by an oscillatory movement between the therapist's hands assisted by rocking the therapist's hips from side to side with a combined forward and side movement of the right side of the pelvis (for this particular patient) – Figure 10.13 for a painful left side.
- During this procedure the near hand on the neck acts as a fulcrum against the articular pillar and thus achieves gapping on the opposite side of the spine.

Non-specific mobilisation

- The position of the hand determines the specificity. For a general non-specific mobilisation it is placed at the base of the neck (Figure 10.14). It is important to produce a true lateral flexion and not simply muscle stretching.

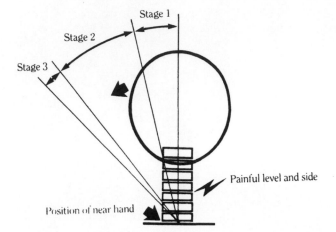

Figure 10.14 Non-specific lateral flexion mobilisation: illustration of this method for the three stages. Note the near hand position at the base of the neck.

Specific mobilisation

- The hand is placed at the painful level directly opposite the painful side.
- The head is laterally flexed in the same way but the soft border of the index finger exerts pressure against the pillar so that the slack is taken up.
- The mobilisation is directed specifically, thus producing intermittent gapping at the affected joint on the far side. The method is illustrated in Figure 10.15.

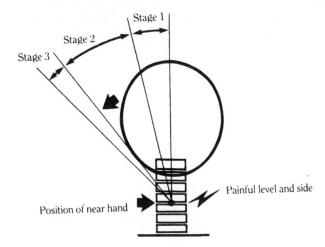

Figure 10.15 Specific lateral flexion mobilisation. Note the near hand position on the affected level.

Time span

- 30 to 60 seconds is a suitable time with one or two repeats in a treatment session, depending on the response. This technique is usually followed by a rotation mobilisation.

6. Longitudinal distraction gliding (traction)

Traction, which is an excellent and safe method, can be administered by machines but can also be applied manually, including by the use of a belt. It is an underrated technique and is often most effective when used manually. Indications include:

- nerve root irritation
- irritable spine
- headache
- wry neck
- severe degenerative changes.

For acute neck pain it is often the first technique used.

Manual traction

Position of the patient

- The patient lies supine, relaxed with arms by the side.
- The head can be supported at the end of the couch or just over the couch.

Position of the therapist

- The therapist stands at the head of the couch facing the patient.
- One hand clasps the occiput just above the atlanto-occipital joint with the thumb wedged under the mastoid process of one side and the middle finger under the opposite mastoid process (Figure 10.16).
- The other hand holds the chin (it may be necessary to use the lower three fingers only, to avoid undue pressure on the upper throat) with the forearm resting alongside the patient's face (Figure 10.17).

Method

- Traction is achieved by using body weight, and not the arms, which quickly fatigue. This implies placing the feet to take a firm and comfortable stance, and leaning back during the traction.
- The steady controlled traction stretches the cervical spine.

Precautions

- Avoid traction to an extended neck.

Note: The traction force should be taken up slowly and released gently – never suddenly. Sudden release will exacerbate an irritable condition.

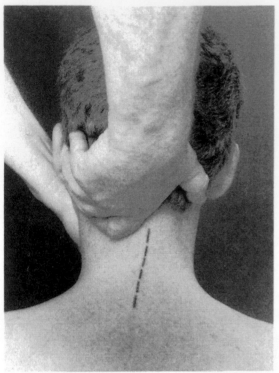

Figure 10.16 Cervical mobilisation technique 6: manual traction. Inferior view showing grip on occiput.

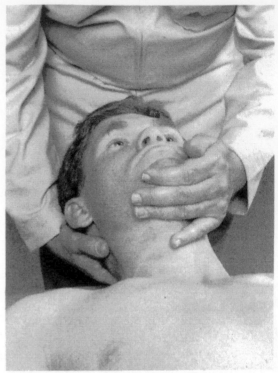

Figure 10.17 Traction: superior view showing grip on chin.

Variations of traction

The method of traction can be semi-specific for the three general areas of the cervical spine – upper, mid and lower. As traction is applied for the lower parts of the spine the neck should be flexed proportionally.

The upper cervical spine (occiput to C2–C3): the head should be in a neutral position for traction (Figures 10.18 and 10.19).

The mid cervical spine (C3–C4 and C4–C5): the head should be lifted off the couch at an angle of 30 degrees (Figures 10.20 and 10.21). The lower cervical spine (C5–C6 and C7–T1): the angle of the neck to the couch should be about 45 degrees (Figures 10.22 and 10.23).

Belt traction

Belt traction is the best manual traction technique. The belt, which can be a modified car seat belt or camping gear belt, enables the application of greater stretch with better control for longer periods. The belt, which is looped over the hands (Figure 10.24), fits comfortably under the occiput as shown and is applied to the therapist's body. The traction is applied by leaning backwards and allowing the body weight to exert the force. The force can be applied to the upper, middle or lower cervical spines.

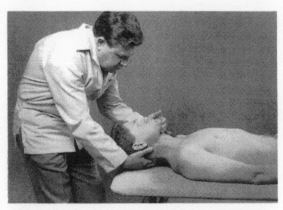

Figure 10.18 Traction for the upper cervical spine: the head is held in a neutral position.

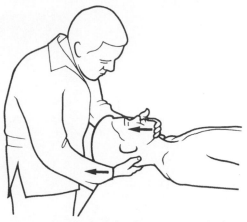

Figure 10.19 Traction for the upper cervical spine showing the line of traction as straight.

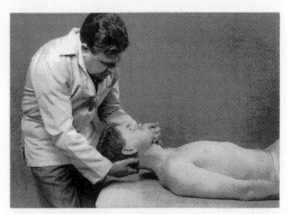

Figure 10.20 Traction for the mid cervical spine: the head is flexed to about 30 degrees.

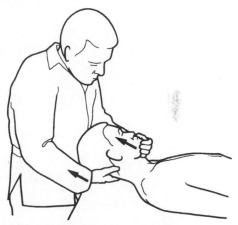

Figure 10.21 Traction for the mid cervical spine showing the line of traction.

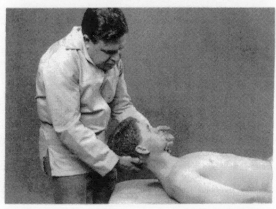

Figure 10.22 Traction for the lower cervical spine: the head is flexed to about 45 degrees.

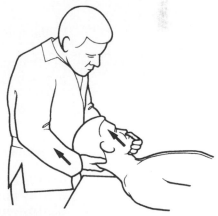

Figure 10.23 Illustration of the direction of traction for the lower cervical spine.

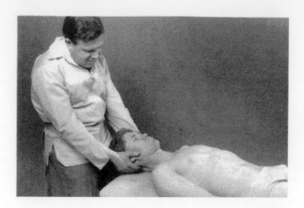

Figure 10.24 Hand position for belt traction.

7. Muscle energy therapy

This is a specialised type of mobilisation involving stretching at the end range and will be described in Chapter 11.

APPLICATION OF MOBILISATION

The choice of technique is determined by the following:

● The area of the spinal problem – upper cervical or lower cervical.
● Whether pain is unilateral or central/bilateral.

Note: There is a limit to the amount of improvement that can be obtained with any one treatment; the treatment method may be altered following re-assessment of the response to the initial method.
   The following sequences are recommended:

Unilateral pain

1. ADG unilateral
2. Rotation
3. Traction
4. Lateral flexion

Upper cervical methods

1. ADG central
2. ADG unilateral
3. ADG unilateral (in rotation)
4. Traction
5. Rotation

Central (or bilateral) pain

1. ADG central
2. Rotation
3. Traction
4. ADG unilateral (both sides)

Lower cervical methods

1. ADG central
2. ADG unilateral
3. Rotation
4. Lateral flexion
5. Traction

Coding: anterior directed central gliding: ADG central
anterior directed unilateral gliding: ADG unilateral

PRACTICE TIPS

- Use mobilisation rather than manipulation as first line technique for cervical problems.
- If in doubt, use mobilisation or use no manual therapy.
- Remember that many patients prefer cervical mobilisation to manipulation.
- Use a belt for manual traction.
- More specificity for a general technique can be obtained by placing the neck in various degrees of flexion: neutral positions for upper with more flexion for lower.
- Always aim to achieve gapping of the painful joint or joints.
- Maintain a uniform rhythm and range of amplitude for all anterior directed (postero-anterior), lateral flexion and rotational techniques.

SUMMARY

Cervical mobilisation is a vital basic skill for the beginner in manual therapy to master. If a therapist does not wish to use cervical manipulation, then mobilisation alone will be very effective. It can be rendered more specific by placement of the therapist's hand at the affected level or by placing the neck in varying degrees of flexion. As for the other techniques, it is essential to rotate or flex away from the painful side and not to aggravate the patient's pain. Anterior directed (postero-anterior) gliding techniques give excellent results and are very specific but may not be possible in the acutely tender neck. Rotation mobilisation is the appropriate first line treatment in these cases.

11
Muscle energy and muscle stretching therapy

'Scant attention has been given to a neglected, major cause of pain and dysfunction in the largest organ of the body – voluntary (skeletal) muscle which accounts for 40 per cent or more of body weight.'

Janet Travell, 1983

Contents

KEY CHECKPOINTS

● If a patient presents with acute torticollis use muscle energy therapy (MET) as first line treatment, because the main presenting feature is altered muscle tone (spasm).
● If a patient responds well to treatment, give instruction in self-administered MET which can be performed several times a day (Chapter 13, page 188).
● Use coordinated breathing and respiration to achieve more effective results. However, it is not essential to outcome.
● If MET in one direction for cervical problems causes pain or is ineffective, attempt a different variation whether it be a contralateral or an ipsilateral method.
● The muscles should not contract to the point of pain – stay just short of this with MET.
● Passive muscle stretching can be simple effective therapy for stiff and tender muscles. This applies particularly for large neck muscles such as sternomastoid, trapezius and the scalenus.

MUSCLE ENERGY THERAPY

The cervical spine is the ideal area in which to apply muscle energy therapy especially for acute or subacute problems involving muscle spasm. It is very effective for problems that have a high level of irritability.

The classic application is for acute torticollis but it can be used for all types of dysfunctional neck problems.

Treatment of acute torticollis

The patient has a very painful left side of the neck with painful spasm of both the left lateral flexors and rotators (especially rotators). Some spasm is present also in the right-sided muscles. The site and degree of muscular spasm can vary in wry necks, with one muscular movement being more affected than the other – sometimes exclusively. However, it is important to direct treatment at that muscular movement which is the most painful. In the authors' experience this is rotation.

The standard contralateral method

The contraction phase

1. The therapist positions the neck at the pathological motion barrier by passively flexing and rotating the head towards the painful side to the absolute extent of comfortable movement.
2. The level of painful joint or joints is determined. During movement towards the painful side this level can be 'fixed' by the free hand in order not to allow movement and thus make the therapy more specific.
3. The therapist places his (or her) hand on the side of the head opposite the painful side and then pushes towards the direction of the pain, at the same time requesting the patient to resist this movement by pushing his or her head moderately hard into the therapist's hand. The patient should thus be producing a moderately strong isometric contraction of the neck in rotation away from the painful side. The counterforce applied by the therapist is firm and moderate, never forceful; it should not hurt, or 'break' through the patient's resistance. During this contraction phase, which occupies five to seven seconds, the patient is asked to inhale and hold his or her breath for the duration. In addition, he or she should look upwards in the direction of the contracting muscles (Figures 11.1 and 11.2).

Relaxation and stretch

After the contraction the patient is requested to 'let go' (relax). As the muscle relaxes in the immediate post isometric contraction phase, the therapist stretches the neck gently yet firmly towards the painful side in the equivalent direction of the contracting movement, namely rotation (in this patient). During this phase the patient is asked to slowly exhale and gaze downwards in the direction of the stretching (Figures 11.3

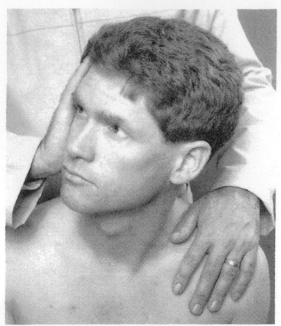

Figure 11.1 Muscle energy therapy: the contraction phase. This shows contraction of the neck in rotation away from the painful (left) side with a resisting counterforce by the therapist.

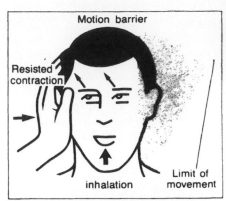

Figure 11.2 Illustration of the contraction phase including the motion barrier and resisted rotation (lateral flexion in other patients) of the head away from the painful side. The patient gazes upwards and outwards during inspiration.

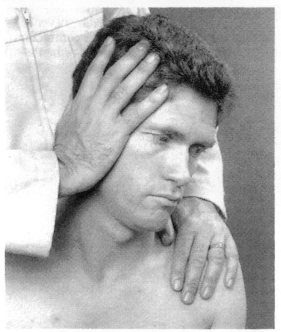

Figure 11.3 Muscle energy therapy: the stretching phase. This shows stretching of the neck towards the painful side.

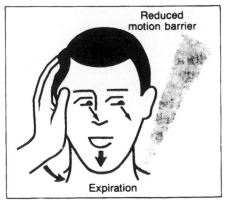

Figure 11.4 Illustration of the stretching phase. The stretch in rotation is towards the painful side with the patient looking downwards in the direction of stretch during exhalation. An improved motion barrier is achieved.

and 11.4). This stretching phase lasts for 10 seconds with the neck being stretched as far as the altered motion barrier will permit. This sequence of events is summarised in Figure 11.5.

The procedure is repeated from the new starting position of the improved motion barrier. The sequence is repeated three to five times and hopefully a full range of pain-free movement of the neck is achieved.

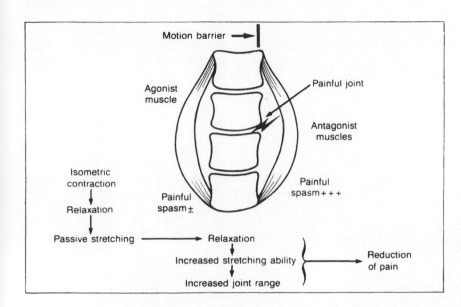

Figure 11.5 Sequence of events in muscle energy therapy for the cervical spine: contralateral method (simplified diagram for purpose of illustration).

This may be accomplished in one visit or over a few (often just two) visits. The patient can be taught self-treatment at home by this method.

The ipsilateral method

A variation of the muscle energy technique, based mainly on the ability to stretch a fatigued muscle in its post isometric contraction relaxation phase, is the 'contraction–relaxation–stretch' method for muscles on the painful side exclusively.

After the neck is positioned to the painful limit the therapist achieves contraction of the muscles on that side by pushing the patient's head **away** from the painful side as the patient resists this movement. This causes the patient to contract the muscles directly responsible for the painful contraction – lateral flexion or rotation (both movements may be used alternately). Surprisingly this does not usually hurt the patient. After five to seven seconds the neck is stretched towards the painful side and the process repeated after the motion barrier has improved.

Whether to use the contralateral or the ipsilateral method is usually decided after a quick therapeutic trial to determine which side causes least discomfort for the patient. This is usually the contralateral side but occasionally it is so uncomfortable that the opposite side may be suitably treated.

Another ipsilateral method

The combination of physiological principles permits various permutations and combinations of treatment methods for the neck, depending on the nature and chronicity of the pain. For less painful and more chronic painful necks, if the motion barrier is not such a problem, the above method can be used to achieve stretching on the painful side by stretching that side away from the painful level after the contraction phase.

This principle is illustrated in the following method which can be performed with the patient lying or sitting. This method demonstrates a specific technique directed at the affected segmental level and which is most suitable for mid cervical problems.

Method

- The patient sits upright in the chair.
- The therapist stands behind the patient and firmly grasps the lower of the two vertebrae (or segments) at the painful level (Figure 11.6).
- The upper hand curves around the patient's face with the fingers resting on the other 'fixing' hand (Figure 11.7).

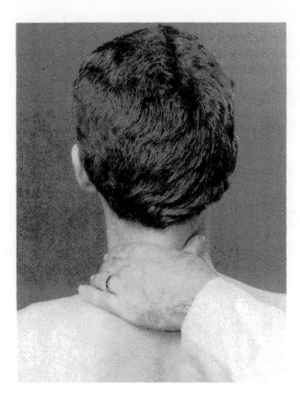

Figure 11.6 Muscle energy therapy (a specific ipsilateral method) 1: fixation of the painful segment.

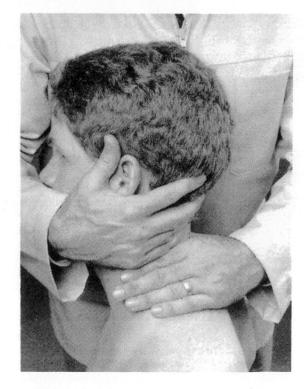

Figure 11.7 Muscle energy therapy (a specific ipsilateral method) 2: contraction of the neck in rotation towards the painful (left) side against the resisting hand.

- The patient attempts to rotate against the upper hand while inhaling and looking up in the direction of contraction. This lasts for about five to seven seconds and only mild pressure is exerted (Figure 11.7).
- The patient now exhales as the therapist stretches the neck by rotating in the opposite direction to the contraction. The lower hand still remains firmly 'fixed' on the neck (Figure 11.8).

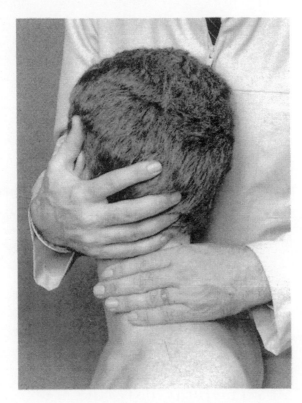

Figure 11.8 Muscle energy therapy (a specific ipsilateral method) 3: the stretching phase away from the painful side (towards the right).

A traction technique for the upper cervical spine

This technique demonstrates the use of longitudinal traction of the neck as a muscular energy therapy. Coordination of breathing is considered to be most effective for the upper cervical spine.

Method

- The patient sits on the chair (sitting is preferable to lying supine) with the head in a 'neutral' position.
- The therapist stands behind the patient and places the palms of the hand on the sides of the face.
- The patient is asked to breathe in and look upwards simultaneously (without extending the neck).
- The therapist holds the neck in a fixed position during this inspiration phase (the neck muscles will contract during the phase) (Figure 11.9).

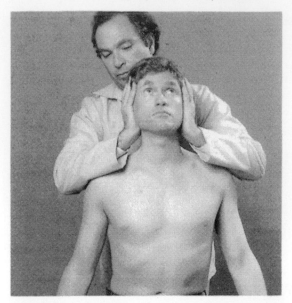

Figure 11.9 Muscle energy therapy (traction method for the upper cervical spine) step 1: the therapist holds the head in a fixed position during inspiration and upward gaze.

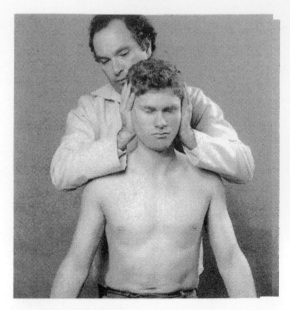

Figure 11.10 Muscle energy therapy (traction method for the upper cervical spine) step 2: the therapist applies traction during expiration and downward gaze.

- The patient then exhales while looking down. The therapist applies a gentle but firm upward stretch (Figure 11.10).
- This procedure is repeated a number of times, with traction being applied during the expiration phase.

MUSCLE STRETCHING THERAPY

Indications

- Taut and tender muscles of the neck.
- Tender 'trigger points'. This implies that the muscles are slightly contracted since they are not at their normal resting length. It manifests as altered function, that is, altered movement pattern.

Trapezius and levator scapulae stretch

Method

- The patient sits in a chair with the head in a neutral position and the therapist stands behind the patient.
- The shoulders are slightly abducted and the elbows flexed to 90 degrees (Figure 11.11).
- The therapist, who stands behind and above the patient, applies firm and steady pressure down on the patient's shoulders.

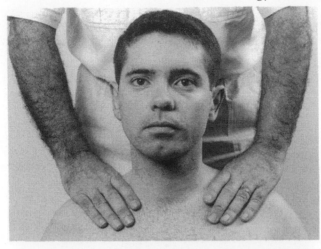

Figure 11.11 Trapezius and levator scapulae stretch: initial position.

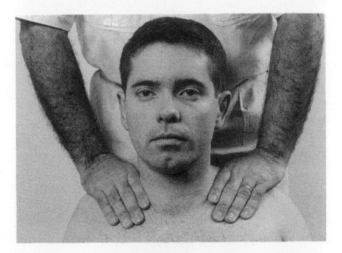

Figure 11.12 Trapezius and levator scapulae stretch: Stage 1: resisted contaction of muscles.

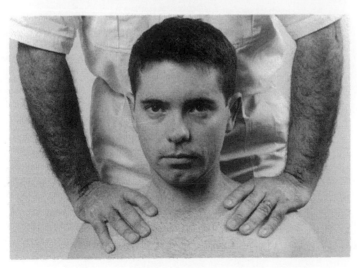

Figure 11.13 Trapezius and levator scapulae stretch: Stage 2: stretching of muscles during relaxation phase.

- The patient resists this by contracting the muscles. (Figure 11.12).
- This is maintained for about five to seven seconds and then the patient relaxes.
- The therapist then stretches the muscles during the relaxation phase (Figure 11.13). This can be repeated.

Sternomastoid stretch

The sternomastoid muscle is responsible for acute torticollis when it contracts. This causes a tilt of the head towards the shoulder of the same side in addition to rotating the head so as to carry the face towards the opposite side.

Method

- The patient can sit in a chair or lie down.
- Resisted rotation on the affected side is performed in a similar way to that described in muscle energy therapy.
- During the relaxation phase the neck is stretched in rotation away from the tender side.

Scalenus muscle stretch

Scalenus muscle stretching is performed in lateral flexion (side bending). It can be performed by the therapist or by the patient as a self-passive stretching exercise. It can be performed following a contraction (as in MET) or by a simple straight stretching. The treatment should be given bilaterally.

Method

- The patient lies on the back in a supine position and a three phase stretch is performed.

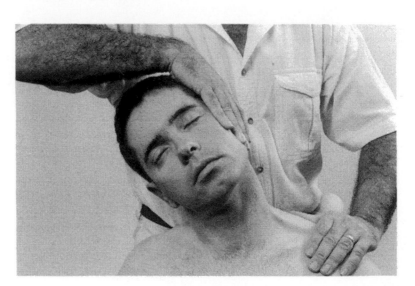

Figure 11.14 Scalenus medius muscle stretch: stretching into side flexion with face looking directly forward.

1. The head is stretched into side flexion with the face looking directly forward (Figure 11.14). This stretches scalenus medius.
2. The face is turned away from the direction of the stretch. This stretches scalenus anterior.
3. The face is turned towards the direction of the stretch. This stretches scalenus posterior.

12
Manipulation of the cervical spine

'In Australia and some other countries ... the tuition of physiotherapy students has concentration on mobilisation. This policy
unhappily leaves them with methods which cannot be compared in
rapid success with "layman's" manoeuvres.'

James Cyriax in
Textbook of Orthopaedic Medicine,
Volume 2, 10th edition, 1980, p. 68.

Contents
☐ An introductory note of caution
☐ Key checkpoints
☐ The pre-manipulation safety examination
☐ Cervical manipulation techniques
    1. Non-specific rotation (supine)
    2. Semi-specific rotation A (supine)
    3. Semi-specific rotation B (supine)
    4. Specific rotation (supine)
    5. Non-specific rotation (the sitting or
        'chair' method)
    6. Semi-specific rotation (the sitting
        method)
    7. Lateral flexion
    8. Traction manipulation
    9. 'Manipulation' under anaesthesia
☐ Practice tips
☐ Summary

AN INTRODUCTORY NOTE OF CAUTION

Manipulation of the cervical spine can be dramatically effective and is
one of the most rewarding areas of manipulative therapy. However, it is
potentially dangerous and has to be approached with appropriate care.
It is a fact that many thousands of manipulations of the cervical spine
are performed each day with relative ease and complete safety. It is also
a fact that high velocity thrust techniques to the cervical spine can
cause instant death and other catastrophes such as cerebrovascular
accidents (CVAs) and quadriplegia.

These incidents can occur even in younger patients. In some of these there may be vascular anomalies but others may have no demonstrable abnormality.

The problem arises from the following circumstances:

1. An inadequate diagnosis.
2. Lack of provocation tests in an individual at risk.
3. Use of brute force or an inappropriate technique.

The most devastating complications are:

- sudden death
- CVAs, usually vertebro-basilar infarction
- quadriplegia, usually following forward dislocation of the atlas
- intracranial haemorrhage such as a tear of a lateral sinus.

Mobilisation techniques should be attempted as first line management, manipulation being reserved for patients not responding to mobilisation.

It is not sufficient to learn just one manipulation technique – have a repertoire of several and then select the most appropriate technique for the individual patient.

This selection will depend on (1) the site of pain; (2) the degree of irritability; and (3) the presence of contra-indications.

KEY CHECKPOINTS

- Take a careful history and perform a proper physical examination prior to treatment.
- X-ray the cervical spine prior to manipulation.
- Perform a provocation test for vertebro-basilar insufficiency prior to manipulation.
- Never manipulate through muscle spasm.
- Use mobilisation in preference to manipulation.
- Take special care with patients with dizziness and migraine and with the elderly patient.
- Never manipulate patients with rheumatoid arthritis, those with significantly narrowed intervertebral foramina on X-ray, those with a history of stroke, drop attacks and vertebro-basilar insufficiency or those on anti-coagulant therapy.
- The joints must be at absolute full stretch (at end range) before the manipulative movement.
- Never use a high velocity rotation technique from a wide arc. Always commence the rotation from the position of the limit of stretch of the neck – that is, at the end of range – the movement should be 2–5 degrees.
- Do not manipulate without having carefully considered mobilisation as a first-line treatment.
- Avoid over-manipulation of the cervical spine.

THE PRE-MANIPULATION SAFETY EXAMINATION

Prior to any cervical manipulation, especially a rotation technique, it is mandatory to perform a proper clinical assessment of the patient, including the all important tests for vertebro-basilar insufficiency.

Clinical assessment of the patient

History

Check for evidence of fainting or drop attacks, subclavian 'steal', migraine and other neurological symptoms. Manipulation is contra-indicated if the patient is on anti-coagulant therapy or has an arthritide affecting the cervical spine, such as rheumatoid arthritis.

Examination

Test subclavian 'steal', blood pressure in both arms, auscultate over the carotids and perform ophthalmoscopy where indicated.

Provocation tests

One of the two tests shown, where the extended head is rotated bilaterally, should be performed with care. Should symptoms be provoked, return the head to the neutral position immediately.

X-ray

Radiology is very important after trauma and with the arthritides. An antero-posterior view taken through the mouth should be included.

Provocation tests for vertebro-basilar insufficiency

The problem of vertebro-basilar insufficiency (VBI) is obviously a high risk factor in the older patient. There are several provocation tests for this condition, which has already been outlined in Chapter 6 (pp. 75–76).

A knowledge of the excursion of the vertebral artery is important. When the head is rotated to one side the blood flow is diminished at the atlanto-axial junction on the opposite side. Sharp rotation to the right results in sharp angulation of the left vertebral artery. Both sides need to be carefully tested.

As well as atherosclerosis of the arteries, the presence of cervical spondylosis can compromise the arterial flow.

VBI provocation test 1

The patient lies supine with the head beyond the couch. The head is firmly supported in full extension (Figure 12.1). The patient must feel the security of this support and the head must not be allowed to suddenly drop free in extension.

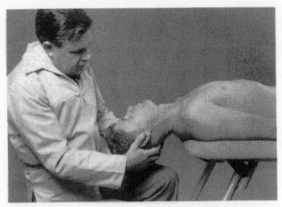

Figure 12.1 Provocation test 1 for vertebro-basilar insufficiency. Step 1: the hanging head is supported in full extension.

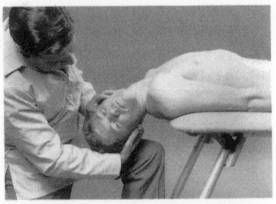

Figure 12.2 Provocation test 1 for vertebro-basilar insufficiency. Step 2: the extended head is passively rotated to the side and held for 20–30 seconds. Watch for nystagmus and ask about unusual symptoms.

The head is now passively rotated slowly to one side and maintained in this combined extension/rotation position for 20 to 30 seconds (Figure 12.2).

Ask the patient to report any subjective symptoms. It is better to ask this general question but later you can enquire about specific symptoms such as visual disturbances (blurred vision, double vision), dizziness and nausea. During this test observe the patient's eyes carefully for nystagmus.

If symptoms are provoked during this procedure return the head to the neutral position immediately.

VBI provocation test 2

This is basically an identical test, but is performed with the patient sitting upright. The head is passively extended (Figure 12.3) and then rotated slowly to both sides and held for 20 to 30 seconds (Figure 12.4).

Test 1, where the patient lies supine with the head over the couch, is considered to be the better method but either test can be used.

If any symptoms of vertebro-basilar insufficiency are present cervical manipulation, especially rotation, must not be attempted.

If there are no symptoms or signs of vertebro-basilar insufficiency or other contra-indications, manipulation may be attempted but only if symptoms such as reproduction of sharp pain and a hard end feel are absent when the joints are taken to the end range.

The manipulation should only proceed if all the slack has been taken up.

Taking up the slack

The important detail of 'taking up the slack' conforms to the basic rule of procedure 'the joint(s) must be at absolute full stretch prior to manipulation'.

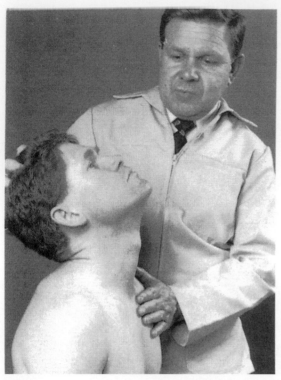

Figure 12.3 Provocation test 2 for vertebro-basilar insufficiency. Step 1: full extension of the head.

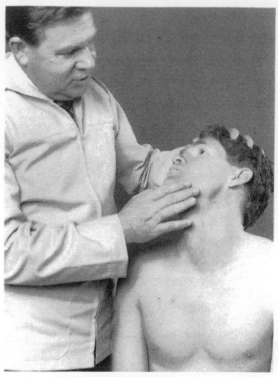

Figure 12.4 Provocation test 2 for vertebro-basilar insufficiency. Step 2: rotation of the extended head.

The method is slowly to approach the end range while searching for the type or quality of feel at the end of normal movement. This end feel can be either hard or soft (see Chapter 4, p. 59–60).

A hard end feel (often referred to as a hard stop) is usually associated with pain, reproduction of the patient's symptoms and protective muscle spasm. This means that there is no elasticity at the end range, that the joint is pathological, that the direction is not pain-free and that manipulation should not proceed. It represents a biomechanical contra-indication for manipulation which may not be evident prior to examining the end range and attempting the procedure.

Principle of manipulation

Manipulation should always achieve a gapping or opening up of the painful side.

This will involve (a) with **rotation** – rotation away from the painful side and (b) in **lateral flexion** – thrusting towards the painful side (from the opposite side). This gapping opens up the intervertebral foramina.

CERVICAL MANIPULATION TECHNIQUES

The techniques can be either general or specific, depending on whether the objective is to manipulate one or more cervical levels. A specific technique should be used whenever possible because it targets one level without affecting other levels. This is particularly desirable in the cervical region, where significant osteoarthritic changes can be present (especially in the lower cervical spine) which may be asymptomatic. Manipulation to such an asymptomatic area may render it symptomatic.

Manipulation of the cervical spine can be performed with the patient either lying or sitting (as described in the following specific techniques) while some very effective techniques can be performed with the patient prone.

Table 12.1 *Manipulation techniques for the cervical spine.*

TECHNIQUE	POSITION	TARGET LEVEL
Rotation		
1. Non-specific	Supine	C0–C1 to C5–C6 mainly upper
2. Semi-specific A	Supine	C1–C2 to C6–C7
3. Semi-specific B	Supine	C2–C3 to C6–C7
4. Specific	Supine	C1–C2 to C6–C7
5. Non-specific	Sitting	C1–C2 to C6–C7 mainly lower
6. Semi-specific	Sitting	C2–C3 to C6–C7 mainly mid
Lateral flexion		
7. Specific	Supine	C2–C3 to C7–T1
Traction		
8. Traction	Supine	C0–C1 to C2–C3

The main cervical manipulation techniques (set out in Table 12.1) are rotation (techniques 1–6), lateral flexion (technique 7) and traction (technique 8).

1. Non-specific rotation (supine)

This manipulation is an extension of the stage 3 mobilisation technique. Full stretch of the neck in rotation is necessary. No traction is applied. It will cover the cervical levels C1–C2 to C5–C6 – that is, upper to middle.

Position of patient

- The patient lies supine with arms relaxed by the side.
- The patient's head can lie on the top of the couch or over the edge for this non-specific technique.

Position of therapist

- The therapist stands at the head of the couch and faces the patient (a higher couch level than usual is preferable).
- The head is cradled in the therapist's arms with the hand near the painful side grasping the base of the occiput with the thumb lying over the mastoid process and just above the angle of the mandible. The other hand and forearm support the patient's head with the fingers embracing the chin.

    It is most important that the head should be cradled comfortably in this arm so that the patient feels confident that the head is firmly supported.

    In addition, the therapist should be close to the patient so that the patient feels the chest touching the vertex of his head (Figure 12.5).

Method

- The neck is rotated into full stretch away from the painful side.
- At absolute full stretch a sharp short rotation is applied using both hands in unison (Figure 12.6). The force is therefore provided by (1) the hand on the chin producing a rotatory force; and (2) the hand on the neck providing rotatory thrust.

Note: The final rotatory range should be barely perceptible to the observer and certainly should be less than five degrees. There is no place for a large amplitude thrust from the central or mid position to the end of range. Such inappropriate wide arc vigorous rotations can cause serious complications.

2.   Semi-specific rotation A (supine)

This method is simply a variation of technique 1 but is rendered more specific by placing the thrusting hand over the affected level. It is most effective for the mid cervical area.

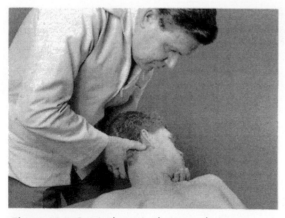

Figure 12.5 Cervical manipulation technique 1: non-specific rotation, showing the neck at full stretch immediately prior to manipulation (right-sided problem).

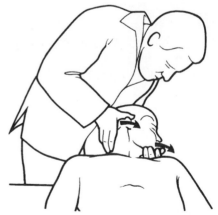

Figure 12.6 Illustration of the direction of forces for non-specific rotation in the supine position.

Position of the patient

● The same as for technique 1.

Position of the therapist

● This is the same as for technique 1 except that the thrusting hand is placed over the painful level of the neck with the soft part of the index finger (formed by the V) resting on the posterior aspect of the articular pillar.

Method

● With the neck at full stretch the usual rotatory movement is applied with the thrust being imparted from the hand on the neck (Figure 12.7).

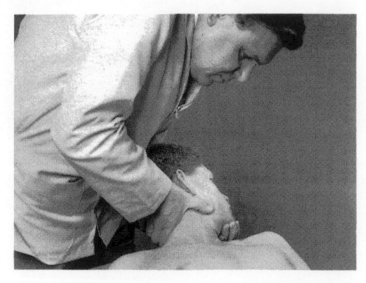

Figure 12.7 Cervical manipulation technique 2: semi-specific rotation A: note the position of the thrusting hand on the affected segment of the neck.

3. Semi-specific rotation B (supine)

Position of the patient

● The patient lies supine with arms relaxed by the side and with their head on a pillow.

Position of the therapist

● The therapist stands behind the patient and cups the patient's head with both hands. The palms are slightly anterior to the occiput (towards the mastoid processes) and the fingers encircle the neck.

Method

● The encircling fingers identify the dysfunctional area by palpation.
● On the painful side the index finger (mid point of proximal phalanx of radial border) is firmly positioned against the relevant vertebra.

- A combined movement is performed simultaneously in which the neck is laterally flexed at the affected level (Figure 12.8) (towards the painful side) and rotated away from the painful side. This is only a small degree of both lateral flexion and rotation and it serves to take up the slack and lock the joint at the available end range prior to manipulation.
- Using both hands perform a sharp short arc of rotation away from the painful side (Figure 12.9).

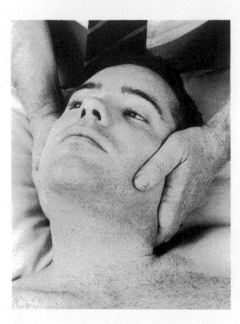

Figure 12.8 Cervical manipulation technique 3: semi-specific rotation B. Stage 1: neck laterally flexed towards the painful side and rotated away from the painful side.

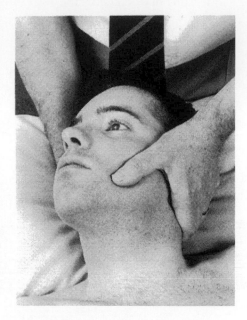

Figure 12.9 Cervical manipulation technique 3: semi-specific rotation B. Stage 2: short rotatory movement away from the painful side.

4.   Specific rotation (supine)

This method is the best of the cervical manipulative techniques and has the advantage of specifically manipulating a particular level without manipulating other levels.

The position of the patient and the therapist is the same as for technique 2 but the method of obtaining greater specificity is quite different and it takes considerable practice to master the technique.

Note: The patient's head should lie over the top edge of the couch.

Method

Step 1 – Determining the position of the hands

The level of the cervical spine which is responsible for the pain has already been generally located and is precisely determined by palpation from behind (Figures 12.10 and 12.11).

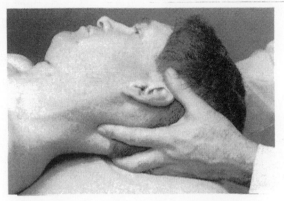

Figure 12.10 Cervical manipulation technique 4: specific rotation. Palpating the affected joint from behind.

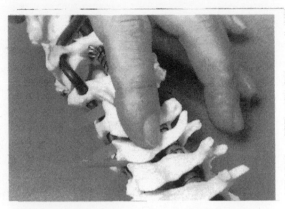

Figure 12.11 Specific rotation method: illustrating palpation on the spinal model.

The index finger is placed behind the apophyseal joint to be treated. The point of contact with this finger should be behind the joint at the level in question, that is, the posterolateral surface of the articular pillar (Figure 12.12).

The point of contact with the finger is the junction of the proximal and middle thirds of the proximal phalanx of the index finger (Figure 12.13).

When the thrusting hand is placed on the tender level of the neck the thumb should rest on the edge of the mandible (not on the soft tissue of the neck). The other hand is placed on the chin so that the head is cradled comfortably in the forearm (as for the previous methods) (Figure 12.14).

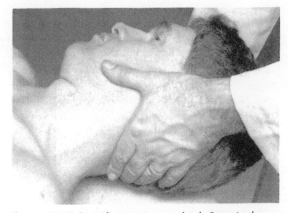

Figure 12.12 Specific rotation method. Step 1: the position of the 'thrusting' finger on the neck.

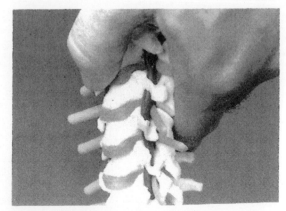

Figure 12.13 Specific rotation method: illustrating the point of contact of the thrusting finger on the neck.

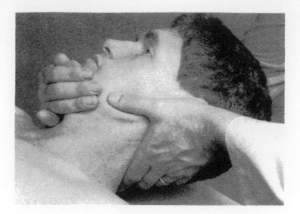

Figure 12.14 Specific rotation method: initial position of the hands.

Step 2 – Initial rotation to stretching level

The neck is now rotated until movement of the articular pillar is felt beneath the thrusting index finger.

At this point rotation is ceased and the head and neck held in this position (Figure 12.15). This rotatory process to the affected level is illustrated in Figure 12.16.

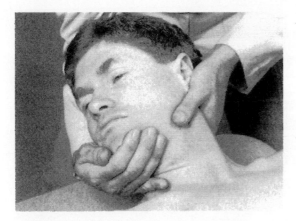

Figure 12.15 Specific rotation method. Step 2: rotation down to the level to be manipulated.

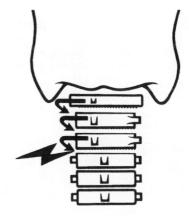

Figure 12.16 Illustration of rotation to the affected level in Figure 12.15. Painful level indicated (posterior view).

Step 3 – Lateral displacement

With the wrist hyperextended, laterally displace the neck with a gliding movement by pushing laterally with the hand towards the opposite shoulder (Figure 12.17). This transverse glide is illustrated in Figure 12.18. This movement is designed to 'fix' the neck at that level.

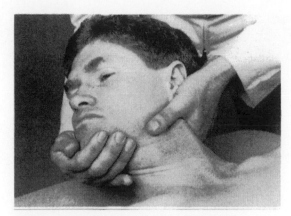

Figure 12.17 Specific rotation method. Step 3: lateral displacement to 'fix' the neck.

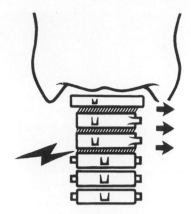

Figure 12.18 Illustration of lateral displacement by transverse gliding to the right side.

Step 4 – Lateral flexion

Now move the neck into lateral flexion by tilting the head towards the painful side (Figure 12.19). This manoeuvre will 'lock' the neck (Figure 12.20).

Step 5 – Rotate to end range and thrust into rotation

Rotate the neck to the absolute end of range so that the joint to be manipulated is completely locked.

Manipulation is achieved by a sharp rotation with one hand rotating while the index finger of the other reinforces the movement with a corresponding thrust against the articular pillar (Figure 12.21). Note that the movement occurs at a specific junction that is taut above and lax below (see Figure 12.20).

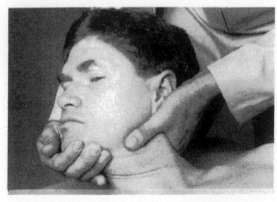

Figure 12.19 Specific rotation method. Step 4: lateral flexion to 'lock' the neck.

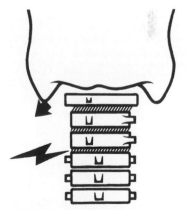

Figure 12.20 Illustration of lateral flexion to the left. This produces a level that is taut above and lax below.

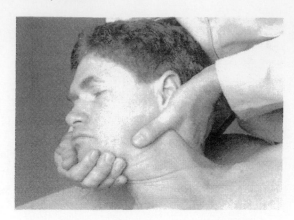

Figure 12.21 Specific rotation method. Step 5: rotation to the right.

5.   Non-specific rotation (the sitting or 'chair' method)

This technique, which employs considerable stretch, is an excellent technique for that stubborn neck problem, especially where the neck feels 'jammed' and rotatory movements are stiff and decreased.

In this technique traction is very important. Often the problem can be relieved during stretching manoeuvres so that the manipulative thrust is not necessary.

It is more effective for problems of the lower cervical spine. Figures 12.22–12.24 show a patient whose problem is right-sided.

Position of the patient

- The patient sits comfortably in a chair.
- The patient's head rests comfortably against the therapist's chest with it turned away from the painful side.

Position of the therapist

- The therapist stands behind the patient as shown and places the upper hand on the head as the left side of the face (in this case) rests against the chest.
- The forearm and hand embrace the face with the fingers being spread over the bony parts of the head (Figure 12.22) so that the pressure from the hand and forearm is widely distributed. Avoid pressure under the mandible – the hand and forearm should embrace the head without hurting (Figure 12.23) or hooking under the chin.
- The other hand steadies the shoulder on the painful side thus ensuring maximum stretch on the neck and stability of the shoulder. At all times the head should be maintained in an erect position without flexion or extension.

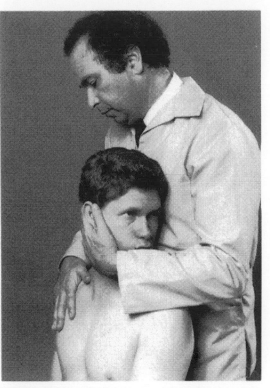

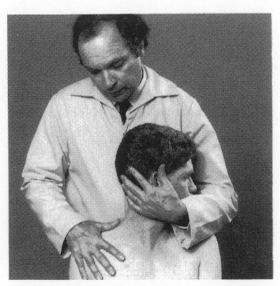

Figure 12.22 Cervical manipulation technique 5: non-specific rotation of the neck while seated in the chair (front view).

Figure 12.23 Cervical manipulation technique 5: (a lateral view).

Method

- The neck is taken into full stretch by combining upward traction and rotation away from the painful side. If sharp pain or other symptoms such as dizziness are produced at the point of full stretch, the procedure should be abandoned.
- When the point of **absolute full stretch** is reached a short sharp rotation is applied with the arm embracing the head. The lines of force are illustrated in Figure 12.24. It is important not to delay the manipulation at this end point – the manipulation should be applied as soon as full stretch is reached.

6.   Semi-specific rotation (the sitting method)

This useful technique has the advantage that it can follow on from a passive movement examination which is most easily performed in sitting. No traction is required. It is most appropriate for mid cervical problems. A left-sided problem is shown in Figures 12.25 and 12.26.

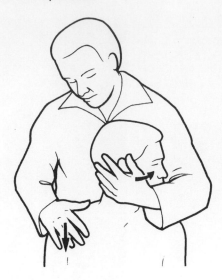

Figure 12.24 Cervical manipulation technique 5: illustration of the direction of forces.

Position of the patient

● The patient sits relaxed in a chair.

Position of the therapist

● The therapist stands behind and slightly to the side of the patient.
● The left hand grips the lower of the two vertebrae at the affected level.
● The right hand curls around the head with the forearm embracing the mandible and the fingers gripping the neck with the lowest finger placed just above the fingers of the left hand to grip the upper vertebra (Figure 12.25).

Method

● The bottom hand holds the neck steady while the upper hand rotates the head and neck to the right and takes up the slack.
● At the end range a rotatory manipulative thrust is applied. The direction of forces is illustrated in Figure 12.26.

7.   Lateral flexion

Lateral flexion is a very useful manipulation and, like rotation, can be specific or general. For specific manipulation the thrusting hand is placed at the level to be manipulated with the line of the forearm in the plane of the joint.

For non-specific (general) manipulation, one hand is placed at the cervico-thoracic junction to both stabilise and block the base of the neck.

The specific method which is described has the following features:

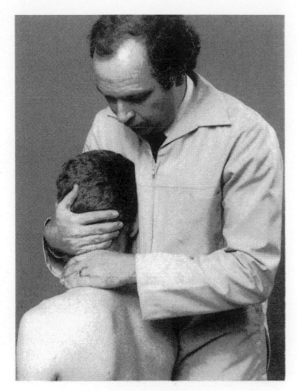

Figure 12.25 Cervical manipulation technique 6: semi-specific method while sitting in the chair.

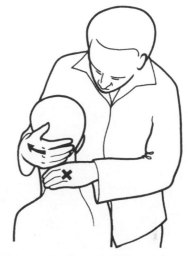

Figure 12.26 Cervical manipulation technique 6: illustration of the direction of forces.

- Manipulation is directed towards the painful side.
- Gapping of the painful joints occurs at the affected level.
- Manipulation is performed at the end of range.

A right-sided problem is illustrated in Figures 12.27–12.29.

Position of the patient

- The patient lies relaxed on the couch with their head resting on a pillow.
- The patient's head can be on the couch (preferably) or held over the edge.

Position of the therapist

- The therapist stands behind the patient.
- With the index finger, the therapist palpates behind the articular pillar to localise the affected level (on RHS).
- The lateral border of the middle third of the index finger of the other hand is applied to the **opposite** side of the neck at the same level (on LHS) (Figure 12.27). The thrust point should be just behind and to the side of the articular pillar.

Method

- Lateral flexion is obtained by laterally flexing the head and neck to the left by using the right hand. At the same time lateral flexion is reinforced by pushing across with the thrusting (left) hand.
- Lateral flexion is increased to the point of elastic stretch and then manipulation is performed by simultaneously sharply increasing lateral flexion of the neck with the right hand while thrusting with the left hand towards the painful side (Figure 12.28).

The direction of forces for this specific lateral flexion technique is shown in Figure 12.29.

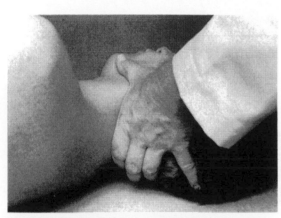

Figure 12.27 Cervical manipulation technique 7: lateral flexion (specific method) – position of the thrusting hand on the non-painful side of the neck. Note the angle of the forearm to the neck.

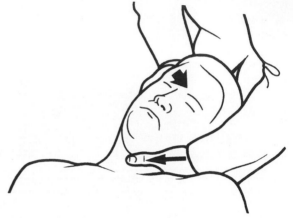

Figure 12.29 Illustration of direction of forces for specific lateral flexion.

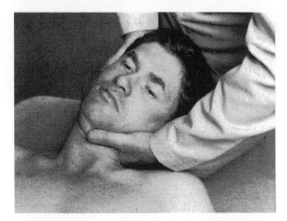

Figure 12.28 Cervical manipulation technique 7: lateral flexion (specific method) – position of the neck prior to manipulation (for right-sided pain).

8.   Traction manipulation

This technique is a traction manipulation for problems of the upper cervical spine which are often relatively inaccessible to other methods.

Position of the patient

● The patient rests supine with the head on the couch and in the midline.

Position of the therapist

● The therapist stands at the head of the couch and slightly towards the painful side.
● The 'knuckle' of the metacarpo-phalangeal joint of the index finger of the thrusting hand rests on the base of the occiput or around the mastoid process.
● The upper hand grips the patient's chin (Figure 12.30).

Method

● Although not essential, a slight degree of rotation is applied away from the painful side. This is mainly to allow more room for hand movements.
● The end range is reached by providing firm traction with the upper hand. There is no end-feel but the technique should be stopped if this traction is painful.
● At this point of stretch a short sharp cephalic thrust is exerted by the lower hand on the base of the skull (occiput or mastoid process). This produces a longitudinal movement with gapping of the stiff joints of the upper cervical spine (Figure 12.31).

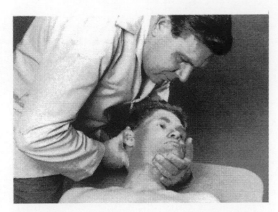

Figure 12.30 Cervical manipulation technique 8: traction manipulation.

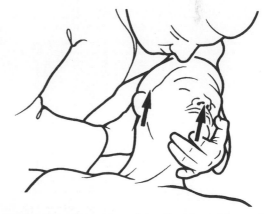

Figure 12.31 Illustration of the direction of forces for traction manipulation.

9.   'Manipulation' under anaesthesia

This procedure is rarely necessary and should be used only as a last resort method. However, it can provide dramatic relief for the patient.

Indications for manipulation under anaesthesia

- Chronic or intermittent cervical pain.
- Patient with a biomechanical vertebral dysfunction problem.
- Patient unable to relax for routine cervical manipulation.
- Normal manipulation (if possible) provides short-term relief only.
- Negative provocation tests.

Method

- The procedure is not actually a manipulation but is a traction or longitudinal stretch which is extremely effective when the patient is fully relaxed. The authors recommend administration of thiopentone only or propofol as the general anaesthetic.
- When the patient is relaxed a steady manual traction (without a belt) is applied in the same manner as for the non-anaesthetised patient (Figure 12.32). Counter traction to the shoulders should be applied by an assistant.

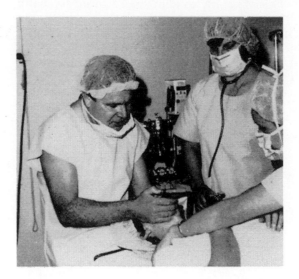

Figure 12.32 Traction of the neck under general anaesthesia.

- The degree of flexion of the neck depends on the level of the problem. If the whole spine is affected, the traction should occupy the three phases as described in Chapter 10, but usually most of the indications are for upper cervical disorders, so that the traction should occur in a neutral position. If considered necessary, a short phase of specific lateral flexion stretching or mobilisation can be given.

PRACTICE TIPS

- Always perform a provocative test prior to any intended cervical manipulation.
- Perfect the specific rotational technique – it is highly effective.
- More than one manipulative technique can be attempted in any one treatment session.
- Should a cracking sound be produced when taking up the slack, a manipulative thrust may not be necessary. Assess the response of the stretching.
- Traction under anaesthetic is a potentially excellent method for the patient with a chronic stiff painful neck (and in whom there are no contra-indications to manipulation or anaesthesia).

SUMMARY

Manipulation of the cervical spine is very effective in the absence of contra-indications, but is potentially hazardous and should not be attempted by the novice. If manipulation is contemplated, the therapist must ask the question 'Would mobilisation suffice in this patient?' If in doubt it is better to mobilise or perform no manual therapy. However, if manipulation is to proceed it is essential to perform a provocation test for vertebro-basilar insufficiency. If no contra-indications exist, manipulation should be administered, but only at full stretch at the end range and provided no sharp pain is produced at this level.

There are dozens of manipulative techniques for the cervical spine, and a select few only are presented here. The therapist is advised to develop special skills with a few proven techniques rather than to try to practise too many methods.

13
Other treatment methods for the cervical spine and shoulder

'Cervical collars are very helpful for a short period for acutely painful necks, but should not be worn for any longer than 7–10 days at a time and not at night. Your neck needs to be mobile and exercised naturally.'

J. Murtagh
Patient Education, 1992

Contents
- ☐ Injection techniques for shoulder disorders
  - ● The subacromial space
  - ● Supraspinatus tendinitis
  - ● Bicipital tendinitis
  - ● Acromio-clavicular joint
  - ● Shoulder joint
- ☐ Treatment for specific disorders
  - ● Adhesive capsulitis
  - ● Polymyalgia rheumatica
- ☐ Exercises for the neck

INJECTION TECHNIQUES FOR SHOULDER DISORDERS

Injections of local anaesthetic and corticosteroid, mainly the latter, produce excellent results for inflammatory disorders of and around the shoulder joint, especially for supraspinatus tendinitis (Richardson, 1975).

The best results are obtained with precise localisation of the area of inflammation, although according to Moran (1984) and McQueen (1987), injections into the subacromial space are all that is necessary to reach inflammatory lesions of the tendons comprising the rotator cuff (including supraspinatus) and the subacromial bursa.

The subacromial space

The recommended approach is from the posterolateral aspect of the shoulder with the patient sitting upright.

Method

● Draw up 1 ml of corticosteroid and 2 to 3 ml of 1% lignocaine (or other agent).
● Sit the patient upright and explain the procedure in general terms.
● Identify the gap between the acromion and the humeral head with the palpating finger or thumb.
● Mark this spot.
● Swab the area with antiseptic.

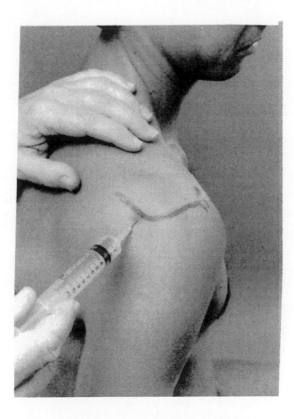

Figure 13.1 The subacromial bursa injection using the posterolateral approach.

● Place the needle (23 G, 32 or 38 mm long) into this gap, just inferior to the acromion.
● Aim the needle slightly medially and anteriorly (Figures 13.1 and 13.2).
● Insert it for a distance of three centimetres. The solution should flow into the subacromial space without resistance.

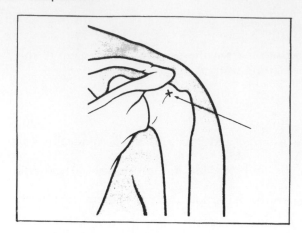

Figure 13.2 Posterior view of subacromial bursa injection site.

Alternative method

The lateral approach to the subacromial space can be used with good effect but it is important to angle the needle into the appropriate anatomical plane.

- Identify the lateral edge of the acromion and select the mid point.
- Insert the needle 4–5 mm below the edge of the acromion and angle it between the head of the humerus and the acromion.

Supraspinatus tendinitis

An injection directed onto the inflamed tendon of supraspinatus is so effective that it is preferable to administer a specific injection rather than a general infiltration into the subacromial space.

The tendon can be readily palpated as a tender cord anterolateral as it emerges from beneath the acromion to attach to the greater tuberosity of the humerus (Figure 13.3).

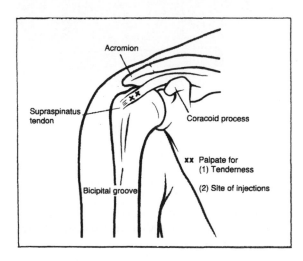

Figure 13.3 Site of tenderness in supraspinatus tendon.

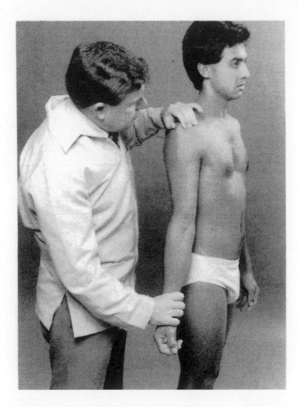

Figure 13.4 Palpating supraspinatus tendon by shoulder depression, arm traction and alternately applying external and internal rotation of the arm.

This identification is assisted by depressing the shoulder by pulling downwards on the arm and then externally and internally rotating the humerus (Corrigan and Maitland, 1983) (Figure 13.4). This manoeuvre allows the examiner to readily locate the tendon.

Method

- Identify and mark the tendon.
- The patient's arm is placed behind the back, with the back of the hand touching the far waistline. This places the arm in the desired internal rotation and forces the humeral head anteriorly.
- A 23 G, 32 mm long needle is inserted under the acromion along the line of the tendon and injected around the tendon just under the acromion (Figure 13.5). If the gritty resistance of the tendon is encountered, slightly withdraw the needle to ensure that it lies in the tendon sheath.
- The recommended injection is 1 ml of long-acting corticosteroid with 2 ml of local anaesthetic.

Bicipital tendinitis

Bicipital tendinitis is diagnosed by finding an abnormal tenderness over the tendon when the arm is externally rotated. The usual site is the bicipital groove of the humeral head.

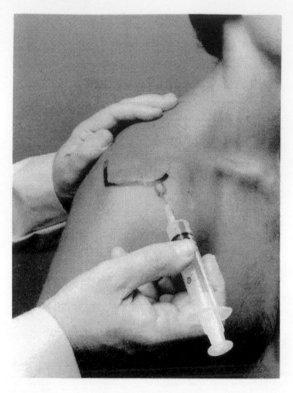

Figure 13.5 Injection for supraspinatuš tendinitis.

Method

- The patient sits with the arm hanging by the side and the palm facing forwards.
- Find and mark the site of maximal tenderness. This is usually in the bicipital groove and more proximal than expected.
- Insert a 23 G needle at the proximal end of the bicipital groove above the tender area.

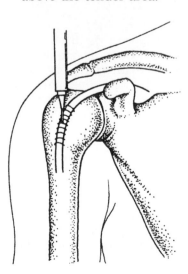

Figure 13.6 Injection for bicipital tenditis.

- Slide the needle down the groove to reach the tender area (Figure 13.6).
- Inject 1 ml of long-acting corticosteroid and 1 ml of local anaesthetic around this site.

Injection into joints

Intra-articular injections of corticosteroids can be very therapeutic for some acute inflammatory conditions, particularly severe synovitis caused by rheumatoid arthritis (especially monarticular rheumatoid arthritis). This use is limited in osteoarthritis but can be very effective for a particularly severe flare up of osteoarthritis such as in the knee or the acromioclavicular joint. (Corticosteroids can cause degeneration of articular cartilage and hence restricted usage is important.) Strict asepsis is essential, using disposable equipment.

Acromioclavicular joint

Method

- The patient sits with the arm hanging loosely by the side and externally rotated. The joint space is palpable just distal (lateral) to the bony enlargement of the clavicle. It is about 2 cm medial to the lateral edge of the acromion.

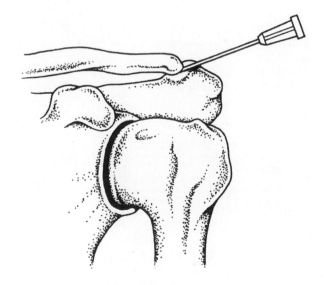

Figure 13.7 Injection into the acromio-clavicular joint.

- Palpate the 'gap' for maximal tenderness.
- Insert a 25 G needle, which should be angled according to the different surfaces encountered (Figure 13.7). It should reach a depth of about 2 cm when it is certainly intra-articule.
- Inject a mixture of 0.25–0.5 ml of corticosteroid with 0.25–0.5 ml of 1 per cent lignocaine.

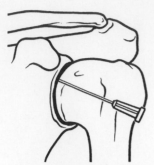

Figure 13.8 Injection into the gleno-humeral joint of the shoulder.

Shoulder joint

Method

- The patient sits in the same position as for the acromioclavicular joint injection.
- Use an anterior approach and insert a 21 G to 23 G needle just medial to the head of the humerus. Feel for the space between the head of the humerus and the glenoid cap. (If in doubt, feel for it by rotating the humerus externally.)
- This insertion should also be 1 cm below and just lateral to the coracoid process (Figure 13.8).
- Inject a mixture of 1 ml of corticosteroid and 1 ml of 1% lignocaine.

TREATMENT FOR SPECIFIC DISORDERS

Adhesive capsulitis

This debilitating problem can present for at least 12 months so an intra-articular injection of corticosteroid was recommended and still can be used. However, the modern approach is to hydrodilate the joint preferably under sedation. Once the acute episode subsides active exercises are important to restore function.

Polymyalgia rheumatica

Corticosteroids give dramatic relief but long-term management can be problematic; regular review and support is essential.

Dosage

- Prednisolone 15 mg initially.
- Taper down gradually to the minimum effective dose (often < 5 mg daily) according to the clinical response and the erythrocyte sedimentation rate. Aim for treatment for two years: relapses are common.

EXERCISES FOR THE NECK

Neck exercises (Figure 13.9 (series)) appear to be very beneficial, especially in those prone to suffer with a postural problem, such as students and typists, and in those who have been involved in an accident, and suffered injury such as 'whiplash'. The earlier the exercises can be instituted the better.

Patients with dysfunction of the cervical spine including apophyseal joint and disc problems can benefit from extension exercises (exercise

1) while the neck retraction exercises (exercise 7) are most appropriate for those who have a problem with relaxing their neck.

Exercises involving movement, especially head rolling exercises, can aggravate some neck problems, particularly in patients with osteoarthritis and rheumatoid arthritis. Isometric exercises are more appropriate for patients with such inflammatory problems and for those with a hypermobile neck.

A variety of isometric exercises which are a form of muscle energy therapy can be prescribed for the patient especially if movement is limited in one or two directions, when they are particularly effective. The isometric contraction should occur in the limited direction, followed by stretching in the same direction. One technique is to use resisted movements against a firm object. This is achieved by getting the patient to lie down, placing the head on a small firm pillow and pushing it down firmly in the affected direction – flexion, extension, rotation or lateral flexion (neck exercise 1). Another technique is for the patient to perform such resisted movements into his or her own hands, either lying down (neck exercise 2) or sitting (neck exercise 3).

The specific muscle energy techniques can be readily adapted for patient exercise programmes. For acute neck problems with muscle spasm the methods shown (exercises 3 and 4) are ideal. For patients with chronic pain and stiffness the better method is to contract against resistance, using the hand from the opposite side, over the head (lateral flexion), so that the muscles on the affected side undergo isometric resisted contraction and are then stretched away from that side.

General advice to patients

If you have neck pain and stiffness, a course of exercises is important because it loosens the stiff joints (all 35 of them) and strengthens the muscles that control the movements of the neck.

If there is pain with a particular exercise you should stop doing it and contact your therapist for advice.

It is best to keep your head in a neutral position with your chin tucked in before you start.

Do the exercises two or three times a day, but exercises 3,4,6,7,8 can be done sitting up many times during the day.

Isometric exercises

Exercise 1: hand press

While lying on your back lock your fingers behind your head and press your forearms against the sides of your head. Take a deep breath in, hold it and press your head down into the locked fingers. Repeat five times.

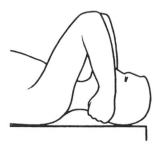

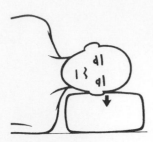

Exercise 2: resisted side bending (left side demonstration)

Lie on your side with your head resting on a small firm pillow. Your head and neck should be in a straight line. Take a deep breath in, hold it and push down hard on the pillow for seven seconds, then breathe out as you relax. Repeat three times. Repeat on the opposite side if this side is tender. It is important to make sure that you press down on your painful side.

This type of exercise can be used for extension (lying face downwards), flexion (lying on back) and rotation (lying on back).

Muscle energy exercises (isometric plus stretching)

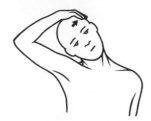

Exercise 3: resisted side bending (right-sided problem)

Sit upright in a chair, tuck your chin in and keep your head straight. Place your right hand over the top of your head to grasp the head just above the ear. Pull your head down until it first begins to feel uncomfortable. Take a deep breath in – hold it – press firmly against your hand for seven seconds (you will be pushing to the left). Breathe out, relax and then pull your head firmly towards the right. Repeat this three to five times.

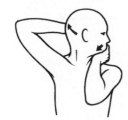

Exercise 4: resisted rotation (left-sided problem)

Sit upright in a chair, tuck your chin in and turn it to the left side to the point of discomfort. Then place your right hand on the back of your head and your left on the chin as shown. Take a deep breath in – now try to turn your head to the right but hold it in place by resistance from your hands. As you relax and breathe out, rotate your head firmly but gently towards the left. Repeat three to five times.

Other exercises

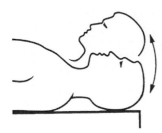

Exercise 5: neck flexion

Lie on your back on a firm surface such as a floor or bed. Tighten the muscles at the front of your neck and touch your chest with your chin. Hold for five seconds. Relax and return to the starting position. Repeat five times.

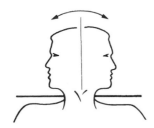

Exercise 6: neck rotation

Lie on your back as for exercise 5. Turn your head firmly (but not quickly) to the side by turning your chin towards your shoulders. Hold for five seconds and then turn to the opposite side. Repeat five times.

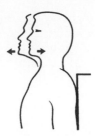

Exercise 7: the 'bird' exercise

Sit upright, tuck your chin in and then thrust it forwards and backwards in a bird-like manner. Repeat five times.

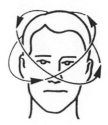

Exercise 8: drawing circles

Sit upright. Rotate your head and neck with a firm steady circular motion (never quickly) drawing circles in the air with your chin, for at least 12 seconds.

   Note: This exercise must not be done if you have dizziness or rheumatoid arthritis.

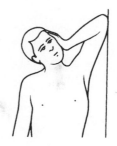

Exercise 9: the wall press

Adopt the position illustrated: elbow touching the wall; hand pushed firmly against your face; and feet fixed firmly on the floor. Your feet should be further away from the wall than your head so that you are on a slight lean against the wall. Turn your face slightly away; slide your elbow up the wall. Ensure you do this on your painful side. Repeat once. Try this on the other side if you have pain on that side as well.

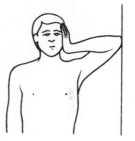

14
The cervical spine: case histories and management problems

The onset of modern transport brought with it the phenomenon of rear end collisions with its effect on the neck. Erichsen coined the term 'railway spine' in 1886 while Harold Crowe introduced the term 'whiplash injury' in 1928.

Contents
- ☐ Cervical spine: manual therapy
- ☐ Case histories
- ☐ Answers to management problems: cervical spine

The following case histories of patients with cervical pain are presented for discussion. For each patient presented make the appropriate decisions according to the following plan:

1. Provisional diagnosis.
2. Level of the lesion.
3. Management plan.
4. Select the appropriate manual therapy (if any) from the mobilisation and manipulation techniques as listed:
   A. First line techniques
   B. Second line techniques.

The main techniques are summarised in list form and also in the coded format:

CMo = cervical mobilisation
CMa = cervical manipulation

CERVICAL SPINE: MANUAL THERAPY

Summary of techniques

Mobilisation techniques		*Code*
1. Anterior directed central gliding: A, B and C		CMo 1
2. Anterior directed unilateral gliding: A, B and C		CMo 2
3. Anterior directed unilateral gliding with head rotation (C1–C2): A, B and C		CMo 3
4. Rotation	A. Initial range	CMo 4
	B. Mid range	
	C. End range	CMo 5
5. Lateral flexion	A. Specific	CMo 6
	B. Non-specific	
6. Longitudinal distraction gliding = traction		CMo 7
	A. Upper	
	B. Mid	
	C. Lower	
7. Muscle energy therapy (various)		CMo 8

Manipulation techniques	*Code*
1. Non-specific rotation (supine)	CMa 1
2. Semi-specific rotation (supine) A	CMa 2
3. Semi-specific rotation (supine) B	CMa 3
4. Specific rotation (supine)	CMa 4
5. Non-specific rotation (sitting)	CMa 5
6. Semi-specific rotation (sitting)	CMa 6
7. Lateral flexion	CMa 7
8. Traction manipulation	CMa 8
9. Manipulation under anaesthesia	CMa 9

CASE HISTORIES

Case 1

A 29-year-old male presents with 10 days of neck pain radiating to the right suprascapular area. This had a gradual onset and is aggravated by turning his head to reverse the car. There is associated neck stiffness.

Inspection

No abnormality.

Palpation

Tender right C4–C5 apophyseal joint.

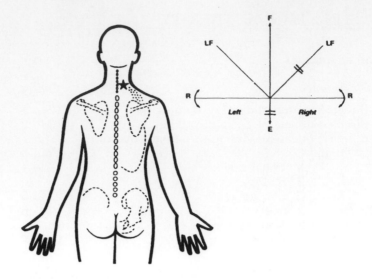

Movements

Restricted right lateral flexion and extension.

X-ray

Normal.

Questions

1. Provisional diagnosis.
2. Spinal level of lesion.
3. Management plan.
4. Selection of manual therapy techniques:
   A. First line techniques
   B. Second line techniques.

Case 2

A 63-year-old male presents with a four month history of generalised neck pain, painful restriction of all movements and 'giddiness'. He has no visual disturbance but does experience headaches 'in the back of the head'.

Inspection

Head held very stiff – tends to move body rather than turn head.

Palpation

Generalised tenderness C3–C7 (central and bilateral).

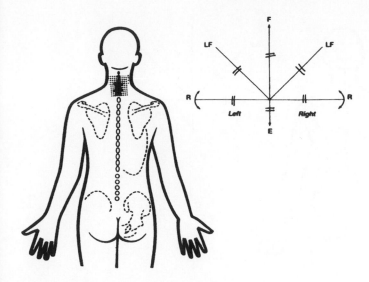

Movements

Restriction of all movements.

General examination

VB1 provocation test – positive.

X-ray

Generalised cervical spondylosis.

Questions

1. Provisional diagnosis.
2. Spinal level of lesion.
3. Management plan.
4. Selection of manual therapy techniques:
   A. First line techniques
   B. Second line techniques.

Case 3

A 35-year-old female presents with three weeks of left-sided neck pain associated with left arm pain and paraesthesia, especially affecting the middle finger. The pain and paraesthesia are associated with coughing and neck rotation to the left.

Inspection

Head held stiff and guarded.

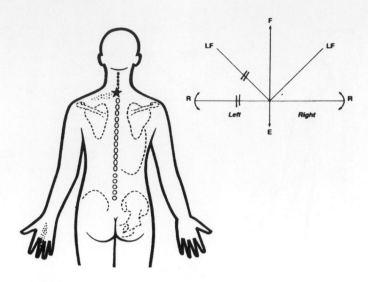

Palpation

Tender over C6 central and C6–C7 to left; associated muscle spasm.

Movements

Restricted left lateral flexion and rotation.

Neurological

Triceps power and reflex decreased.

X-ray

Normal.

Questions

1. Provisional diagnosis.
2. Spinal level of lesion.
3. Management plan.
4. Selection of manual therapy techniques:
   A. First line techniques
   B. Second line techniques.

Case 4

A 19-year-old female presents with a left-sided acute wry neck characterised by intense pain at times.

Inspection

Neck held stiff and in lateral flexion to the right.

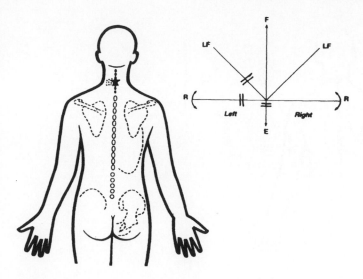

Palpation

Very tender over C3, C4 centrally and C3–C4, C4–C5 unilaterally (left).

Movements

Restricted lateral flexion and rotation to the left; loss of extension.

Neurological

Normal.

X-ray

Normal.

Questions

1. Provisional diagnosis.
2. Spinal level of lesion.
3. Management plan.
4. Selection of manual therapy techniques:
    A. First line techniques
    B. Second line techniques.

Case 5

A 43-year-old female presents with 12 months of neck stiffness and headaches related to a blow to the head from an overhead bar. She has received sporadic massage and mobilisation, with only minimal relief. She is apprehensive about manipulation and cannot relax during therapy.

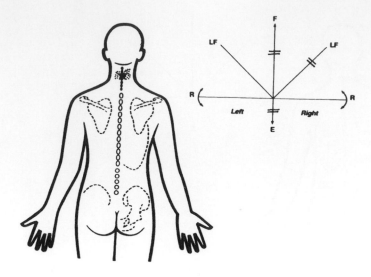

Inspection

Normal movements.

Palpation

Tenderness centrally over C2, C3, C4 and unilaterally at these levels and C1–C2 on right and left sides.

Movements

Restricted flexion, extension and right lateral flexion.

X-ray

Early degenerative changes of apophyseal joints C1–C2, C2–C3 on right.

Questions

1. Provisional diagnosis.
2. Spinal level of lesion.
3. Management plan.
4. Selection of manual therapy techniques:
   A. First line techniques
   B. Second line techniques.

Case 6

A 45-year-old female presents with a six month history of retro-orbital frontal headaches with associated neck pain. The headaches are worse in the morning and following reading. There is associated stiffness and

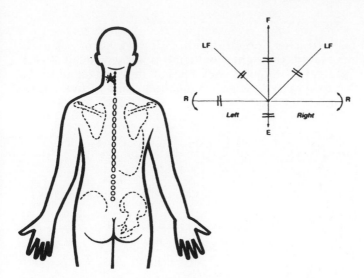

'grating' in the neck. She relates the headaches to a minor motor accident four weeks previously.

Inspection

Head held stiffly.

Palpation

Stiff and tender C2–C3 lateral (on left) and central C2.

Movements

Restricted and tender flexion, extension, lateral flexion (R and L) and L rotation.

Neurological

Normal.

X-ray

Normal.

Questions

1. Provisional diagnosis.
2. Spinal level of lesion.
3. Management plan.
4. Selection of manual therapy techniques:
    A. First line techniques
    B. Second line techniques.

Case 7

A 29-year-old male (teacher) presents with a 10 week history of neck pain that radiates towards the right shoulder. It is not severe but affects his driving of the car as looking over his left or right shoulder is difficult. He has received massage, mobilisation and acupuncture without significant benefit.

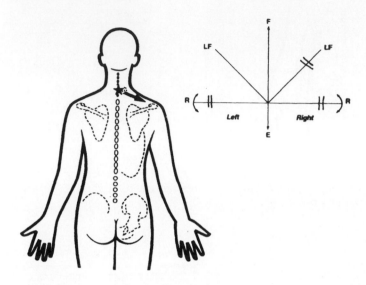

Inspection

Normal.

Palpation

Tender over C5 and C6 central and C5–C6, C6–C7 lateral (R).

Movements

Limited bilateral rotation (L and R) lateral flexion to R.

X-ray

Normal.

Questions

1. Provisional diagnosis.
2. Spinal level of lesion.
3. Management plan.
4. Selection of manual therapy techniques:
   A. First line techniques
   B. Second line techniques.

Case 8

A 23-year-old female presents with right-sided upper neck pain and headaches which are occipital and radiate to the right temporal area. At times the headaches are severe. She attributes the problem to sleeping awkwardly in a chair four weeks previously.

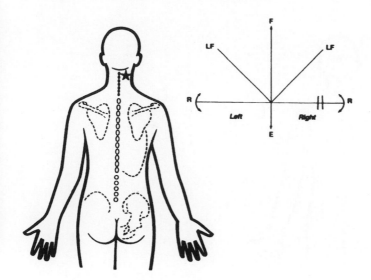

Inspection

Normal.

Palpation

Tender over the right lateral area at C1–C2 level.

Movements

Restricted right rotation only.

X-ray

Normal.

Questions

1. Provisional diagnosis.
2. Spinal level of lesion.
3. Management plan.
4. Selection of manual therapy techniques:
   A. First line techniques
   B. Second line techniques.

Case 9

A 45-year-old female (cleaner) presents with a six week history of intermittent pain of the right shoulder which is gradually becoming worse and at times radiates to the base of the neck and the right elbow. In the past three days the throbbing pain has been constant and wakes her at night.

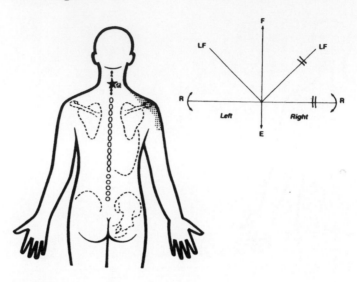

Inspection

Right shoulder held stiffly.

Palpation

Tenderness anterolateral to the tip of the acromion; tender over C4 centrally and C4–C5 lateral (R).

Movements

Shoulder – painful on active abduction; painful on resisted abduction; 'impingement test' positive.
Neck – restricted and tender right lateral flexion and rotation.

General

Normal.

X-ray

Normal.

Questions

1. Provisional diagnosis.
2. Spinal level of lesion.
3. Management plan.
4. Selection of manual therapy techniques:
   A. First line techniques
   B. Second line techniques.

Case 10

A 39-year-old female presents 10 days after a 'whiplash' injury due to a rear end motor vehicle collision. She is complaining of severe neck pain, occupital headache, neck stiffness, feelings of nausea and depression and occasional pains in the right arm.

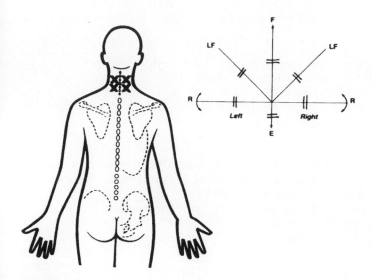

Inspection

Neck held very stiffly: in cervical collar.

Palpation

Generalised tenderness – central and bilaterally C2–C6; moderate muscle spasm.

Movements

All movements restricted.

Neurological

Normal.

X-ray

Normal.

Questions

1. Provisional diagnosis.
2. Spinal level of lesion.
3. Management plan.
4. Selection of manual therapy techniques:
    A. First line techniques
    B. Second line techniques.

ANSWERS TO MANAGEMENT PROBLEMS: CERVICAL SPINE

In your management plan for each patient, follow the following general rules:

● Provide appropriate reassurance, information and support.
● Monitor the patient's progress without over-treatment.
● Prescribe basic analgesics for pain.
● Prescribe tranquillisers/muscle relaxants in cases where there is considerable pain.
● Prescribe NSAIDs if inflammation is present (a two week course may be an optimal trial).
● Provide general rules to live by, including advice regarding sleeping, and advice on pillows, activities involving prolonged flexion and extension and other aggravating factors.
● Prescribe an exercise programme as early as possible.
● Avoid the use of cervical collars wherever possible and advise on judicious use when appropriate.

Case 1

1, 2. This patient has vertebral dysfunction, presumably of the apophyseal joint at the right C4–C5 level.
3.   As in introduction.
4.   The appropriate first line techniques are the mobilisation techniques CMo 2 (anterior directed unilateral gliding), and CMo 5 (rotation at the end range – if possible).

       Second line techniques (should the first line techniques fail to relieve symptoms) are the manipulation techniques CMa 4 (specific rotation) and CMa 2 or 3 (semi-specific rotation). All the other techniques except CMa 8 could also be used if necessary.

Case 2

1, 2. This patient has widespread degenerative osteoarthritis affecting the apophyseal joints from C3 to C7 particularly C5–C6 and C6–C7.

3.   The patient requires pain relief and a course of NSAIDs would be advisable for his arthritis. Gentle mobilising exercises should be prescribed if tolerated.

4.   This patient has too much stiffness and inflammation to be considered for manipulation. In addition, he has vertebro-basilar insufficiency which precludes manipulation.

    The choice of first line mobilisation techniques is open, with little to choose between some techniques, but CMo 4 (rotation – mid to end range) and CMo 7 (traction) would be suitable starting techniques.

    Second line techniques include CMo 1 (central) and CMo 2 (unilateral) anterior directed gliding techniques.

Case 3

1, 2.   This patient has nerve root irritation or compression due to vertebral dysfunction at the C6–C7 level. This is likely to be a disc prolapse of C6–C7 affecting the C7 nerve root.

3.   The patient requires careful supervision and relatively intensive treatment to relieve the pressure from the C7 nerve root.

4.   The first line technique should be carefully applied traction (mobilisation technique CMo 7).

    The second line techniques should be rotation at the end range to the right (technique CMo 5) as this maximally gaps the left intervertebral foramen.

    Spinal manipulation is to be avoided.

Case 4

1, 2.   The patient has acute torticollis caused by acute vertebral dysfunction at the C3–C4 level presumably due to acute dysfunction of the left C3–C4 apophyseal joint, although a disc lesion (C3–C4) could be responsible.

3.   Management includes pain relief, reassurance that the problem will settle in two or three days and that treatment is effective.

4.   The first line technique is CMo 8 – muscle energy therapy (as outlined in Chapter 11).

    Second line techniques include the mobilisation techniques CMo 7 (traction), CMo 6 (lateral flexion) and CMo 4 (rotation).

    Should the condition improve sufficiently during this therapy, manipulation techniques can be considered, namely CMa 4 (a specific rotation at C3–C4); and/or CMa 7 (lateral flexion – specific for C3–C4). However, manipulation initially is not recommended.

Case 5

1, 2.   This patient has apophyseal joint dysfunction of upper cervical joints from C1–C2 to C3–C4.

3, 4.   The management of this patient is difficult and if she cannot relax sufficiently for routine manipulation she should be offered 'manipulation' under general anaesthesia. This is basically a longitudinal distraction gliding CMa 9 (Chapter 12) which can be dramatically effective in such a patient.

Case 6

1, 2.   The patient has left C2–C3 apophyseal joint dysfunction causing referred headache.

3, 4.   The first line manual therapy techniques are the mobilisation techniques – CMo 2 (unilateral ADG), CMo 4/CMo 5 (rotation) and CMo 7 (traction).   Manipulation cannot be attempted initially as there is a biomechanical contra-indication (five movements restricted).

The second line techniques are manipulations – CMa 4 (specific rotation) or CMa 2 or 3 (semi-specific rotation) – provided that mobilisation is effective in producing at least three free movements. If the symptoms are not relieved then CMa 7 (lateral flexion) should be considered.

Case 7

1, 2.   The patient has lower cervical dysfunction resulting in right C5–C6 and C6–C7 apophyseal joint pain.

3, 4.   Since mobilisation techniques have failed, manipulation must be considered. However, there is biomechanical restriction in rotation bilaterally and lateral flexion to the right – all other movements are free.

As there are three degrees of freedom, the most appropriate technique is left lateral flexion (CMa 7), which maximally gaps the C5–C6 and C6–C7 foramen and joints on the right.

This may result in freedom of left rotation. If so, then either a semi-specific rotation (CMa 2 or 3) to the left or a specific rotation (CMa 4) to the left can be performed.

Case 8

1, 2.   The patient has upper cervical dysfunction resulting in right C1–C2 apophyseal joint pain with referred occipital and temporal headaches.

3, 4.   The initial technique should be a mobilisation by applying CMo 3 – anterior directed unilateral gliding, with the head rotated to the right.   In addition, CMo 7 – traction (in neutral position) or muscle energy – CMo 8 (a traction technique for the upper cervical spine – Chapter 11) – can be applied.

The most appropriate second line technique is CMa 8 – traction manipulation.

Case 9

1, 2.   The provisional diagnosis implicates dual pathology, namely mid cervical dysfunction and right supraspinatus tendinitis, both of which can cause pain referable to C5.

3, 4.   The first line management plan includes treatment for the supraspinatus tendinitis with a specific injection of corticosteroid and local anaesthetic. The cervical problem is managed with the mobilisation techniques CMo 5 (rotation) and CMo 6 (lateral flexion) towards the left side.

The second line techniques for the cervical problem are the manipulation techniques CMa 4 (specific rotation) and CMa 7 (lateral flexion).

Case 10

1, 2.   This patient has the 'whiplash' syndrome which has been described in Chapter 7. It affects many levels of the cervical spine, especially affecting the apophyseal joints.

3.   Management of the 'whiplash' syndrome is such a common and difficult problem that it will be considered in considerable detail.

The objective of treatment is to obtain (gradually) a full pain-free range of free movement of the neck. It is essential to focus equally on the physical and psychological components of the problem, as ignoring either will impair management. Other objectives include an early return to work and discouragement of unnecessary reliance on legal action.

Explanation and reassurance

An appropriate empathy will be achieved by demonstrating a caring and responsible approach in addition to an understanding of the injury. Explanation with the use of a patient education leaflet to supplement the discussion would be appropriate. Explain that the majority of such injuries settle rapidly. Discussion of anticipated emotional responses (usually frustration) is appropriate with those who have more severe injuries.

Medication

- *Analgesics.* Use simple analgesics initially; do not prescribe narcotics.
- *Non-steroidal anti-inflammatory drugs.* These have a place in the short-term treatment of whiplash by minimising the adverse effects of the inflammatory response to injury.
- *Tranquillisers and muscle relaxants.* These are useful in the short term.

Cervical collar

For painful necks a soft cervical collar should be worn during the day for the first one or two weeks. The method rests the injured part and helps healing. Ideally, the neck should be placed in a non-painful posture, usually that of slight forward flexion. A soft collar that is wider at the back achieves this objective.

Table 14.1 *Guidelines for treatment of whiplash.*

PHASE	OBJECTIVE	METHOD
Acute	Promote healing Reduce inflammation of injury	Patient education X-ray Rest Collar (2 weeks) NSAIDs (2 weeks) Analgesics Tranquillisers (mild)
Sub-acute	Encourage healing in a functional manner	Neck exercises (early as possible) Heat and massage 'Spray and stretch' Heat and massage Mobilisation
Chronic	Reverse effects of chronic inflammation and poor healing. Minimise patient's discomfort, and any deterioration of condition	Injection of trigger sites Deep friction massage Muscle energy techniques Manipulation Antidepressants Facet joint block (consultant) Acupuncture Manipulation under general anaesthesia Consider discography/discectomy

Be alert for the patient who regards it as a psychological (as well as physical) crutch. It is best to discard the collar after two weeks and start mobilising the neck.

Mobilisation techniques

Early mobilisation

Encourage early mobilisation even if it is uncomfortable. A graduated series of exercises should be prescribed after the acute pain subsides. Use only gentle mobilisation initially to allow full healing of ligaments. Healing time for a muscle tear is two to three weeks, and for ligamentous tears six to eight weeks. Manipulation or vigorous mobilisation earlier than eight weeks is contra-indicated.

Massage

Massage can promote relaxation and decrease muscle spasm. Gentle therapeutic massage is useful and may help the all important exercise programme.

'Spray and stretching'

The use of topical freezing spray in conjunction with stretching by lateral flexion is an appropriate technique for gradual restoration of normal neck movements. Gradual stretching techniques can be continued to the end range of movement.

Manipulation

Cervical manipulation is contra-indicated in the early stages and should be reserved for patients who do not respond to gentler and more active techniques of physical therapy. It should be performed by a skilled therapist in the chronic phase of the problem and when no contra-indications exist for its use.

Coarse or rough manipulation of the cervical spine, especially in the acute or subacute phase, will usually aggravate or prolong symptoms.

As a last resort, manipulation of the cervical spine under general anaesthesia by traction can be dramatically effective. It should be performed by a skilled therapist.

4. The appropriate first line techniques are the mobilisation techniques CMo 4, CMo 5 (if possible) and CMo 7 – rotation and traction.

The second line techniques are the anterior directed gliding techniques CMo 1 and CMo 2.

This can be slow and rather laborious but, in many cases, both patient and therapist must accept a slow response.

Section 3
The Thoracic Spine and Chest Wall

15
Thoracic back pain and chest wall pain

'Since learning about the various causes of chest wall pain I am continually amazed about the number of pain syndromes that I am now diagnosing as originating from the thoracic spine. I wonder what I was thinking beforehand.'

Comments from past course participants, 1985–1994

Contents
- ☐ Key checkpoints
- ☐ Functional anatomy
- ☐ Referred pain
- ☐ A diagnostic approach
- ☐ The clinical approach
- ☐ Clinical syndromes
- ☐ Practice tips
- ☐ Summary

Thoracic (dorsal) back pain is common in people of all ages including children and adolescents. Dysfunction of the joints of the thoracic spine, with its unique costo-vertebral joints, which are an important source of back pain, is very commonly encountered in medical practice, especially in people whose lifestyle creates stresses and strains through poor posture and heavy lifting. Muscular and ligamentous strains may be common, but rarely come to light in practice because they are self-limiting and not severe.

This dysfunction can cause referred pain to various parts of the chest wall and can mimic the symptoms of various visceral diseases such as angina, biliary colic and oesophageal spasm. In similar fashion, heart and gall bladder pain can mimic spinal pain.

KEY CHECKPOINTS

- The commonest site of pain in the spine is the costo-vertebral articulations, especially the costo-transverse articulation (Figure 15.1).
- Pain of thoracic spinal origin may be referred anywhere to the chest wall, but the commonest sites are the scapula region, the paravertebral region 2–5 cm from the midline, and anteriorly, over the costo-chondral region.
- Thoracic (also known as dorsal) pain is more common in patients with abnormalities such as kyphosis and Scheuermann's disorder.
- Trauma to the chest wall (including falls on the chest such as those experienced in body contact sport) commonly lead to disorders of the thoracic spine.
- Patients recovering from open heart surgery, when a longitudinal sternal incision is made and the chest wall is stretched out, commonly experience severe thoracic back pain.
- Unlike the lumbar spine the joints are quite superficial and it is relatively easy to find the affected (painful) segment.
- The intervertebral disc prolapse is very uncommon in the thoracic spine.
- The older patient presenting with chest pain should be regarded as having a cardiac cause until proved otherwise.
- If the chest pain is non-cardiac, then the possibility of referral from the thoracic spine should be considered.

FUNCTIONAL ANATOMY

The functional unit of the thoracic spine is illustrated in Figure 15.1. It appears that pain from the thoracic spine originates mainly from the apophyseal joints and rib articulations. Any one thoracic vertebra

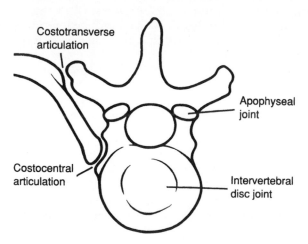

Figure 15.1 The functional unit of the thoracic spine.

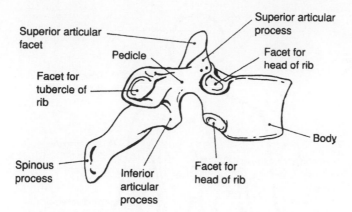

Figure 15.2 Typical thoracic vertebra: lateral view.

has 10 separate articulations so the potential for dysfunction and the difficulty in clinically pinpointing the precise joint at a particular level are apparent. A lateral view of a typical thoracic vertebra (Figure 15.2) highlights the characteristic features to accommodate the rib articulations.

The 12 thoracic vertebrae have slightly wedged shaped bodies that result in the familiar thoracic curvatures. The orientation of the apophyseal joints is such that the characteristic thoracic rotation occurs in addition to extension, flexion and lateral flexion. The intervertebral discs of the thoracic spine are relatively thin compared with cervical and lumbar discs. Disc disruption from T1 to T10 is rare.

The costo-vertebral joints

The costo-vertebral joints are synovial joints unique to the thoracic spine and have two articulations – costo-transverse and costo-central. Together with the apophyseal joints, they are capable of presenting with well localised pain close to the midline or as referred pain, often quite distal to the spine, with the major symptoms not appearing to have any relationship to the thoracic spine.

The thoracic cage

The bony components of the thoracic cage are the ribs, sternum and thoracic spine which forms its posterior boundary. Ribs 1 to 7 articulate with the sternum via the costal cartilages at the sterno-costal joints which are subject to traumatic injury and to inflammation. The costal cartilages of ribs 8 to 10 articulate with the costal cartilages above. Ribs 1 and 10 articulate with the corresponding vertebrae only while ribs 2 to 9 articulate with two vertebrae and ribs 11 and 12 are described as 'floating' because they have no anterior articulation and no costo-transverse joints.

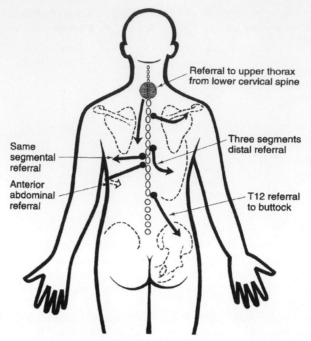

Figure 15.3 Examples of referral patterns for the thoracic spine.

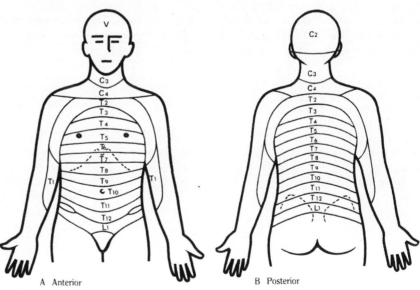

Figure 15.4 Dermatomes for the thoracic nerve roots indicating possible referral areas.

REFERRED PAIN

Generalised referral patterns are presented in Figure 15.3, while the dermatome pattern is outlined in Figure 15.4.

The pain pattern acts as a guide only because there is considerable dermatomal overlap within the individual and variation from one person to another. It has been demonstrated that up to five nerve roots may contribute to the innervation of any one point in the anterior segments of the trunk dermatomes, a fact emphasised by the clinical distribution of herpes zoster.

Lower cervical referred pain

Disorders of the lower cervical segments can cause referred pain in the upper thoracic area, as evidenced clinically by pain in this region following a 'whiplash' injury. The C4 dermatome is in close proximity to the T2 dermatome which appears to represent the cutaneous areas of the lower cervical segments, as the posterior primary rami of C5, C6, C7, C8 and T1 innervate musculature and have no significant cutaneous innervation.

Cervical causation of interscapular pain can be confirmed by manipulative correction of the cervical lesion, following which the painful interscapular area resolves. Furthermore, injection of local anaesthetic at the T2 level, which coincides with the superficial exit of the posterior branch of T2, results in disappearance of the interscapular pain (Figure 15.5).

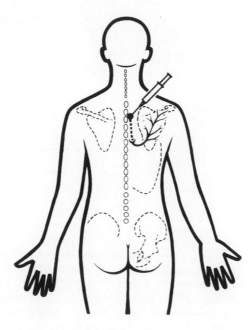

Figure 15.5 The estimation of the 'cervical point of the back'.

The pain from the lower cervical spine can also refer pain to the anterior chest, and mimic coronary ischaemic pain. The associated autonomic nervous system disturbance can cause considerable confusion in making the diagnosis.

Upper thoracic pain

Dysfunction of the joints of the upper thoracic spine usually gives rise to localised pain and stiffness posteriorly but also can cause distal symptoms, probably via the autonomic nervous system.

A specific syndrome called the T4 syndrome (McGuckin, 1986) has been shown to cause vague pain in the upper limbs and diffuse, vague head and posterior neck pain. However, most of the pain, stiffness and discomfort arises from dysfunction of the upper and middle thoracic segments with patients presenting with the complaint of pain 'between my shoulder blades'.

Costo-vertebral joint dysfunction

The unique feature of the thoracic spine is the costo-vertebral joint. It is frequently responsible for referral pain ranging from the midline, posterior to the lateral chest wall, and even anterior chest pain. When the symptoms radiate laterally, the diagnosis is confirmed only when movement of the rib provokes pain at the costo-vertebral joint. This examination will simultaneously reproduce the referred pain.

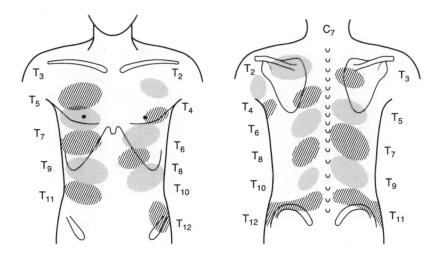

Figure 15.6 Kellegren's (1939) pain referral patterns after stimulation of deep joints of the thoracic spine.

Figure 15.6 presents the pattern of referred pain from these joints and highlights the capacity of the thoracic spine to refer pain centrally to the anterior chest and upper abdomen. Confusion arises for the clinician when the patient's history focuses on the anterior chest pain and fails to mention the presence of posterior pain, should it be present. The shaded areas in Figure 15.6 represent those areas where the patient experiences pain following the injection of hypertonic saline into the posterior elements of the spine.

The lower thoracic spine and thoraco-lumbar junction

Dysfunction of joints in the thoraco-lumbar region can cause pain presenting primarily as iliac crest or buttock pain. The initial impression is that the symptoms are arising from lower lumbar spine but, as shown in Figure 15.7, the skin over the iliac crest and the upper

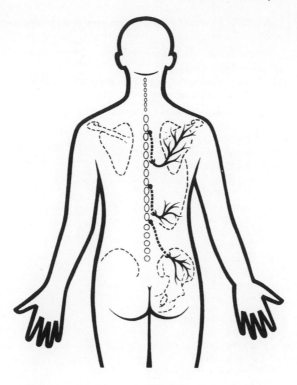

Figure 15.7 Illustration of the painful subcutaneous syndromes of sites distal to the causative nerve. Note how the posterior branch from T12 to L1 causes pain over the iliac crest and buttock.

outer buttock area is supplied by the posterior primary rami of nerves arising from the thoraco-lumbar junction (T12 and L1).

Similarly, anterior groin pain can arise from this region as the nerve supply is from the anterior rami of the spinal nerves T12 and L1) (Figure 15.8).

The cutaneous branches of the posterior primary rami usually exit three to four levels lower than the vertebral level where dysfunction exists. For example, a patient with apophyseal joint dysfunction at T8 will present with skin pain opposite T12. The examiner can reproduce the patient's pain laterally at the T12 level, but palpation of the vertebral segment by pressure on the spinous process and apophyseal joint will not reproduce the symptoms. It is important to be aware that the affected level is usually three or four segments proximal (Figure 15.7).

The patient's dermatomal symptoms can be present in either the posterior or anterior branches of the dorsal rami. Consequently, with anterior abdominal symptoms it is necessary to palpate the thoracic spine.

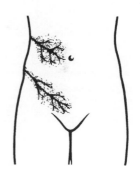

Figure 15.8 Anterior abdominal wall pain syndromes with pain caused by a lesion of the distal nerve. T9 and T12 involvement is illustrated. The pinch roll test of the skin reproduces considerable local pain.

A DIAGNOSTIC APPROACH

A diagnostic approach based on the history, is essential for the patient with thoracic back pain or chest wall pain. A reference table is presented in Table 15.1 (Murtagh, 1994).

Table 15.1 *Thoracic back pain: summary of diagnostic strategy model.*

Q.   *Probability diagnosis*
A.   Musculoligamentous strains (mainly postural)
     Vertebral dysfunction

Q.   *Serious disorders not to be missed*
A.   Cardiovascular
         myocardial infarction
         dissection aneurysm
         pulmonary infarction
     Neoplasia
         myeloma
         lung (with infiltration)
         metastatic disease
     Severe infections
         pleurisy
         infectious endocarditis
         osteomyelitis
     Pneumothorax
     Osteoporosis

Q.   *Pitfalls (often missed)*
A.   Angina
     Gastrointestinal disorders, e.g. oesophageal dysfunction
     Herpes zoster
     Spondyloarthropathies
     Fibromyalgia syndrome
     Polymyalgia rheumatica
     Chronic infection
         tuberculosis
         brucellosis

Q.   *Is this patient trying to tell me something?*
A.   Yes, quite possible with many cases of back pain

Probability diagnosis

The commonest cause of thoracic back pain is musculoskeletal, commonly due to musculoligamentous strains due to poor posture. However, these pains are usually transitory and present rarely to the practitioner. The problems that commonly present are those caused by dysfunction of the lower cervical and thoracic spinal joints especially those of the mid thoracic (interscapular) area.

Arthritic conditions of the thoracic spine are not relatively common, although degenerative osteoarthritis is encountered at times while the inflammatory spondyloarthropathies are uncommon.

Not to be missed

A special problem with the thoracic spine is its relationship with the many thoracic and upper abdominal structures which can refer pain to the back. These structures are listed in Table 15.2, but in particular myocardial infarction and dissecting aneurysm must be considered.

Table 15.2 *Non-musculoskeletal causes of thoracic back pain.*

Heart	Myocardial infarction
	Angina
	Pericarditis
Great vessels	Dissecting aneurysm
	Pulmonary embolism (rare)
	Pulmonary embolus/infarction
	Pneumothorax
	Pneumonia/pleurisy
Oesophagus	Oesophageal rupture
	Oesophageal spasm
	Oesophagitis
Subdiaphragmatic Disorders of	Gall bladder
	Stomach ⎫
	Duodenum ⎬ including ulcers
	Pancreas ⎭
	Subphrenic collection
Miscellaneous infections	Herpes zoster
	Bornholm's disease
	Infective endocarditis
Psychogenic	

Cardiopulmonary problems

The acute onset of pain can have sinister implications in the thoracic spine where various life threatening cardiopulmonary and vascular events have to be kept in mind. The pulmonary causes of acute pain include spontaneous pneumothorax, pleurisy and pulmonary infarction. Thoracic back pain may be associated with infective endocarditis due to embolic phenomena. The ubiquitous myocardial infarction or acute coronary occlusion may, uncommonly, cause interscapular back pain, while the very painful dissecting or ruptured aortic aneurysm may cause back pain with hypotension.

Osteoporosis

Osteoporosis, especially in elderly women, must always be considered in such people presenting with acute pain which can be caused by a pathological fracture. The association with pain following inappropriate physical therapy such as spinal manipulation in the older person should also be considered.

Acute infections

Infective conditions that can involve the spine include osteomyelitis, tuberculosis, brucellosis, syphilis and salmonella infections.

Such conditions should be suspected in young patients (osteomyelitis), farm workers (brucellosis) and migrants from South East Asia and third world countries (tuberculosis). The presence of poor general health and fever necessitates investigations for these infections.

Neoplasia

Fortunately, tumours of the spine are uncommon. Nevertheless, they occur frequently enough for the full time practitioner in back disorders to encounter some each year, especially metastatic disease.

The three common primary malignancies that metastasise to the spine are those originating in the lung, breast and the prostate (all paired structures). The less common primaries to consider are the thyroid, the kidney and adrenals and malignant melanoma.

Reticuloses such as Hodgkin's disease can involve the spine. Primary malignancies that arise in the vertebrae include multiple myeloma and sarcoma.

The symptoms and signs that should alert the clinician to malignant disease are:

- back pain occurring in an older person
- unrelenting back pain, unrelieved by rest (this includes night pain)
- rapidly increasing back pain
- constitutional symptoms – for example, weight loss, fever, malaise
- a history of treatment for cancer – for example, excision of skin melanoma.

A common trap for the thoracic spine is carcinoma of the lung such as mesothelioma which can invade parietal pleura or structures adjacent to the vertebral column.

Pitfalls

Pitfalls include ischaemic heart disease presenting with interscapular pain, herpes zoster at the pre-eruption stage and the various gastro-intestinal disorders. Two commonly misdiagnosed problems are a penetrating duodenal ulcer presenting with lower thoracic pain and oesophageal spasm which can cause thoracic back pain.

Inflammatory rheumatological problems are not common in the thoracic spine but occasionally a spondyloarthropathy such as ankylosing spondylitis manifests here although it follows some time after the onset of sacro-iliitis.

Psychogenic considerations

Psychogenic or non-organic causes of back pain can present a complex dilemma in diagnosis and management. The causes may be apparent from the incongruous behaviour and personality of the patient, but often the diagnosis is reached by a process of exclusion. There is obviously some functional overlay to everyone with acute or chronic pain – hence the importance of appropriate reassurance to these patients that their problem invariably subsides with time and that they do not have cancer.

THE CLINICAL APPROACH

The history

The history of a patient presenting with thoracic back pain should include a routine pain analysis which usually provides important clues for the diagnosis. The age, sex and occupation of the patient are relevant. Pain in the thoracic area is very common in people who sit bent over for long periods especially working at desks. Students, secretaries and stenographers are therefore at risk, as are nursing mothers, who have to lift their babies.

People who are kyphotic or scoliotic or who have 'hunchbacks' secondary to disease such as tuberculosis and poliomyelitis also suffer from recurrent pain in this area.

Older people are more likely to present with a neoplastic problem in the thoracic spine and with osteoporosis. Senile osteoporosis is usually a trap because it is symptomless until the intervention of a compression fracture. Symptoms following such a fracture can persist for three months.

Pain that is present day and night indicates a sinister cause.

Features of the history that give an indication that the pain is arising from dysfunction of the thoracic spine include:

- Aggravation and relief of pain on trunk rotation. The patient's pain may be increased by rotating (twisting) towards the side of the pain but eased by rotating in the opposite direction.
- Aggravation of pain by coughing, sneezing or deep inspiration. This can produce a sharp catching pain which if severe, tends to implicate the costo-vertebral joint.
- Relief of pain by firm pressure. Patients may state that their back pain is eased by firm pressure such as leaning against the corner of a wall.

It is very important to be able to differentiate between chest pain due to vertebral dysfunction and that caused by myocardial ischaemia.

The physical examination

The examination of the thoracic spine is straightforward with the emphasis being on palpation of the spine – centrally and laterally. This achieves the basic objective of reproducing the patient's symptoms and finding the level of pain. The 'look, feel, move, X-ray' clinical approach is the most appropriate for the thoracic spine. A more detailed presentation of the physical examination will be presented in Chapter 16.

Investigations

The main investigation is a plain X-ray which may exclude the basic abnormalities and diseases such as osteoporosis and malignancy. If serious disease such as malignancy or infection is suspected and the plain X-ray is normal a radionuclide bone scan or CT scan may detect these disorders.

Other investigations to consider are:

- Full blood examination and ESR
- Alkaline phosphatase
- Serum electrophoresis for multiple myeloma
- Bence Jones protein analysis
- Brucella agglutination test
- Blood culture for pyogenic infection and bacterial endocarditis
- Tuberculosis studies
- HLA B_{27} antigen for spondyloarthropathies
- ECG or ECG stress tests (suspected angina)
- Gastroscopy or barium studies (peptic ulcer).

CLINICAL SYNDROMES

There are several pain disorders referable to the thoracic spine. Dysfunction of the thoracic spine is the most common cause. 'Postural backache' also known as 'TV backache' which is typically found in adolescent girls is a common problem.

Although vertebral dysfunction still occurs but less commonly in the elderly (over 65 years), it is important to carefully search for organic disease.

Special problems to consider in the elderly are:

- Malignant disease, e.g. multiple myeloma, lung, prostate
- Osteoporosis
- Vertebral pathological fractures
- Polymyalgia rheumatica
- Paget's disease (may be asymptomatic)
- Herpes zoster
- Visceral disorders, e.g.
      ischaemic heart disease
      penetrating peptic ulcer
      oesophageal disorders
      biliary disorders.

Scheuermann's disorder

This common disorder which is spinal osteochondritis typically affects adolescent males in the lower thoracic spine (around T9) and the thoracolumbar spine. It may be asymptomatic but can be associated with back pain especially as the patient grows older.

Typical features

- Age 11–17
- Males > females
- Lower thoracic spine
- Thoracic pain or asymptomatic
- Increasing thoracic kyphosis over 1–2 months
- Wedging of the vertebrae

- Pain in the wedge especially on bending
- Short hamstrings
- Cannot touch toes
- Diagnosis confirmed by X-ray.

Treatment

- Explanation and support
- Extension exercises
- Postural correction
- Avoidance of sports involving lifting and bending
- Consider bracing or surgery if serious deformity.

Idiopathic adolescent scoliosis

A degree of scoliosis is detectable in 5 per cent of the adolescent population (Stephens, 1984). The vast majority of curves, occurring equally in boys and girls, are mild and of no consequence. 85 per cent of significant curves in adolescent scoliosis occurs in girls (Kane and Moe, 1970). Such curves appear during the peripubertal period usually coinciding with the growth spurt.

The screening test (usually in 12–14 year olds) is to note the contour of the back on forward flexion (Figure 15.9).

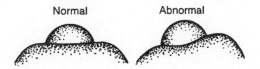

Normal   Abnormal

Figure 15.9 Screening for idiopathic adolescent scoliosis: testing asymmetry by forward flexion.

Investigation

- A single erect PA spinal X-ray is sufficient (Easter Seal Guide, 1982).
- The Cobb angle (Figure 15.10) is the usual measurement yardstick.

Management

Aims are to:

- Preserve good appearance – level shoulders and no trunk shift
- Prevent increasing curve in adult life: less than 50 degrees
- **Not** to produce a straight spine on X-ray.

Methods

Braces

- Milwaukee brace
- Trial contact brace
- To be worn for 20–22 hours each day until skeletal maturity is reached.

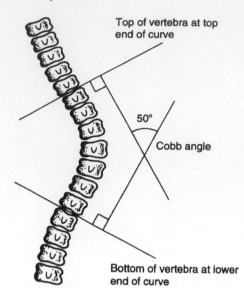

Top of vertebra at top end of curve

50°

Cobb angle

Figure 15.10 Scoliosis: the Cobb method of curve measurement.

Bottom of vertebra at lower end of curve

Surgical correction

Depends on curve and skeletal maturity.

Guidelines for treatment

Still growing	>20°	Observe (repeat examination + X-ray)
	20–30°	Observe, brace if progressive
	30–45°	Brace
	≥45–50°	Operate
Growth complete	<45°	Leave alone
	>45°	Operate

Dysfunction of the thoracic spine

This is the outstanding cause of pain presenting to the practitioner, is relatively easy to diagnose and usually responds dramatically to a simple spinal manipulation treatment.

Other musculoskeletal causes of thoracic wall pain are presented in Table 15.3.

A typical profile

Age:	Any age, especially between 20 and 40.
History of injury:	Sometimes slow or sudden onset.
Site and radiation:	Spinal and paraspinal – for example, inter-scapular, arms, lateral chest, anterior chest, sub-sternal, iliac crest.

Type of pain:	Dull, aching, occasionally sharp; severity related to activity, site and posture.
Aggravation:	Deep inspiration, postural movement of thorax, slumping or bending, walking upstairs, activities – for example, lifting children, making beds, beds too hard or soft, sleeping or sitting for long periods.
Association:	Chronic poor posture.
Diagnosis:	Examination of spine, therapeutic response to manipulation.

Management

- Explanation and reassurance
- Analgesics for a painful episode
- Spinal mobilisation and manipulation
- Exercise programme
- Preventive programme.

Table 15.3 *Musculoskeletal causes/origins of thoracic pain.*

Spinal origin	Cervical spine, esp. C4–C7
	Cervicothoracic junction
	Thoracic spine, including joints
	   costo-vertebral
	   apophyseal
	   intervertebral with disc
	Thoraco-lumbar junction

Other thoracic joints	Sternoclavicular Manubriosternal Costo-chondral Sternocostal Scapulothoracic

Disorders of:	Ribs, including
	   12th rib syndrome
	   rib tip syndrome
	   slipping rib syndrome
	Muscles
	Ligaments

Other	Costo-chondritis Tietze's syndrome Xiphoidalgia Myofascial syndrome Mondor's syndrome

Thoracic disc protrusion

Fortunately, a disc protrusion in the thoracic spine is uncommon. This reduced incidence is related to the firm splintage action of the rib cage.

Most disc protrusions occur below T9, with the commonest site, as expected, being T11–T12.

The commonest presentation is back pain and radicular pain which follows the appropriate dermatome.

However, disc lesions in the thoracic spine are prone to produce spinal cord compression manifesting a sensory loss, bladder incontinence and signs of upper motor neurone lesion. The disc is relatively inaccessible to surgical intervention, but over the past decade there has been a significant improvement in the surgical treatment of thoracic disc protrusions due to the transthoracic lateral approach.

Vertebral compression fracture

A vertebral collapse fracture of the thoracic spine can occur under the following circumstances:

- direct trauma
- indirect trauma – for example, fall from a height onto the feet
- osteoporosis
- other diseased vertebrae – for example, myeloma, metastases.

Initially the pain is severe with great discomfort on trunk movements, especially rotation. Girdle pain may be present and referred pain to two to three distal segments may be noticed. The pain tends to improve so that after two or three weeks the patient is moving and breathing with reasonable comfort.

Muscle injury

Muscular injuries such as tearing are uncommon in the chest wall. The strong paravertebral muscles do not appear to be a cause of chest pain, but strains of intercostal muscles, the serratus anterior and the musculotendinous origins of the abdominal muscles can cause pain. Injuries to these muscles can be provoked by attacks of violent sneezing or coughing or overstrain – for example, lifting a heavy suitcase from an overhead luggage rack.

Fibromyalgia, fibrositis and myofascial trigger points

Fortunately fibromyalgia is relatively uncommon but when encountered presents an enormous management problem. It is not to be confused with so-called fibrositis or tender trigger points.

Fibrositis is not a diagnosis but a symptom indicating a localised area of tenderness or pain in the soft tissues especially of the upper thoracic spine. It is probably almost always secondary to upper thoracic or lower cervical spinal dysfunction.

Myofascial trigger points

As described by Travell and Rinzler (1952) a trigger point is characterised by:

- circumscribed local tenderness
- localised twitching with stimulation of juxtaposed muscle
- pain referred elsewhere when subjected to pressure.

Trigger spots also tend to correspond to the acupuncture points for pain relief.

Treatment is by local injections of local anaesthetic into the painful point.

Fibromyalgia syndrome

The main diagnostic features are:

1. A history of widespread pain (neck to low back).
2. Pain in 11 of 18 tender points on digital palpation.

These points must be painful, not tender.

Smyth and Moldofsky (1977) have recommended 14 of these points on a map as a guide for management (Figure 15.11).

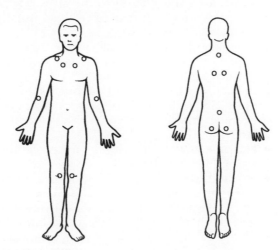

Figure 15.11 Fibromyalgia syndrome: typical tender points (the tender point map represents the 14 points recommended for use as a standard for diagnostic or therapeutic studies).

Other features

- Female:male ratio 4:1.
- Usual age: 29–37: diagnosis 44–53.
- Poor sleep pattern.
- Fatigue (similar to chronic fatigue syndrome).
- Psychological disorders – for example, anxiety, depression, tension, headache, irritable digestive system.

This disorder is very difficult to treat and is usually unresponsive in the long term to passive physical therapy or injections. The patients require considerable explanation, support and reassurance.

Treatment

- Explanation and reassurance.
- Attention to sleep disorders, stress factors and physical factors.
- Rehabilitation exercise programme – for example, walking, swimming or cycling.

Medication

- Anti-depressants (of proven value), **or**
- Clonazepam (Rivotril) 0.5 mg twice daily.

PRACTICE TIPS

- Feelings of anaesthesia or paraesthesia associated with thoracic spine dysfunction are rare.
- Thoracic back pain is frequently associated with cervical lesions.
- Upper thoracic pain and stiffness is common after 'whiplash'.
- The T4 syndrome of upper to mid thoracic pain with radiation (and associated paraesthesia) to the arms is well documented.
- Symptoms due to fractured vertebra usually last three months and a fractured rib six weeks.
- The pain of myocardial ischaemia, from either angina or myocardial infarction, can cause referred pain to the interscapular region of the thoracic spine.
- Beware of the old trap of herpes zoster in the thoracic spine, especially in the older person.
- Consider multiple myeloma as a cause of an osteoporotic collapsed vertebra.
- Examine movements with the patient sitting on the couch and hands clasped behind the neck.
- Spinal disease of special significance in the thoracic spine includes osteoporosis and neoplasia, while disc lesions, inflammatory diseases and degenerative diseases (spondylosis) are encountered less frequently than with the cervical and lumbar spines.
- Always X-ray the thoracic spine following trauma, especially after motor vehicle accidents, as wedge compression fractures (typically between T4 and T8) are often overlooked.

SUMMARY

Dysfunction of the joints of the thoracic spine, with its unique costo-vertebral joints, which are an important source of back pain, is very commonly encountered in medical practice, especially in people whose lifestyles create stresses and strains through poor posture and heavy lifting. Muscular and ligamentous strains may be common, but rarely come to light in practice because they are self-limiting and not severe.

Spinal disease of special significance in the thoracic spine includes osteoporosis and neoplasia, while disc lesions, inflammatory diseases and degenerative diseases (spondylosis) are encountered less frequently than with the cervical and lumbar spines.

It is imperative to differentiate between spinal and cardiac causes of chest pain: either cause is likely to mimic the other. A working rule is to consider the cause as cardiac until the examination and investigations establish the true cause. Sometimes the pain of vertebral dysfunction will be confused with angina when it causes anterior chest tightness, but examination of the thoracic spine will locate stiffness and tenderness. The problem will be relieved virtually instantly by manipulation which gives outstanding results with the thoracic spine.

16
Examination of the thoracic spine

'The skilful doctor knows by observation, the mediocre doctor by interrogation, the ordinary doctor by palpation.'

Chang Chung-Ching
AD 180

Contents
☐ Key checkpoints
☐ Inspection
☐ Movements
☐ Palpation
☐ Neurological examination
☐ X-rays
☐ Practice tips
☐ Summary

The objective is to reproduce the patient's symptoms and this is usually achieved by palpation. The time-honoured 'look, feel, move, X-ray' clinical approach is most appropriate for the thoracic spine. It is important to assess all the spine by inspection so appropriate exposure of the patient is necessary. Neck movements should be performed where referred pain from the lower cervical spine to the upper chest is a possibility. However, it should be emphasised that neck flexion may provoke any thoracic pain originating in the upper thoracic spinal joints.

KEY CHECKPOINTS

- Scheuermann's disease, which affects the lower thoracic spine in adolescents, is often associated with kyphosis and recurrent thoracic back pain. Always inspect the thoracic spine of the younger patient for kyphosis and scoliosis.
- The most useful movements to detect hypomobile lesions and painful levels in the thoracic spine are lateral flexion and rotation. The application of overpressure at the active end range is useful to detect the painful segment.
- Palpation is the most important component of the physical examination. Of all techniques transverse palpation is the most effective.

INSPECTION

Careful inspection is important since it may be possible to observe at a glance why the patient has thoracic pain. Note the symmetry, any scars, skin creases and deformities, 'flat spots' in the spine, the nature of the scapulae or evidence of muscle spasm. Note the overall posture of the patient. Look for kyphosis and scoliosis.

Kyphosis may be generalised, with the back having a smooth uniform contour, or localised where it is due to a collapsed vertebra such as occurs in an older person with osteoporosis. Generalised kyphosis is common in the elderly, especially those with degenerative spinal disease. The so-called 'dowagers hump' is seen in elderly women following osteoporotic wedge fractures. In the young it may reflect the important Scheuermann's disorder.

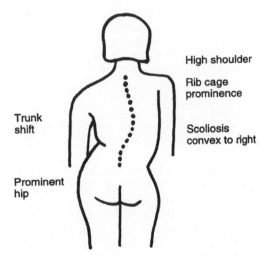

Figure 16.1 Screening for idiopathic adolescent scoliosis: configuration of the thoracic spine.

The younger person in particular should be screened for scoliosis (Figure 16.1) which becomes more prominent on forward flexion (Figure 15.9). Look for any asymmetry of the chest wall, inequality of the scapulae and differences in the levels of shoulders. A useful sign of scoliosis is unequal shoulder levels and apparent 'winging' of scapula. When viewed anteriorly a difference in the levels of the nipples indicates the presence of scoliosis, or other problems causing one shoulder to drop. Inspection should therefore take place with posterior, lateral (side) and anterior views.

MOVEMENTS

There are four main movements of the thoracic spine to assess, the most important of which is rotation, as this is the movement that so frequently reproduces the patient's pain whether it is apophyseal or costo-vertebral in origin. The movements and their normal ranges are presented in Table 16.1.

Table 16.1 *Movements of the thoracic spine with normal ranges.*

MOVEMENT	NORMAL RANGE (DEGREES)
Extension	30
Lateral flexion L and R	30
Flexion	90
Rotation L and R	60

Check these four active movements noting any hypomobility, the range of movement, reproduction of symptoms and function and muscle spasm.

Passive movement, superimposed on active movements, is needed to stress the joints and reproduce pain if it had not been elicited by normal active movement. An auxillary test in the form of passive 'overpressure' can be applied at the end range of each movement, especially with rotation. This is a sensitive method to stress the joint and reproduce the patient's pain.

Method

- Ask the patient to sit on the couch and place the hands behind the neck. This has the effect of winging the scapula along with the medial scapulae musculature away from the midline, and thus facilitates an uninhibited view of the mid and upper thoracic spine during active movement.
- Ask the patient to indicate the site of the pain, because it is important to observe if movement occurs through this allegedly painful region during active movement or whether this area is being 'guarded' and presents as a hypomobile segment.

Figure 16.2 illustrates active extension of the thoracic spine. The spinous processes of the thoracic vertebrae of this patient have been marked to facilitate inspection during movement. Figure 16.3 illustrates active left lateral flexion. Lateral flexion should be tested on both right and left sides. It is the best movement to test the hypomobile lesion. Figure 16.4 illustrates active (forward flexion).

Rotation of the thoracic spine is the key movement that requires close scrutiny on examination. Ask the patient to cross arms with the hands resting on opposite shoulders for this movement. The patient can usually rotate to about 60–70 degrees (Figure 16.5).

If the patient's pain is not reproduced, apply gentle overpressure by placing a hand on each shoulder and applying further pressure towards the end range (Figure 16.6). Note not only the range but also the end feel of the movement, observing whether it is 'healthy' (that is, springy and elastic) or 'pathological' (that is, a firm hard stop).

Record the patient's direction of movement, degree of restriction and presence of pain on the DOM diagram. An example is presented in Figure 16.7.

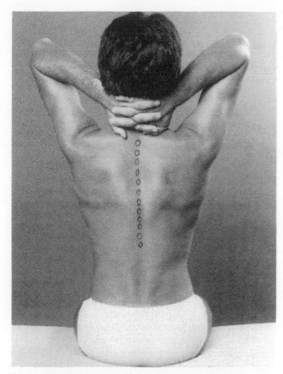

Figure 16.2 Extension of the thoracic spine.

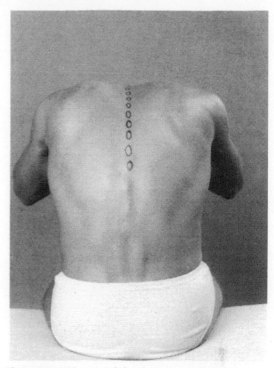

Figure 16.4 Flexion of the thoracic spine.

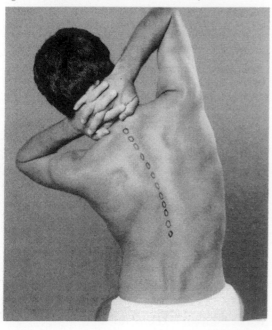

Figure 16.3 Left lateral flexion of the thoracic spine.

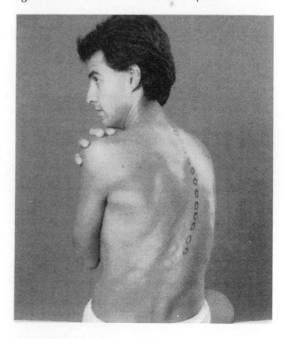

Figure 16.5 Left rotation (active) of the thoracic spine.

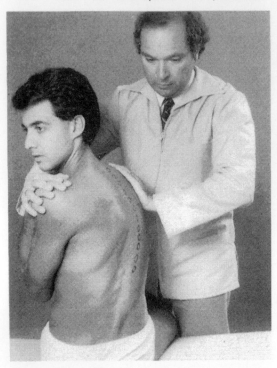

Figure 16.6 Left rotation with passive overpressure applied at the end range of active rotation.

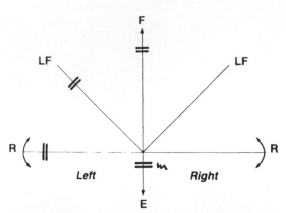

Figure 16.7 DOM for a patient with thoracic back pain. This indicates severe restriction (with pain) on extension, restriction by one-third of left lateral flexion and left rotation, decreased movement only at the end range of flexion and free movement on right rotation and lateral flexion.

PALPATION

Palpation is the key to examination and treatment. It is the means whereby the site and origin of the pain can be identified and it is the basis of the technique for specific mobilisation.

With the patient prone, test passive extension of each joint with firm pressure from the pad of the thumbs or the bony hand (either the 'pisiform' prominence or the lateral border of the fifth metacarpal). Ask the patient if the pressure reproduces the pain.

Apart from asking the patient 'Is that the pain?' note:

● the distribution of pain and its change with movement
● the range of movement
● the type of resistance in the joint
● any muscle spasm.

Palpation must follow a set plan in order to reproduce the patient's pain. The sequence is as follows:

1. Central – over spinous processes.
2. Unilateral – over apophyseal joints (2–3 cm from midline).
3. Transverse – on side of spinous processes.
4. Unilateral – costo-transverse junctions (4–5 cm from midline).
5. Unilateral – over ribs.

Patient position for palpation

The most commonly used position is that with the patient lying prone. Although this is an acceptable position it is less effective because the anterior directed movement is examined with the thoracic spine in slight extension.

The preferable position (Figure 16.8) is for the thoracic spine to be in slight flexion and with the arms over the side of the couch. This is achieved by lowering the top of the examination couch. The position opens up the apophyseal joints, thus enhancing palpation and reproduction of the symptoms. This method is illustrated diagrammatically in Figure 16.9.

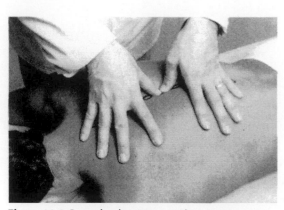

Figure 16.8 Central palpation over the spinous processes. The most suitable method for palpation of the thoracic spine with the patient's head and upper trunk slightly flexed.

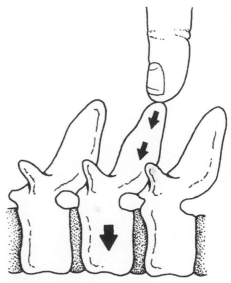

Figure 16.9

Central palpation

With the tips of the thumbs applied to the spinous process, rhythmic pressure is directed anteriorly (Figure 16.8). Some therapists may prefer to spring the spinous processes using the pisiform process on the leading hand. This is applied gently to begin with, and then more firmly in order to reproduce pain if it is present.

The pathological level is characterised by reproduction of pain and restriction of movement. This central pressure method is most useful when the patient complains of central pain. The precise anatomical location is determined by identifying the prominent C7 and T1 spinous processes. However, central pressure does not usually localise this level precisely. This is due to the fact that the examiner may find several painful levels on palpation, with two or more levels being equally painful and restricted. This also applies to adjacent regions. The problem is illustrated in Figure 16.10. One must remember that the spinous processes of the thoracic spine are long and angulated.

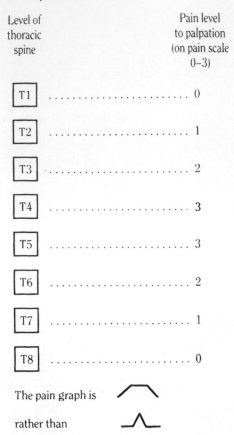

Figure 16.10 Example of painful response to palpation at specific levels of the upper to mid thoracic spine in a patient complaining of interscapular pain.

Unilateral palpation

Unilateral palpation is employed at two sites, namely, 2–3 cm from the midline to provoke the apophyseal joints and 4–5 cm from the midline to provoke the costo-transverse joints. This section will concentrate on the first method, where direct pressure is applied with the pads of the thumbs 2–3 cm from the midline of the spinous processes systematically alongside the vertebral column on either side (Figure 16.11).

Unlike central palpation this method can determine quite localised symptoms and, if found at a specific level, the examination should carefully assess the segment immediately above and below and then on the opposite side at the same level (Figure 16.12).

It is surprising how sensitive and tender palpation in this paravertebral 'gutter' can be so it is appropriate to commence gently using light pressure initially and then gradually increasing the pressure to provoke underlying pathology.

Transverse palpation

Transverse palpation can be considered to be the definitive palpation technique for localisation of segmental dysfunction in the thoracic spine.

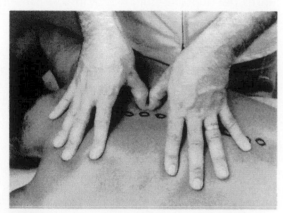

Figure 16.11 Unilateral palpation. Direct pressure from the thumbs is applied over the apophyseal joints 2–3 cm from the midline.

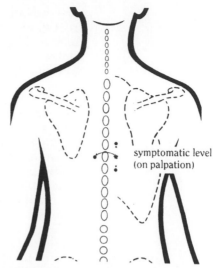

symptomatic level (on palpation)

Figure 16.12 Rule of procedure for unilateral palpation if a symptomatic level is found. Palpate above, below and opposite this site.

It involves exerting pressure on the side of the spinous processes. Although it may appear that a transverse glide is being produced, in fact a rotatory movement is being produced at that segmental level. At a specific level the range of oscillatory rotation is very small but if this range is lost there is a hard end feel and a sharp reproduction of pain with transverse pressure. This is an excellent method of reproducing the pain as the pressure is transmitted through all the joints at that segment.

Method

With the hands relaxed and lying flat across the curvature of the thoracic wall (Figure 16.13) gently sink the opposed thumbs into the

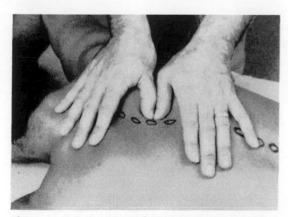

Figure 16.13 Transverse palpation: pressure is applied with the thumbs against the spinous processes from the side.

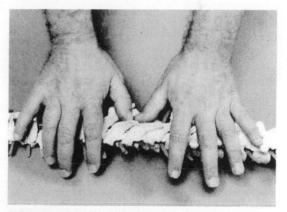

Figure 16.14 Transverse palpation, demonstrating the position of the thumbs on the side of the spinous process.

paravertebral gutter so they they press against the side of the spinous process, away from the tip. This position is shown on the model of the skeleton (Figure 16.14). When the slack is taken up, gently push the spinous process directly towards the opposite side. Repeat this at each level until the painful segment is located.

Location of painful site

The great benefit of this technique is that it enables the examiner to determine which side (left or right) is causing the symptoms. This is significant since the patient may complain of central thoracic pain radiating bilaterally, and central palpation will only determine the level without pinpointing the side of the lesion. Furthermore, some manual techniques require knowledge of which side is affected so that the appropriate direction of mobilisation and manipulation can be determined. This localisation of pain involves the same principles as outlined for transverse palpation of the lumbar spine (p. 365). The side on which the thumbs are applied to the transverse process is the side responsible for the pain. For example, if palpation from the right towards the left elicits pain but palpation from the left is painless, the painful lesion is right-sided. Figure 16.15 illustrates the mechanics of movement with the axis of rotation being in the spinal canal.

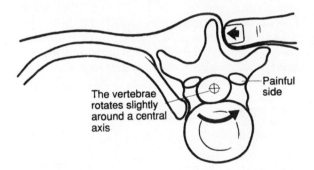

The vertebrae rotates slightly around a central axis

Painful side

Figure 16.15 Illustration of the effect of transverse palpation on the painful side at one level of the thoracic spine.

Palpation of ribs

There are two methods of provoking pain at the costo-vertebral joints, namely (1) direct pressure over the costo-vertebral joint, and (2) springing the ribs thus producing an indirect stretching of the joint.

Unilateral palpation over costo-vertebral joint

Direct localised pressure over this joint is achieved by palpation with the thumbs or pisiform border of the hand unilaterally about 4–5 cm from the midline (Figure 16.16). If the costo-vertebral joint is affected it is very painful to pressure since it is relatively superficial and also produces soft tissue irritation in its vicinity.

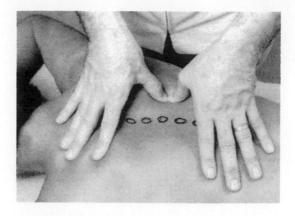

Figure 16.16 Unilateral palpation over the costo-vertebral joint 4–5 cm from the midline.

Unilateral dorso-medial rib palpation

Provocation of the costo-vertebral articulation is achieved by exerting firm pressure over the rib, just distal to its vertebral articulation. This is achieved by applying a soft medial (ulnar) border of the hand over the rib as it curves around the posterior wall and applying a firm (but controlled and never heavy) pressure (Figure 16.17). Figure 16.18 illustrates how springing the ribs produces indirect stretching of the joints.

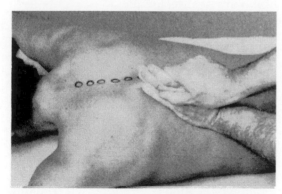

Figure 16.17 Unilateral dorso-medial rib springing, along the line of the ribs.

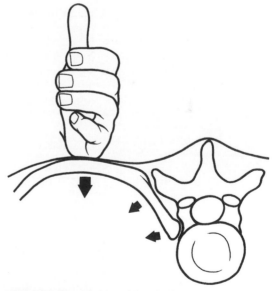

Figure 16.18 Palpation of the rib showing how springing with the ulnar border of the hand or pisiform produces an indirect stretching of the costo-vertebral joints.

NEUROLOGICAL EXAMINATION

Disc lesions in the thoracic spine are prone to produce spinal cord compression manifesting as sensory (e.g. paraesthesia of feet), bladder incontinence and upper motor neurone signs (e.g. spastic gait, hyper-reflexia). If this is suspected a neurological examination including sensory and motor assessment, reflexes and Babinski response should be performed.

X-RAYS

X-rays of the painful thoracic spine are often normal procedures but remember that tuberculosis and malignant disease (especially metastases from lung and breast) can appear in the thoracic spine.

Suspect serious disease if both rotations are free but there is painful and limited lateral flexion away from the painful side. Also suspect serious disease if overpressure to the end of passive movement causes a sharp increase in pain. If the plain X-ray is normal and you strongly suspect serious disease a bone scan is mandatory.

Always X-ray the thoracic spine following trauma, especially after motor vehicle accidents, as wedge compression fractures (typically between T4 and T8) are often overlooked.

PRACTICE TIPS

● Examine movements with the patient sitting on the couch and hands clasped behind the neck.
● Flexion of the thoracic spine by lowering the upper part of the couch helps locate the painful lesion by palpation.
● Transverse palpation is the key palpatory method to detect the site, and side, of the painful joint. The palpatory techniques are an important forerunner of mobilisation techniques.
● Keep to a basic system for the physical examination (Table 16.2).

SUMMARY

The time-honoured orthopaedic method of 'look, feel, move, X-ray' has important clinical application for the thoracic spine. Inspection, movements and palpation must be linked closely to determine the level of the problem by reproducing the patient's symptoms. The key to this, however, is palpation. Central palpation may not localise the painful lesion precisely; hence unilateral and transverse palpation is essential to achieve localisation. The examination should be supported by appropriate radiological investigation.

Table 16.2 *Physical examination of the thoracic spine: a summarised guide.*

1. **Inspection**

2. **Palpation**
   1. Central – over spinous processes.
   2. Unilateral – over apophyseal joints (2–3 cm from midline).
   3. Transverse – on side of spinous processes.
   4. Unilateral – costo-transverse junctions (4–5 cm from midline).
   5. Unilateral – over the ribs (spring over posterior rib curve with ulnar border of hand, along axis of rib).

3. **Movements**

Extension	30°
Lateral flexion L and R	30°
Flexion	90°
Rotation L and R	60°

   Check these four active movements noting any hypomobility, the range of movement, reproduction of symptoms and function and muscle spasm. Passive movement, superposed on active movements, is needed to stress the joints and reproduce pain if it has not been elicited by normal active movement. A passive 'overpressure' can be applied at the end range of each movement, especially with rotation.

17
Mobilisation of the thoracic spine

'When an elderly lady has localised vertebral dysfunction in her thoracic spine I resort to gentle mobilisation of the affected part, lest I fracture a rib or vertebrae which sometimes does not require much force.'

Experienced practitioner, 1986

Contents
□ Key checkpoints
□ Mobilisation versus manipulation
□ Lumbar spine differences
□ Thoracic mobilisation techniques
    1. Anterior directed central gliding
    2. Anterior directed unilateral gliding
    3. Transverse directed rotational gliding
    4. Anterior directed costo-vertebral gliding
    5. Rib mobilisation – direct
    6. Rib mobilisation in rotation (sitting position)
□ Practice tips
□ Summary

Mobilisation of the thoracic spine is a useful technique that is an extension of palpation. Thoracic problems are invariably hypomobile lesions, and manipulation is the most effective technique; some patients, however, do not tolerate the application of forceful techniques to the thorax, and mobilisation is appropriate for these patients.

KEY CHECKPOINTS

- The methods and principles of mobilisation of the thoracic spine are almost identical to those used for the lumbar spine.
- The transverse directed method of mobilisation is probably the most effective method for unilateral pain.
- Rib mobilisation methods which stretch the costo-vertebral articulations are special techniques unique to the thoracic spine.
- Thoracic cage/rib mobilisation by rotation with the patient in the sitting (straddling chair or couch) position is very effective.

MOBILISATION VERSUS MANIPULATION

Although mobilisation is widely used, the authors regard manipulation as being so superior at achieving the desired result rapidly that mobilisation should be performed only when contra-indications to manipulation exist.

Mobilisation is used where the condition is too irritable or too stiff to manipulate, and can gradually release this stiffness to the point where manipulation can be attempted.

LUMBAR SPINE DIFFERENCES

Because the apophyseal joint articulations lie in a slightly different plane from those in the lumbar spine, different manipulation techniques are used for the thoracic spine in order to effect distraction of these joints. The mobilisation techniques, however, are virtually identical.

THORACIC MOBILISATION TECHNIQUES

The various techniques of thoracic mobilisation are summarised in Table 17.1.

Table 17.1 *Classification of mobilisation techniques for the thoracic spine.*

TECHNIQUE	TARGET JOINT	SYMPTOMS
Anterior directed central gliding	Apophyseal	Central or bilateral pain
Anterior directed unilateral gliding	Apophyseal	Unilateral pain
Transverse rotational gliding	Apophyseal Costo-vertebral	Unilateral pain
Anterior directed costo-vertebral gliding	Costo-vertebral	Unilateral or central pain
Rib mobilisation – direct	Costo-vertebral	Unilateral pain
Rib mobilisation – rotational	Costo-vertebral	Unilateral pain

1. Anterior directed central gliding

This widely used extension technique is suitable for midline or bilateral pain and follows the same guidelines as those used for central mobilisation of the lumbar spine.

Position of the patient

- The patient lies prone and relaxed.
- If possible the top of the couch should be lowered so that partial forward flexion of the thoracic spine can be achieved.

- The arms should lie over the side of the couch or abducted with the hands resting at the head of the couch or under the patient's head.

Position of the therapist

- The therapist stands by the patient's side and places the pisiform prominence or lateral border of the bone of the fifth metacarpal over the spinous process or processes at the affected joint. Alternately, the pads of the thumbs can be used. The grip is exactly the same as for the lumbar spine (p. 397).
- It is important to be well above the patient so that the arms are straight and the shoulders directly above the spine.

Method

- A firm controlled oscillatory pressure is applied by transmitting the body weight through the arms to the hands (Figure 17.1).
- As for mobilisation of the lumbar spine, this method can be used in the three stages – namely, early, mid or end range techniques.

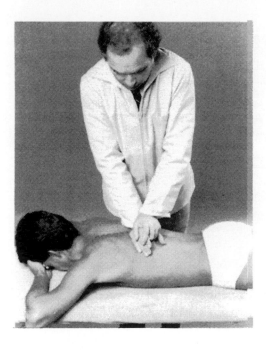

Figure 17.1 Anterior directed central gliding: the pisiform method. *Note*: This position can be used for manipulation (if desired) by applying a firm downward thrust of very small amplitude towards extension.

Time span

- The mobilisation should be applied for approximately 30 to 60 seconds, with two or three repeats in one treatment session.

2. Anterior directed unilateral gliding

The technique is similar to that of the central method but is used for unilateral pain where the painful lesion is located lateral to the spinous process. It is usually directed to a painful apophyseal joint which is 2–3 cm from the midline.

Positions of the patient and therapist

- The positions of the patient and the therapist are the same as for anterior directed gliding.

Method

- The oscillatory pressure is applied to the tender point with the thumbs (Figures 17.2 and 17.3) or with the lateral border of the hand (similar to that in Figure 17.1).

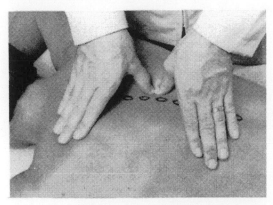

Figure 17.2 Anterior directed unilateral gliding: this is located 2–3 cm from the midline and is usually applied at right angles to the body with the thumbs.

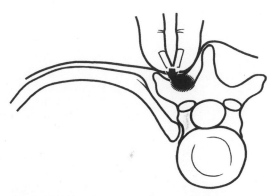

Figure 17.3 Diagrammatic illustration of the point of application of the thumbs for unilateral mobilisation.

3. Transverse directed rotational gliding

This method is used for unilateral pain and produces a rotational mobilisation via pressure applied to the side of the spinous process at the affected vertebral level. There is minimal free movement in this technique and it is therefore most useful at the end range (stage 3). The direction of the pressure should always be towards the painful side.

Position of the patient

- The patient lies prone with the head facing towards the painful side, preferably with the head of the couch lowered.
- The arms should be over the side of the couch or elevated with the hands placed under the forehead.

Position of the therapist

- The therapist stands on the pain-free side.
- The thumbs are applied against the side of the spinous process at the painful level (Figures 17.4 and 17.5).

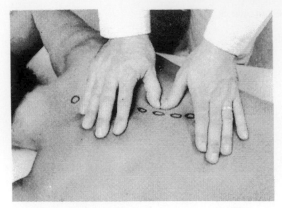

Figure 17.4 Transverse directed rotational gliding: the position of the thumbs is the same as for palpation (refer to Figure 16.14).

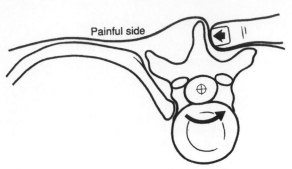

Painful side

Figure 17.5 Diagramatic illustration of the forces involved for transverse directed rotational gliding.

Method

- Allow the thumb to fit deeply into the groove beside the spine.
- The thumbs can be placed side by side or placed one over the other to generate reinforcement.
- The thumbs apply a firm rhythmic oscillating force directed towards the painful side.
- The firm pressure is actually achieved by movement of the therapist's body which transmits the force to the thumbs.
- A degree of pressure is required to achieve satisfactory movement in some patients. If considerable discomfort is felt in the thumbs, the pisiform of the hand can be applied, but this is a relatively crude method and harder to control.

Time span

- Mobilise for 30–60 seconds (maximum two minutes) with two or three repeats.

4. Anterior directed costo-vertebral gliding

This is obviously a unilateral method and is directed at the costo-transverse joint approximately 4–5 cm from the midline. The tip of the transverse process lies superficially and can be felt as a small firm 'bump' at this point (refer to Figure 15.1). Palpation of the thoracic spine is the key to locating this point. This area is tender, so careful palpation and mobilisation is required. Immediately lateral to the 'bump' of the transverse process lies the rib. This is the focus for mobilisation (Figure 17.6).

Position of the patient

- The patient lies prone with the head facing towards the painful side, preferably with the head of the couch lowered.

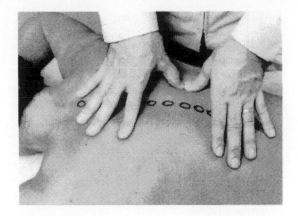

Figure 17.6 Anterior directed costo-vertebral gliding: the thumbs are located 4–5 cm from the midline.

- The arms should be over the side of the couch or elevated with the hands placed under the forehead.

Position of the therapist

- The therapist stands on the painful side.
- The thumbs are applied against the prominent aspect of the rib at the painful level.

Method

- With the pads of the thumb applied over the rib at the appropriate level, apply a rhythmic oscillating force at the rate of about 1 to 2 movements per second (Figure 17.6). This produces a gapping or stretching of the costo-transverse joint.
- The pressure should be directed at right angles or slightly medially.
- The point of application of the thumbs is shown in Figure 17.7.

Time span

- Mobilise for 30–60 seconds (maximum two minutes) with two or three repeats.

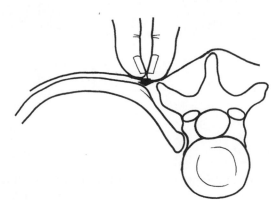

Figure 17.7 Anterior directed costo-vertebral gliding: diagrammatic illustration of the point of application of the thumbs for mobilisation.

5. Rib mobilisation – direct

This technique is very similar to the palpation technique used for the examination of the thoracic spine (Figure 16.18). It is ideally a large amplitude (stage 2) technique. Obviously, caution would have to be exercised in the elderly or frail person as a fracture could be produced by an over-zealous method.

Position of the patient

- The patient lies prone with the head facing towards the painful side, preferably with the head of the couch lowered.
- The arms should be over the side of the couch or elevated with the hands placed under the forehead.

Position of the therapist

- The therapist stands on the painful side distal to the rib to be mobilised and facing the patient's head.
- The medial (ulnar) border of the hand is placed over the affected rib as it curves around the posterior wall.
- The lower hand is reinforced with the upper hand as shown in Figure 17.8.

Time span

- Mobilise for 30–60 seconds (maximum). This can be repeated once.

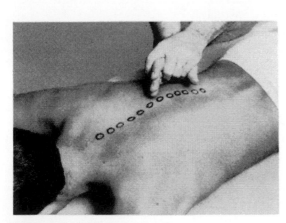

Figure 17.8 Mobilisation of a rib.

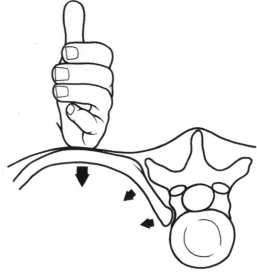

Figure 17.9 Diagrammatic illustration of the forces involved in rib mobilization.

6. Rib mobilisation in rotation (sitting position)

This very effective technique is very similar to that used for manipulation (technique 9, pages 288–290) but is simply a stretching method using gentle oscillatory movements, devoid of any thrusting. It is used for unilateral costo-vertebral joint pain from about T4 or T5 to T12 and can cover several levels.

Position of the patient

- The patient straddles the end of the low couch and sits firm and erect. Alternatively (and perhaps a more practical position) the patient can straddle a chair, facing the back of the chair with a pillow used against the chair to protect the thighs.
   Note: The chair must be a standard open kitchen chair without arm rests. A carpeted floor should be used.
- The patient crosses the arms and rests the hands on opposite shoulders. The arm to be grasped must be uppermost.

Position of the therapist

- The therapist stands directly behind the patient and adopts a firm wide-based stance.
- One hand passes around in front of the patient (coming in from the non-painful side) and grasps the patient's forearm just above the elbow.
- The heel of the other hand is placed over the posterior angle of the ribs at the painful level to be mobilised.

Method

- The patient is rotated to the comfortable level of stretch by rotating away from the painful side. This is done by pulling the trunk across with the encircling arm and pushing with the hand on the trunk. (Figure 17.10). These two movements complement each other to achieve rotation of the thoracic cage.

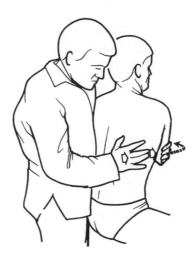

Figure 17.10 Rotational mobilisation of costo-vertebral joints of the thoracic spine using the seated position.

Time span

- At full stretch perform gentle oscillatory rotation of the trunk at this end range for 10–20 seconds.

PRACTICE TIPS

- Mark the painful level with a marking pen prior to mobilisation methods.
- Mobilisation can be used in elderly female patients with thoracic back pain but should be used gently and should not involve a direct rib mobilisation method. A gentle indirect rib mobilisation in rotation can be used.
- Always explain your proposed method to the patient.
- Always stand on the painful side for mobilisation techniques except for the transverse method when the therapist stands on the pain-free side.

SUMMARY

Mobilisation of the thoracic spine is a safe and very easy method to apply, especially if a careful palpatory method has preceded it. The general principles of central, unilateral and transverse gliding techniques are almost identical to those employed with the lumbar spine.

However, mobilisation is not as effective as manipulation for the thoracic spine and in general has a limited clinical application.

18
Manipulation of the thoracic spine

'One of the joys of manual therapy is to experience the virtual instant relief of the patient seized with immobilising posterior chest pain. The "clunk" of a successful deft manipulation heralds being able to indulge in a deep breath without severe pain and rapid relief of discomfort. One of the magic moments of medicine.'

Medical practitioner and patient!
Brisbane, 1988

Contents
□ Key checkpoints
□ Postero-anterior indirect thrust (PAIT) techniques
  ● Hand positions
  ● Thoracic manipulation techniques
    1. PAIT – neutral position
    2. PAIT – into flexion
    3. PAIT – into extension
    4. PAIT – over rib
    5. PAIT – thigh extension
□ Postero-anterior direct thrust techniques
    6. Crossed pisiform technique
    7. Sternal thrust (Nelson hold)
    8. Sternal thrust (crossover technique)
  Other techniques
    9. Thoracic rotation in sitting position
    10. Cervico-thoracic junction distraction
    11. Upper rib technique
□ Practice tips
□ Summary and cautionary advice

Problems of the thoracic spine, which are invariably hypomobile lesions, respond extremely well to spinal manipulation, the preferred treatment in most cases.

A tendency to recurrence is one major problem, but these patients can usually be maintained virtually pain-free by attending for manipulative correction with each relapse. Manipulation of the thoracic spine can be performed with the patient lying prone or supine, or sitting. Although there are numerous effective techniques for the thoracic spine, only a small number of basic techniques, which the authors recommend, will be described. It is better to be familiar and adept with

Table 18.1 *Some thoracic spine manipulation techniques.*

TECHNIQUE	PATIENT POSITION	PAIN SITE	SUITABLE LEVEL
Postero-anterior indirect thrust techniques			
1. Postero-anterior indirect thrust (neutral)	Supine	Central* Bilateral	T3–T8
2. Postero-anterior indirect thrust into flexion	Supine	Central* Bilateral	T5–T12
3. Postero-anterior indirect thrust into extension	Supine	Central* Bilateral	T2–T7
4. Postero-anterior indirect thrust over rib	Supine	Unilateral	T5–T10
5. Postero-anterior thigh extension technique	Supine	Central* Bilateral	T1–T8
Postero-anterior direct thrust techniques			
6. Crossed pisiform technique	Prone	Central* Bilateral	T4–T10
7. Anterior directed sternal thrust ('NELSON hold')	Sitting	Central* Bilateral	T3–T8
8. Anterior directed sternal thrust (crossover technique)	Sitting	Central Bilateral	T4–T8
Other techniques			
9. Thoracic rotation	Sitting	Unilateral	T5–T12
10. Cervico-thoracic junction distraction	Sitting	Central Unilateral	C7–T1–2
11. Upper rib technique	Sitting	Central Unilateral	T1

* May be used for unilateral pain.

a few effective techniques than try to learn all the various permutations and combinations.

A summary of the recommended manipulative techniques for the thoracic spine is presented in Table 18.1. The contra-indications to manipulation are disease of the spine (including osteoporosis), anti-coagulant therapy, and symptoms and signs of a severe disc prolapse, especially with spinal cord compression.

KEY CHECKPOINTS

- Explain to the patient what you intend to do.
- Always coordinate thrusting movements to the thoracic spine with the patient's breathing.
- Use the most specific technique wherever possible.
- Manipulation must occur at absolute full stretch.
- Take care not to injure the rib cage and arms.
- A firm padded couch is essential for all techniques where the patient is supine or prone.

POSTERO-ANTERIOR INDIRECT THRUST (PAIT) TECHNIQUES

The most effective manipulative technique for the thoracic spine, especially for the central spine, is the indirect (or reverse) technique, whereby the patient lies supine and the therapist works from above. A firm couch or base is essential.

A key factor for these techniques is the position and grip of the therapist's lower hand.

Hand positions

Manipulation is achieved by placing the hand between the couch and the spine so that the thrust achieves the appropriate spinal movement at the level of the hand. The effectiveness of the manipulation together with its degree of specificity is determined largely by the lower hand grip position. For this reason three variations of the grip will be presented.

Grip No. 1

The thumb and index finger are extended to make a V while the third, fourth and fifth fingers are flexed (Figure 18.1).

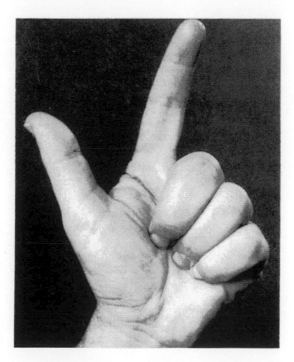

Figure 18.1 Hand grip 1: thumb and index finger extended.

The hand is placed on the spine so that the vertical line of the spinous processes 'bisect' the V and run in the groove between the clenched fingers and the thenar muscles of the thumb.

The position is such that the one transverse process lies across the thumb and the transverse process of the level below lies over the flexed middle or ring finger (Figure 18.2).

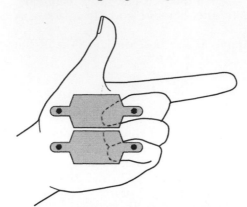

Figure 18.2 Hand grip 1: illustration of the relative position of the vertebrae on the hand with the spinous processes bisecting the V and occupying the hollow of the hand.

The effect of this grip is to create a *block* whereby the movement of these vertebrae are restricted so that when a thrust is applied movement will occur between these two levels. The force transmitted to the hand can be cushioned and thus rendered more comfortable for the therapist by using a small rolled up towel or half a roll of 10 cm soft cotton bandage.

Grip No. 2

In this grip all the fingers are flexed and, with the thumb extended, the spinous processes bisect the V made between the thumb and the index finger. The transverse processes of the same vertebra rest on the flexed

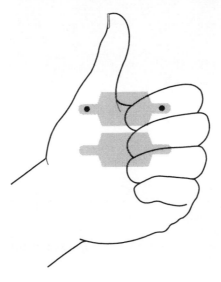

Figure 18.3 Hand grip 2: illustration of the position of the vertebrae on the hand.

index finger and the base of the thumb (Figure 18.3). This creates a different effect as it serves to block one level and facilitates manipulation of the superior and inferior facets of that vertebra.

Grip No. 3

A favoured grip is to use a hyperflexed (curled up) index finger to provide the 'block' over the affected level of the thoracic spine (Figure 18.4). The spinous processess run in the line indicated (Figure 18.5).

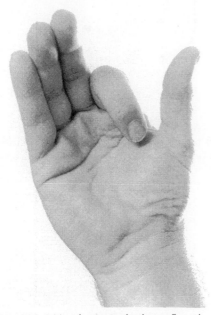

Figure 18.4 Hand grip 3: the hyperflexed index finger grip.

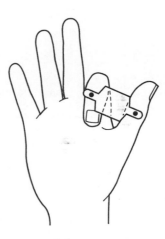

Figure 18.5 Hand grip 3: illustration of the position of the vertebrae on the hand.

Grip No. 4

Another widely used grip which is more comfortable for the patient but does not provide such a specific manipulation is the cupped hand grip. The hand is cupped as shown (Figure 18.6) so the spinous processes lie in the hollow of the hand.

The first and fifth metacarpals engage the transverse processes or ribs on opposite sides of the spine (Figure 18.7). The same manipulative thrust is applied for all hand grips.

THORACIC MANIPULATION TECHNIQUES

1. PAIT – NEUTRAL POSITION

This is an excellent technique for gapping the thoracic spine especially between the third and eighth thoracic vertebrae.

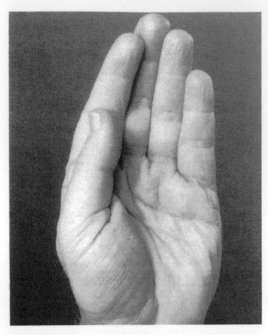

Figure 18.6 Hand grip 4: the cupped hand grip.

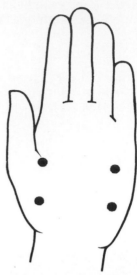

Figure 18.7 Hand grip 4: illustration of the position of the vertebrae on the hand. Note how the spinous processes run along the long axis and occupy the hollow of the hand.

Position of the patient

● The patient lies supine and close to the edge of the couch near the therapist, with a pillow to support the head.
● The patient folds the arms across the body in an X shape so that the hands rest on the opposite shoulders.
● The uppermost forearm should be the one furthest away from the therapist.

Position of the therapist

● The therapist can stand on either side of the patient, depending on his or her own comfort and dexterity.
● The therpist must be able to lean well over the patient, so either a low couch or elevation of the therapist, on a stool, is necessary.

Method

● Request the patient to relax and then roll the patient towards you.
● The hand (illustrating Grip 1) is placed on the spine at the painful level (Figure 18.8).
● The patient is rolled back onto the hand which is then wedged firmly onto the couch. The hand must feel comfortably placed and not be uncomfortable for either. If a spinous process is felt to be impinging against a bony part of the hand the process should be repeated until the hand position is comfortable.

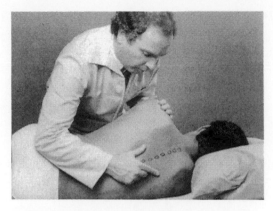

Figure 18.8 Thoracic manipulation technique 1: placement of the hand on the spine.

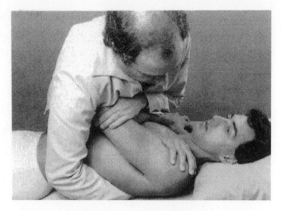

Figure 18.9 Thoracic manipulation technique 1: position immediately prior to thrusting.

- Lean well over the patient and place your upper arm on the patient's upper arm so that your forearm rests directly on top of his or hers, and grasp the patient's far elbow with your hand.
- Now rest your chest over your uppermost arm so that your chin is approximately level with your hand (Figure 18.9).
- Ask the patient to inhale and exhale fully.
- As the patient commences to exhale, lean down to take up the slack on your lowermost hand.
- Just short of full exhalation a sharp downward thrust is applied with your chest and upper arm, directly through the patient's chest onto your hand (Figures 18.10 and 18.11).

Note: This method, using Grip 1, is held by many to be the most effective of all the thoracic manipulative techniques.

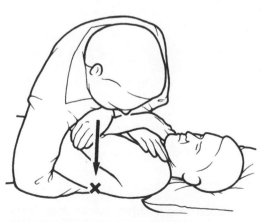

Figure 18.10 Thoracic manipulation technique 1: illustration of the direction of the applied forces.

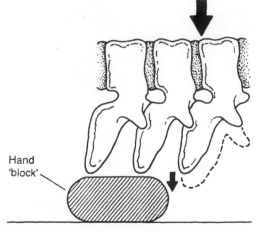

Hand 'block'

Figure 18.11 Thoracic manipulation technique 1: illustration of the manner of movement of the hypomobile segment against the fixed block.

2. PAIT – INTO FLEXION

This technique is very similar to the preceding technique except that the patient clasps the hands behind the neck, a position that permits more flexibility of the thoracic spine, especially flexion, and thus more specificity. It is effective for access to the lower thoracic spine and can be used to treat the T5 to T12 levels.

Position of the patient

- The patient lies supine as for technique 1.
- The patient is asked to interlock the hands behind the neck and bring the elbows forward so that they touch in front of the face, preferably below the chin level.

Position of the therapist

- The therapist adopts the same position and employs the same grip as for technique 1.
- The therapist places the forearm across the patient's forearms/elbows and grasps the furthermost elbow as shown (Figure 18.12).

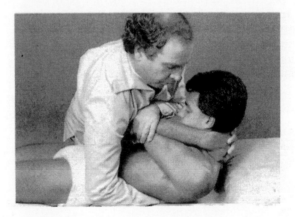

Figure 18.12 Thoracic manipulation technique 2: the therapist achieves more flexion and thus convexity of the thoracic spine by levering the forearms downwards.

- This grip can be used as a lever: pushing down on the patient's arms, which brings the spine into flexion, enables the degree of flexion to be controlled to achieve the best possible contact with the hand on the couch.

Method

- Manoeuvre the thoracic spine so that the appropriate painful level rests on your hand.
- Coordinate the patient's breathing by taking up the slack during exhalation.
- Using hand, arm and chest, transmit a sudden controlled thrust directly downwards by thrusting on the patient's arms. The line of forces is illustrated in Figure 18.13. Once again, the thrust is timed just before full exhalation.

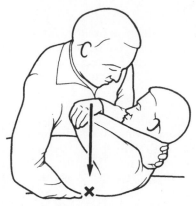

Figure 18.13 Thoracic manipulation technique 2: illustration of the direction of the applied forces.

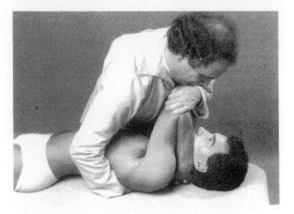

Figure 18.14 Thoracic manipulation technique 3: the spine is extended by lifting the forearms upwards prior to manipulation.

3. PAIT – INTO EXTENSION

This method is a variation of the previous technique in which the trunk is 'levered' into extension to permit manipulation of the upper thoracic spine from T2 to T7.

Position of the patient

- The patient lies supine as for technique 1.
- The patient is asked to interlock the hands behind the neck and bring the elbows forward so that they touch in front of the face, preferably below the chin level.

Position of the therapist

- The therapist adopts the same position but uses a different grip of the patient's forearm to achieve extension.
- The therapist's upper arm is placed across the patient's forearms/elbows to grip the furthermost arm.

Method

- Lift up the patient's arms so that the elbows move in an upward arc around the head. This has the effect of arching (moving into extension) the thoracic spine. (It is important for the patient to keep the elbows close together and the chin above, not between, the forearms to assist this leverage.)
- The slack is taken up as before and a sharp thrust directed through the patient's arms towards the hand at the painful level of the upper thoracic spine (Figure 18.14).

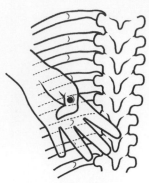

Figure 18.15 Thoracic manipulation technique 4: position of the hand on the thoracic spine (viewed from the posterior direction for a left-sided problem). Note how the rib crosses the proximal phalanx of the thumb (palmar surface shown for purpose of illustration).

4. PAIT – OVER RIB

This technique is designed specifically for manipulating a costo-vertebral joint when palpation over the rib elicits pain at that joint.

The method is very similar to technique 1 except for the nature of the grip and the position of the hand on the back.

The grip and hand position

- The thumb is flexed across the open palm. When the hand is placed in position the posterior angle of the rib lies across the proximal phalanx of the thumb at right angles to it (Figure 18.15). This is quite comfortable for both patient and therapist as the rib fits into the groove of the proximal phalanx.

Position of the patient and therapist

- This is the same as for technique 1, the only difference being the position of the hand, which moves laterally off centre to the angle of the rib.

Method

- As for technique 1, a postero-anterior thrust is applied after the slack is taken up at the end range.

5. PAIT – THIGH EXTENSION TECHNIQUE

This highly effective technique permits extension of the upper to mid thoracic spine over the therapist's thigh. It has a versatile range and can be used for problems from T1 to about T8.

Position of the therapist

- The therapist stands at the head of the couch and flexes the thigh and knee on the couch as shown (Figure 18.16). For a high couch, a stool or chair will be necessary to adopt this position.

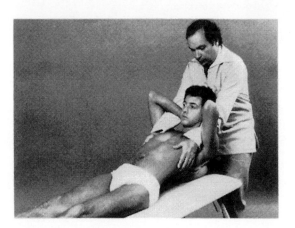

Figure 18.16 Thoracic manipulation technique 5: the position of the thigh extension technique.

Position of the patient

- The patient lies supine on the couch and positions his or her thoracic spine onto the thigh so that the affected area lies just above the knee (Figure 18.17).
- The patient clasps the hands behind the neck.

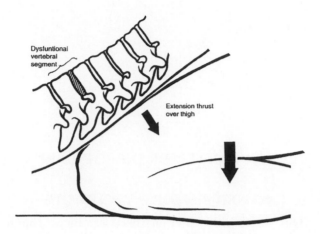

Dysfuntional vertebral segment

Extension thrust over thigh

Figure 18.17 Thoracic manipulation technique 5: illustration of the level of the spinal problem in relation to the therapist's knee.

Method

- Insert your arms through the patient's arms as shown and grasp the patient around the posterolateral aspects of the mid thorax bilaterally. (The further the arms can be inserted the better. Sometimes it is necessary to allow patients with short arms to interlock the tips of the fingers onto the neck rather than interlocking the hands because this allows more room for insertion of the arms.)
- The slack is taken up by gently stretching the patient over your thigh while the patient adducts the arms to ensure that a firm (but not tight) application is made against your arms.
- Now firmly (never forcibly) extend the patient's thoracic spine over your thigh by simultaneously:
  - dropping your body back and down so that your shoulders and buttock drop towards the floor;
  - thrusting with your forearms directly downwards across the patient's shoulder/axilla region.

The direction of forces is illustrated on Figure 18.18. It is important to understand that the main force comes from thrusting directly down with your arms on the patient as you extend his or her thoracic spine with your thigh.

Note: This method should be gentle and controlled without the need to have a lifting and dropping action of the thorax and without unnecessary flexion of the neck.

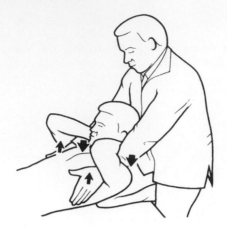

Figure 18.18 Thoracic manipulation technique 5: illustration of the direction of the applied forces.

POSTERO-ANTERIOR DIRECT THRUST TECHNIQUES

6. CROSSED PISIFORM TECHNIQUE

This commonly used method produces rotation in two adjacent thoracic vertebrae by a direct postero-anterior thrust with the pisiforms on these vertebrae at different levels. The key to this technique is to have the pisiforms placed at different levels on either side of the spine – not the same level.

A sharp thrust will therefore cause the two vertebrae to rotate in opposite directions and thus free the locked joint. This method is suitable for lesions from about T4 to T10.

Position of the patient

- The patient lies prone with the head turned to a comfortable position.

Position of the therapist

- The therapist stands at the patient's side opposite the painful level of the thoracic spine.
- The therapist leans over the back well above the patient and *crosses the hands* so that the pisiform bone of one engages the transverse process of the vertebra at the level of the lesion and the pisiform of the other hand engages the transverse process of the vertebra *below* this level on the opposite side (Figure 18.19). The wrists need to be kept well extended so the pisiform makes as close a contact as possible with the transverse processes.

Method

- Bending well over the patient, lean vertically downwards – shoulders directly above the spine, elbows fully extended.

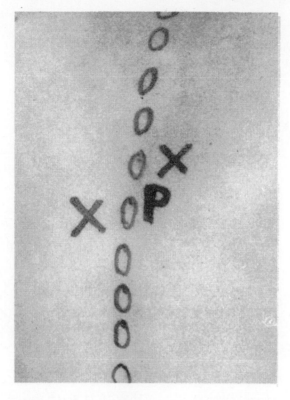

Figure 18.19 Thoracic manipulation technique 6: points on the thoracic spine at which to place the pisiforms. The painful level is indicated with a 'P'.

- Maintain a firm downward pressure in slight rotation to produce a torque effect.
- Instruct the patient to take a deep breath and then completely exhale.
- Just before the end of exhalation take up the rest of the slack by leaning firmly on your hands and then apply a sharp rotatory thrust with a tendency to push your hands in opposite directions (Figure 18.20). The direction of the applied forces in indicated in Figure 18.21.

The effect

- Because the arms are crossed and the thrust is applied at different levels, a rotatory effect is produced, causing gapping of the blocked segment with the upper vertebra rotating anticlockwise on the lower, thus restoring rotation to that side (Figure 18.22).

Significant points

- For a small patient the pisiforms may be over the posterior aspect of the ribs adjacent to the transverse process. This is quite acceptable.
- Although a direct downward thrust will achieve rotation this is reinforced by a corkscrewing or rotation action of the hands immediately before the final thrust.

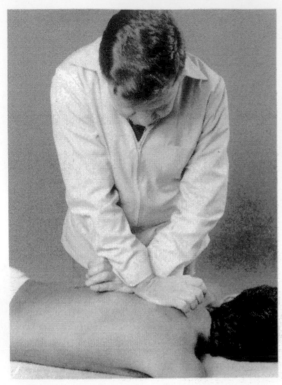

Figure 18.20 Thoracic manipulation technique 6: the crossed pisiform technique. Note how the arms are crossed.

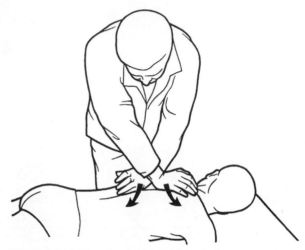

Figure 18.21 The crossed pisiform technique: illustration of the direction of the applied forces.

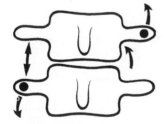

Figure 18.22 Diagrammatic representation of the direction of forces on the vertebrae with the crossed pisiform technique.

● To ensure a controlled manipulation with a direct thrust from the shoulders it may be necessary to stand on a stool and kneel with one knee on the side of the couch.

Precaution

● This technique can generate considerable force which can be painful so tend to use less force if doubtful. It is contra-indicated if the anterior chest wall is painful and in the elderly, especially women. It is usually unsuitable above T4 and should not be attempted above this level.

7. STERNAL THRUST (NELSON HOLD TECHNIQUE)

This time-honoured method is useful for almost all patients with upper to mid thoracic lesions (T3–T8) and suitable for those with tender rib cages.

It is another direct postero-anterior manipulation in extension (similar in principle to the thigh technique) but relies on a sternal (chest) thrust from the therapist. It is a non-specific technique which directs the applied force as near as possible at right angles to the thoracic spine. As the thrust is applied through the locked intervertebral joint, a loud 'popping' noise may indicate successful manipulation.

Position of the patient

- The patient sits across the couch with his or her back to the side (buttocks to the edge) nearest the therapist, preferably with the head at the same level as the therapist.
- The patient locks the hands behind the neck with the elbows pointing outwards.

Position of the therapist

- The therapist stands behind the patient and places either a small rolled up towel or a similar object between the patient's back and the chest, so that the upper edge is just below the painful level (Figure 18.23).

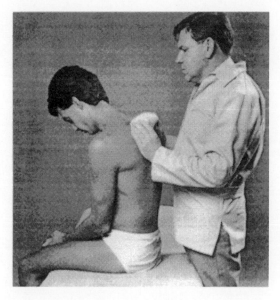

Figure 18.23 Thoracic manipulation technique 7: placement of rolled up towel on the back with upper edge just below the painful level.

Method

- Slide your hands in front of the patient's axillae and grasp the patient's wrists to adopt the traditional 'Nelson hold'. The palms of your hands face outwards.
- Request the patient to slightly adduct the arms to allow snug apposition so that the arms are not too 'winged' during the lift, as this can hurt their arms.
- Gently yet firmly extend the patient's back against your chest in a lifting movement – that is, lifting and pulling the patient as you slightly extend your back. This is performed with a smooth rocking movement ensuring that the patient is relaxed.

- The patient is asked to breath in and breath out and to relax.
- When the patient is relaxed, take up the slack, increase the stretching lift and backward extension and apply a sharp forward thrust with your upper chest (Figures 18.24 and 18.25).

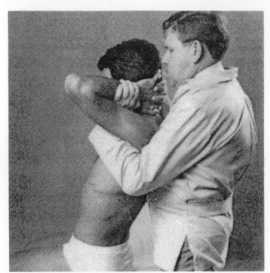

Figure 18.24 Thoracic manipulation technique 7: the 'Nelson hold' technique. The thrust comes from pushing the sternum sharply forwards as the scapulae are brought together.

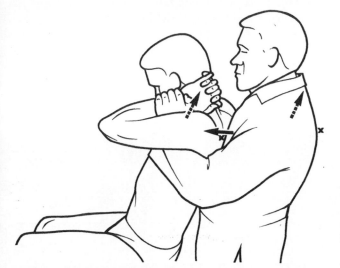

Figure 18.25 Diagrammatic representation of the direction of forces with the 'Nelson hold' technique. Broken lines indicate initial movement. Complete lines and crosses indicate final thrust and blocks.

Variations of technique

- The patient can be standing for this rather than sitting, but it is less strenuous for the therapist if the patient sits across the couch.
- Taller therapists may have to use their epigastrium to thrust, but it is preferable to use the mid sternum.
- This method can be used without the intervening pad; but the pad allows more specificity.

Precautions

- Avoid hurting the upper arms of the patient during stretching and lifting. This is overcome to some extent by getting him or her to approximate the arms without too much tension.
- Avoid jerky sharp lifting movements. The manoeuvre should be controlled and smooth, never jerky.
- Avoid sharp flexion of the patient's neck.
- Avoid straightening of the patient's knees while sitting.

– for costo-vertebral (rib) disorders, the heel is placed more laterally onto the posterior aspect of the rib.
● The other hand passes in front of the patient and grasps the opposite shoulder thus facilitating rotation of the trunk.

Method

● The patient is rotated to full stretch by pulling with your arm on the shoulder or upper arm and pushing with your hand on the thoracic spine.
● At full stretch and towards the end of expiration a short sharp thrust is applied with a combination of both hands increasing rotation (Figures 18.29 and 18.30). The impulse is transmitted through the affected segment or segments.

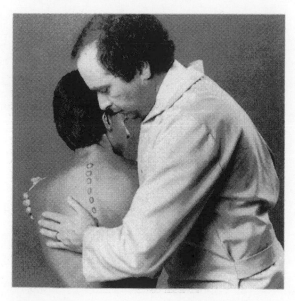

Figure 18.29 Thoracic manipulation technique 9: thoracic rotation in sitting.

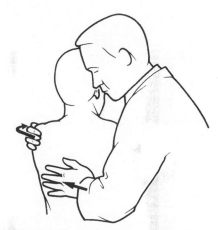

Figure 18.30 Diagrammatic illustration of the direction of forces with the thoracic rotation technique.

10. CERVICO-THORACIC JUNCTION DISTRACTION

This technique is for pain or dysfunction at the cervico-thoracic junction – for example, C7 on T1 or T1 on T2 with tension at the thoracic outlet.

Positions of the patient and therapist

● The patient sits on a low couch or across a chair.
● The therapist stands behind the patient and places a foot on the couch or adjacent chair alongside the side to be treated.
● The patient drapes an arm over the thigh of the therapist and leans across to that side (Figure 18.31).

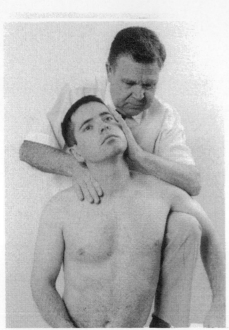

Figure 18.31 Thoracic manipulation technique 10: position of the therapist and patient for the cervico-thoracic junction specific technique (left sided problem).

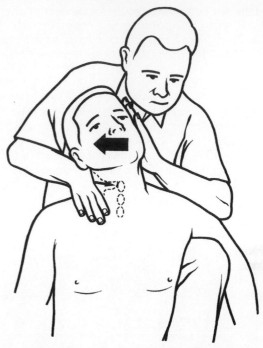

Figure 18.32 The above technique ((for a left sided problem) illustrated): the thumb of the lower hand pushes against the lateral aspect of the spinous process while the upper hand thrusts against the head in the opposite direction.

Method

- The therapist spreads a hand on the opposite side around the neck and firmly holds the thumb onto the spinous process of the lower vertebrae to be treated – for example, on T1 if C7–T1 is to be treated. This hand acts as a fulcrum.
  Position of the head
  The cervico-thoracic spine must be kept erect: the neck is held in slight extension and slightly rotated away from the affected side.
- Use the lower hand to side bend the neck towards the painful side and with the upper hand laterally flex the neck away from the painful side.
- The manipulative thrust is applied by simultaneously thrusting with both hands to gap the affected side (Figure 18.32). The thumb of the lower hand pushes against the lateral spinous process during this thrust.

11. UPPER RIB TECHNIQUE

This technique is used for thoracic outlet discomfort with dysfunction of the first rib which articulates with T1.

Position of the patient and therapist

- The patient sits on a low couch or across a chair or stool.
- The therapist stands behind the patient and places a foot on the couch or adjacent chair on the opposite side to that to be treated.
- The patient drapes an arm over the thigh of the therapist and leans to that side so that the axilla is supported. The knee is used to control sideways translation of the patient's trunk.

Method

- The therapist places a hand on the non-affected side and laterally flexes (side bends) the neck towards the side to be treated.
- Place the other hand on the thoracic outlet with the fingers palpating the rib in front of the trapezius. The thumb is used to fix the posterior aspect of the rib through the trapezius.
- Stretch the ribs of the thoracic outlet downwards with your lower hand and then apply a sharp low amplitude thrust to gap the outlet (Figure 18.33). The thrust from the lower hand is directed at the nipple of the breast on the opposite side.

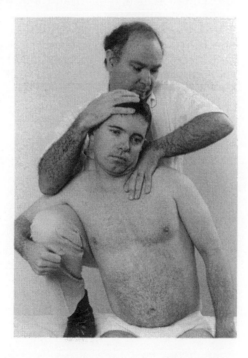

Figure 18.33 Thoracic manipulation 11: upper rib technique (left sided problem).

PRACTICE TIPS

- A low couch is important for techniques with the patient lying prone or supine.
- A higher couch is better for techniques involving the patient sitting.

- A firm (but not hard) padded couch is essential for techniques involving the patient lying prone or supine.
- These techniques can be performed on a carpeted floor.
- Hand grip no. 1 is the most effective grip for postero-anterior indirect thrusting techniques.
- The most effective techniques for the thoracic spine are the postero-anterior indirect thrust techniques 1, 2 and 5.
- Time your manipulative thrust just before the end of expiration.
- For the 'Nelson hold' technique use a rolled object such as a 10–15 cm long door 'sausage'.

SUMMARY AND CAUTIONARY ADVICE

Ensure that organic disease, especially malignant disease, is not present in the spine that you are manipulating. Be careful of the patient with osteoporosis, which is usually asymptomatic – hence a small-framed elderly woman should not be subjected to thrusting techniques.

Fortunately disc prolapse is very uncommon, but take care with the uncommon radicular pain and any symptoms or signs suggestive of cauda equina pressure.

It is possible to fracture or dislocate ribs and costal cartilage using direct thrusting techniques with the patient lying prone; to cause pain under the arms with traction methods such as the 'Nelson hold' technique and to injure the lower neck if the patient's neck grip is too loose for the relevant techniques.

19
Patient education and exercise programmes for the thoracic spine

'Not less than two hours per day should be devoted to exercise.'

Thomas Jeffersen, 1786

Contents
☐ General advice to patients
☐ Prevention
☐ Exercises for the thoracic spine
    1. Shoulder brace
    2. Shoulder lift
    3. 'Sea lion' lift and sway
    4. 'Broom handle' swing
    5. The 'cat back' on elbows

GENERAL ADVICE TO PATIENTS

Pain in the thoracic area of the back is common in people who sit bent forwards for long periods, especially students and typists, and those who lift constantly, such as nursing mothers.

There appear to be two main causes:

1. Chronic strain of the ligaments binding the vertebrae together due to poor posture; and
2. Stiff or 'jammed' joints where the ribs join the spine – usually due to injury including lifting and falls.

PREVENTION

Maintain a good posture by observing the following hints:

● Keep your head erect.
● Brace your shoulder blades together and then release – practice many times a day.

- Look after your posture at the office; have a good chair with a firm back support. If you are typing use a special stand to hold the copy in order to keep your head upright and straight.
- If possible stretch your upper spine by hanging suspended from an overhead bar for several seconds each day or less frequently. Brace your shoulder blades together as you do this.

EXERCISES FOR THE THORACIC SPINE

Select at least three exercises that suit you and perform them two or three times a day for five to ten minutes. Exercise 4 is generally regarded as the most beneficial.

Exercise 1: shoulder brace

Brace the shoulder blades as you sit or stand by swinging your clasped hands behind your back, extending back your head at the same time. Hold for three seconds. Repeat ten times.

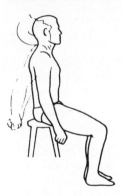

Exercise 2: shoulder lift

Lie face downwards, lift your shoulders, hold for seven seconds, relax. Repeat five to ten times.

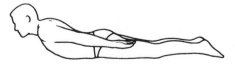

Exercise 3: 'sea lion' lift and sway

Lie face downwards, lift from waist, and rotate your upper trunk from side to side so that you feel a tight stretch in your back. Repeat five to ten times.

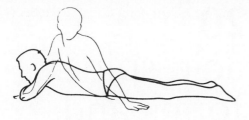

Exercise 4: 'broom handle' swing

Place a long rod, such as a broom handle or golf stick, behind both shoulders and rotate your body from side to side, reaching maximum stretch.

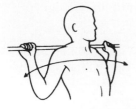

Exercise 5: the cat back

Arch your back like a cat in the way illustrated. Support yourself on both knees and elbows. If you need to exercise the upper part of the spine place your elbows forward and lower your chest. For the lower part of the back perform the exercise on your hands and knees. Hunch your back as you breathe in and then arch it as you fully breathe out. Repeat five to ten times.

20
The thoracic spine: case histories and management problems

'Practice should always be based upon a sound knowledge of theory.'

Leonardo da Vinci (1452–1519)

Contents
☐ Thoracic spine: manual therapy
☐ Case histories
☐ Answers to case histories: thoracic spine

The following ten case histories of patients with thoracic back pain are presented for discussion in courses or for individual deliberation. For each patient, make the decisions according to the plan.

1. Provisional diagnosis
2. Select the appropriate manual therapy (if any) from the mobilisation and manipulation techniques as listed:
   A. First line technique/techniques
   B. Second line technique/techniques

The main techniques for the thoracic spine (as presented in this book) are summarised in list form. Once again a coded format is presented:

TMo = thoracic mobilisation
TMa = thoracic manipulation

THORACIC SPINE: MANUAL THERAPY

Summary of techniques

Mobilisation techniques	*Code*
1. Anterior directed central gliding	TMo 1
2. Anterior directed unilateral gliding	TMo 2
3. Transverse directed rotational gliding	TMo 3
4. Anterior directed costo-vertebral gliding	TMo 4
5. Rib mobilisation	TMo 5
6. Rib mobilisation in rotation	TMo 6

Manipulation techniques	*Code*
1. Postero-anterior indirect thrust (neutral)	TMa 1
2. Postero-anterior indirect thrust (flexion)	TMa 2
3. Postero-anterior indirect thrust (extension)	TMa 3
4. Postero-anterior indirect thrust over rib	TMa 4
5. Postero-anterior thigh extension thrust	TMa 5
6. The crossed pisiform method	TMa 6
7. Anterior directed sternal thrust (Nelson hold)	TMa 7
8. Anterior directed sternal thrust (crossover technique)	TMa 8
9. Thoracic rotation in sitting position	TMa 9
10. Cervico-thoracic junction distraction	TMa 10
11. Upper rib technique	TMa 11

CASE HISTORIES

Case 1

A 23-year-old male (draftsman) presents with two weeks of pain under the left 'shoulder blade' and left breast. The pain, which appeared to develop spontaneously, has a deep dull quality and comes on soon after lifting. It is aggravated by deep breathing or left rotation. He feels as though his chest is stiff.

Inspection

Slight thoracic kyphosis.

Palpation

Tender over T6 central and (left) unilateral.

Movements

Restricted and tender extension, left rotation and left lateral flexion.

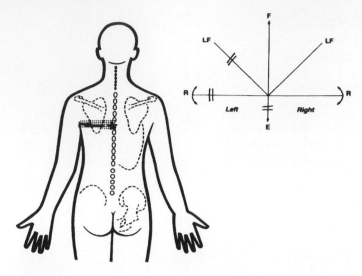

General

Chest examination normal.

X-ray

Normal.

Questions

1. Provisional diagnosis
2. Selection of manual therapy techniques
   A. First line techniques
   B. Second line techniques.

Case 2

A 32-year-old housewife presents with a three day history of constant central and bilateral upper thoracic pain that is deep, dull and can be felt in the front of the chest when the pain is maximal. It is aggravated by knitting and reading and feels better lying on a hard surface.

Inspection

Normal.

Palpation

Tender to central palpation T3 and T4.

Movements

Restricted flexion.

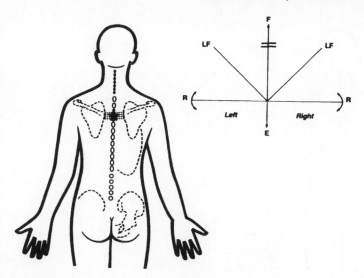

General

Chest and cardiac status normal.

X-ray

Slight degenerative changes T3 and T4 levels.

Questions

1. Provisional diagnosis
2. Selection of manual therapy techniques
   A. First line techniques
   B. Second line techniques.

Case 3

A 40-year-old male (farmer) presents with two weeks of low right-sided thoracic pain after a fall from a fence. The dull pain radiates around the right costal margin to the epigastrium when he is lifting.

Inspection

No abnormality.

Palpation

Tender to right unilateral palpation at T7 and T8 levels and on springing right 7th and 8th ribs.

Movements

Restricted and tender lateral flexion and rotation (to right).

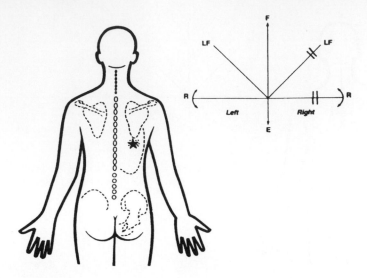

General

No clinical fracture of rib, chest normal.

X-ray

Chest and thoracic spine normal.

Questions

1. Provisional diagnosis
2. Selection of manual therapy techniques
   A. First line techniques
   B. Second line techniques.

Case 4

A 45-year-old housewife presents with a three week history of a 'painful left shoulder'. A careful history indicates that she is referring to upper thoracic pain from the midline to the left suprascapular area. It is aggravated by activities involving neck extension such as hanging out the clothes. She is otherwise well.

Inspection

No abnormality.

Palpation

Tender 2–3 cm unilaterally to the left at T2 with a trigger point 10 cm laterally above the scapula.

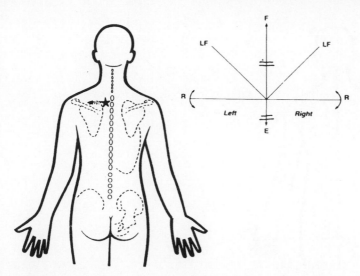

Movements

Slightly restricted extension, restricted and tender flexion.

General

No abnormalities.

X-ray

Normal.

Questions

1. Provisional diagnosis
2. Selection of manual therapy techniques
    A. First line techniques
    B. Second line techniques.

Case 5

A 19-year-old female (computer operator) presents with 24 hours of acute tenderness 'between the shoulder blades' causing her extreme discomfort, an inability to take a deep breath and finding it impossible to work. She claimed that it developed soon after lifting a heavy typewriter. She has been aware of a niggling pain in that site for weeks.

Inspection

Stiff thoracic spine.

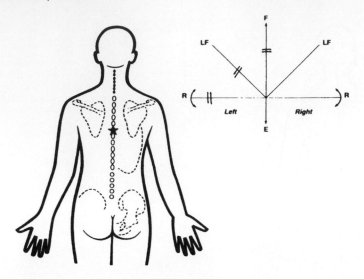

Palpation

Extremely tender over T6 centrally and transversely from left.

Movements

Restricted flexion, L rotation and L lateral flexion.

General

No other abnormality.

X-ray

Normal.

Questions

1. Provisional diagnosis
2. Selection of manual therapy techniques
   A. First line techniques
   B. Second line techniques.

Case 6

A 62-year-old housewife presents with a three month history of mid thoracic pain aggravated by lifting and bedmaking. The pain does not radiate from its central dorsal position.

Inspection

Very thin woman with kyphosis.

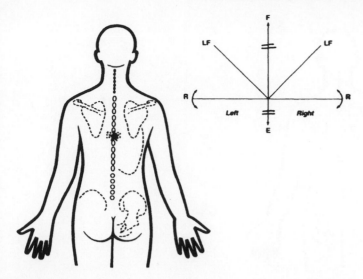

Palpation

Tender T7 centrally and unilaterally; positive to transverse palpation bilaterally.

Movements

Restricted flexion and extension.

General

Bronchospasm with chronic obstructive airways disease.

X-ray

Generalised osteoporosis in thoracic vertebrae; no evidence of fracture.

Questions

1. Provisional diagnosis
2. Selection of manual therapy techniques
   A. First line techniques
   B. Second line techniques.

Case 7

A 51-year-old male (bus driver) presents with low thoracic back pain which 'moves around a bit' but is mainly central. The pain tends to move to either side and can move under the ribs towards the 'area of the appendix' and occasionally in the 'kidney area' on the right side. He has noticed the pain on and off for a month and it usually appears after long trips. His general health is good but he is worried about kidney trouble, including 'stones' which 'run in the family'.

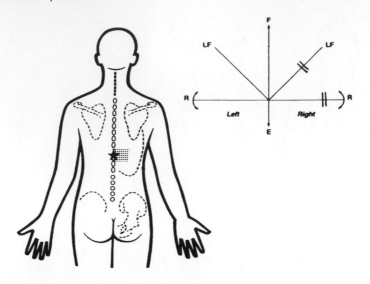

Inspection

Moves lower thoracic spine stiffly.

Palpation

Tender over T9 and T10 centrally and unilaterally to the right; skin rolling test positive under right twelfth rib 12 cm laterally.

Movements

Restricted and tender R lateral flexion and right rotation.

General

No abnormality (including urine analysis).

X-ray

Normal.

Questions

1. Provisional diagnosis
2. Selection of manual therapy techniques
   A. First line techniques
   B. Second line techniques.

Case 8

A 35-year-old female (secretary) presents with a vague history of headaches, pain in the back of the head and between the shoulder blades – high up, 'pains, and pins and needles' in the forearms,

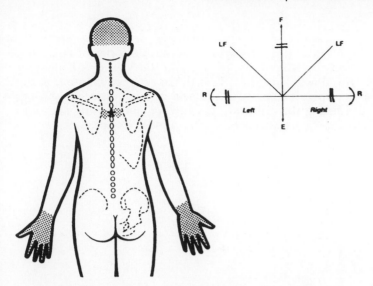

especially the hands ('long glove'-like distribution). She has been feeling unwell for several weeks with these symptoms and wonders whether it is 'nerves'.

Inspection

Depressed looking patient, otherwise normal.

Palpation

Tenderness and stiffness T3–T4, central and bilateral.

Movements

Restricted flexion, bilateral rotation.

Neurological

Normal.

General

No other abnormality.

X-ray

(Thoracic and cervical spines) normal.

Questions

1. Provisional diagnosis
2. Selection of manual therapy techniques
    A. First line techniques
    B. Second line techniques.

Case 9

A 29-year-old housewife presents with recurrent episodes of epigastric pain, but previous investigations for a peptic ulcer and gall bladder disease have proved negative. She relates the onset of pain (more to the right side of the epigastrium) with physical activity, especially lifting, vacuuming and lifting the children. On further questioning she does recall experiencing vague backache in the middle of her back.

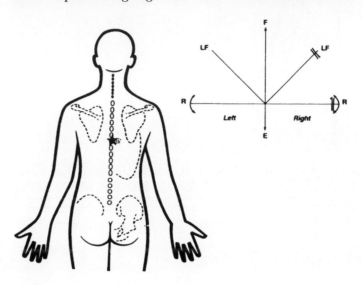

Inspection

Normal.

Palpation

No tenderness or skin rolling tenderness in epigastrium; tenderness to transverse palpation on right side T7 and unilaterally at T7 level.

Movements

Normal; overpressure to R lateral flexion and R rotation reproduces back pain.

General

No abnormality.

X-ray

Normal.

Questions

1. Provisional diagnosis
2. Selection of manual therapy techniques
   A. First line techniques
   B. Second line techniques.

Case 10

A 25-year-old male (athlete) presents with pain in the low back, the right inguinal region and the 'hip' three weeks after a heavy fall in a steeplechase event. It has been quite severe at times and prevents him training. It is aggravated by twisting to the right, sleeping in a soft bed and reclining in a soft chair.

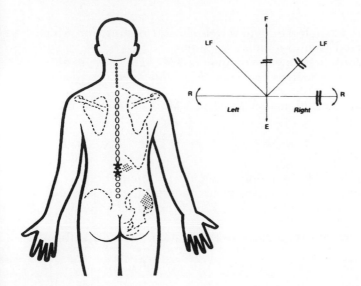

Inspection

Guarded movements at thoraco-lumbar junction.

Palpation

Tender over T12 and L1 centrally and T12–L1 unilaterally on right. Pinch roll test over upper gluteal area very tender.

Movements

Restricted flexion, lateral flexion (R) and R rotation.

General

Inguinal region, lower lumbar spine and hips normal.

X-ray

Normal.

Questions

1. Provisional diagnosis
2. Selection of manual therapy techniques
   A. First line techniques
   B. Second line techniques.

ANSWERS TO CASE HISTORIES: THORACIC SPINE

Case 1

1. This patient has left T6 costo-vertebral joint dysfunction which is giving referred pain in a radicular pattern.
2. The preferred first line technique is TMa 4 – postero-anterior indirect thrust over the rib, followed by TMa 1 – postero-anterior indirect thrust (in neutral).

   Second line technique is TMa 9 or TMo 6 – rotation in sitting position.

Case 2

1. This patient has T3–T4 apophyseal joint dysfunction.
2. The most appropriate first line techniques are the postero-anterior indirect thrust in extension (TMa 3) and the postero-anterior thigh extension (TMa 5) techniques.

   The recommended second line technique is the sternal thrust or Nelson hold (TMa 7).

   These patients usually respond extremely well to any one of these techniques.

Case 3

1. This patient has costo-vertebral dysfunction of the right seventh and eighth articulations due to the traumatic 'springing' of the ribs with his fall.
2. First line techniques include the mobilisations TMo 4 – anterior directed costo-vertebral gliding and TMo 5 – rib mobilisation.

   Second line techniques are the manipulations TMa 4 – postero-anterior indirect thrust over the involved ribs and TMa 9 – rotation (to the left).

Case 4

1. This patient has vertebral dysfunction at T2, most likely due to the left T1–T2 or T2–T3 apophyseal joints, with referred pain to the suprascapular area.

2. The first line techniques are TMa 5 – the postero-anterior thigh extension technique and TMa 7 – the sternal thrust technique.

Second line technique is TMa 3 – postero-anterior indirect thrust into extension.

The slight restriction into extension is not a contra-indication to manipulation in this direction.

Case 5

1. This patient has vertebral dysfunction at T6, most likely due to apophyseal joint dysfunction on the left.
2. Although gentle (stage 1 or 2) mobilisation techniques would be logical in such a patient, the area is often too tender to withstand any direct applied pressure. If the patient can tolerate the pressure, TMo 1 and TMo 3 (transverse directed rotational gliding) would be suitable.

Otherwise an indirect manipulation technique, carefully applied, such as TMa 1 (postero-anterior indirect thrust in the neutral position) or TMa 7 (sternal thrust) or TMa 9 (rotation) can be dramatically effective.

Of all these techniques, the most indirect TMo 6 or TMa 9 (rotation in sitting towards the right) would be the first recommendation.

Case 6

1. This patient has vertebral dysfunction at the T7 level, probably due to dysfunction of the apophyseal joints or the costo-vertebral joints. It is unlikely that the osteoporotic vertebra would be responsible for the pain. It usually requires a compression fracture to be painful.
2. The first line technique is one (or more) of the mobilisation techniques TMo 1 (central), TMo 2 (unilateral) applied bilaterally, or TMo 3 (transverse gliding).

Spinal manipulation is contra-indicated in the presence of osteoporosis. Thrusting techniques in these frailer patients are fraught with danger. However, if the problem is resistant to mobilisation treatment, a gently applied sternal thrust technique (TMa 7) which achieves gapping by traction should be a reasonably safe procedure.

Case 7

1. This patient has vertebral dysfunction at the T9 and T10 levels, especially on the right. Although a disc prolapse is more likely in the lower thoracic area, it is unlikely in this patient. He presumably has a right T9–T10 apophyseal joint disorder with referred pain three to four segments below via the cutaneous branches of the posterior primary rami; also referred pain anteriorly in the vicinity of the umbilicus.
2. The best first line techniques would be TMa 2 – postero-anterior indirect thrust into flexion and TMa 9 – rotation to the left using the thrusting hand to the T9–T10 area to achieve more specificity.

The second line techniques would be TMa 6 – the crossed pisiform – and possibly TMa 5 – the thigh extension technique – both of which may just reach this low level.

Case 8

1. This patient has the so-called T4 syndrome due to vertebral dysfunction at the T3 and T4 levels. There is invariably stiffness and tenderness at T4.
2. The first line technique is the thoracic manipulation (TMa 1) – postero-anterior indirect thrust.

   Second line techniques include the crossed pisiform (TMa 6), and the thigh extension (TMa 5) or the sternal thrust (TMa 7).

Case 9

1. This patient in this interesting case has vertebral dysfunction at the T7 level with reference to the epigastrium (between the costal margin and the midline on the right along the distribution of T7 – see Chapter 15). Many patients present with anterior chest or abdominal symptoms mainly because they tend to overlook their back discomfort, which usually has less sinister implications than anterior pain.
2. The first line techniques would be the manipulation techniques TMa 2 – postero-anterior indirect thrust into flexion – and TMa 6 – the crossed pisiform.

   Second line techniques include the manipulation techniques TMa 1 – postero-anterior indirect thrust in neutral; TMa 5 – thigh extension; and TMa 9 – rotation. The mobilisation techniques, especially TMo 3 – transverse rotational gliding, can certainly be used in this patient.

Case 10

1. This patient has vertebral dysfunction at the thoraco-lumbar junction, at T12 and L1, with the apophyseal joint (R) T12–L1 being obviously involved. Pain is referred to the inguinal region from T12 or L1 or both, while skin pain is experienced in the upper outer buttock area via the posterior primary ramus of T12–L1. This accounts for the sensitive pinch roll test. Intervertebral disc lesions are more common at T11–T12 and T12–L1 so an MID could also be responsible for the symptoms.
2. The first line technique is thoracic rotation in the sitting position (TMa 9). Second line techniques include the non-specific rotation manipulation techniques for the lumbar spine.

Section 4
The Lumbosacral Spine and Lower Limb

21
Low back pain: clinical features

'Last Wednesday night while carrying a bucket of water from the well, Hannah Williams slipped upon the icy path and fell heavily upon her back. We fear her spine was injured for though she suffers acute pain in her legs she cannot move them. The poor wild beautiful girl is stopped in her wildness at last.'

Francis Kilvert, 1874

Contents
- ☐ Key checkpoints
- ☐ Causes of low back pain
- ☐ The diagnostic approach
- ☐ Acute low back pain
- ☐ Chronic low back pain
- ☐ The diagnosis of non-organic back pain
- ☐ Summary

Low back pain, which is one of the most difficult conditions to manage, accounts for at least 5 per cent of the problems seen in general practice. The most common cause is minor soft tissue injury but such patients do not usually seek medical help because the problem settles quickly within a few days.

Most back pain presenting in general practice is due to dysfunction of elements of the mobile segment – that is, the two apophyseal joints, the intervertebral joint (with its disc) and the ligamentous and muscular attachments. This problem, often referred to as mechanical pain or traumatic joint derangement, will be referred to as vertebral dysfunction – a general term, which, while covering radicular and non-radicular pain, mainly includes dysfunction of the joints of the spine.

It is important for practitioners to bear in mind that every patient with a pain syndrome has anxiety about its significance. Does it imply malignant disease, an impending catastrophe, or a complete change in lifestyle or occupation? Pain in the back can, however, sometimes represent a patient's opportunity to 'escape' from an unwanted lifestyle or occupation; hence the practitioner can be faced with the difficult management of a malingering or 'hysterical' patient.

```
KEY CHECKPOINTS
```

- The most common cause of low back pain is vertebral dysfunction invariably originating from the joints.
- Inflammatory disorders characterised by pain at rest and relieved by activity must not be missed.
- A lumbar nerve root is typically compressed by the disc above it – for example, L5 is compressed by the L4–L5 lesion.
- Not all cases of spondylolisthesis are symptomatic.
- Discomfort in the legs on walking can be due to neurogenic (spinal) or vascular (arterial obstruction) claudication.
- Plain X-rays are of limited use, especially in younger patients, and may appear normal in disc prolapse.
- Sacro-iliitis plus involvement of the spine (clinical or radiological) adds up to ankylosing spondylitis, psoriasis, Reiter's disease or inflammatory bowel disorders.

CAUSES OF LOW BACK PAIN

In order to have a rational diagnostic approach to the patient, the practitioner must have a basic knowledge of the possible causes of low back pain, including a perspective of their relative frequency and clinical presentations.

Table 21.1 *Major causes of low back ± leg pain presenting in general practice.*

CAUSE	PATIENTS (%)
Vertebral dysfunction	71.8
Lumbar spondylosis	10.1
Depression	3.0
Urinary tract infection	2.2
Spondylolisthesis	2.0
Spondyloarthropathies	1.9
Musculo-ligamentous strains/tears	1.2
Malignant disease	0.8
Arterial occlusive disease	0.6
Other	6.4

Table 21.1 shows the major causes of low back pain (as the primary presenting symptom) in patients seen by one of the authors. These figures are based on approximately fifteen hundred individual patient presentations.

THE DIAGNOSTIC APPROACH

At the initial consultation for low back pain the practitioner should consider the five leading questions posed in Chapter 2. A summary of the diagnostic model is presented in Table 21.2.

Table 21.2 *Low back pain: diagnostic strategy model.*

Q. Probability diagnosis
A. Vertbral dysfunction esp. facet joint and disc
   Spondylosis (degenerative OA)

Q. Serious disorders not to be missed
A. Cardiovascular
      ruptured aortic aneurysm
      retroperitoneal haemorrhage (anti-coagulants)
   Neoplasia
      myeloma
      metastases
   Severe infections
      osteomyelitis
      discitis
      tuberculosis
      pelvic abscess/PID
   Cauda equina compression

Q. Pitfalls (often missed)
A. Spondyloarthropathies
      ankylosing spondylitis
      Reiter's disease/reactive arthritis
      psoriasis
      bowel inflammation
   Sacro-iliac dysfunction
   Spondylolisthesis
   Claudication
      vascular
      neurogenic
   Prostatitis
   Endometriosis

Q. Seven masquerades checklist
A. Depression   ✓
   Diabetes   –
   Drugs   –
   Anaemia   –
   Thyroid disease   –
   Spinal dysfunction ✓
   UTI   ✓

Q. Is this patient trying to tell me something?
A. Quite likely. Consider lifestyle, stress,
   work problems, malingering, conversion reaction

Note: Associated buttock and leg pain included.

1. What is the probability diagnosis?

The answer, of course, is vertebral dysfunction, which then has to be further analysed. Muscle or ligamentous tears or similar soft tissue injuries are uncommon causes of back pain alone: they are generally associated with severe spinal disruption and severe trauma such as that following a motor vehicle accident.

In the lumbar spine most problems originate from the joints of the spine, either the apophyseal joints or the intervertebral discogenic joint, or from both simultaneously. The disc can cause pain, either intrinsically from internal disruption or extrinsically by pressure on adjacent pain-sensitive structures, leading to radicular pain (if the nerve root is involved) or non-radicular pain. However, disc prolapse is not the common cause of back pain it was once believed to be.

Muscle spasm is often incorrectly considered to be the cause of pain but the spasm is usually secondary to a disruption of the joints.

Degenerative changes in the lumbar spine (lumbar spondylosis) are commonly encountered in the older age group (over 50 years).

2. What serious disorder must not be missed?

It is very important to consider malignant disease, especially in an older person. However, with the lumbar spine it is essential to be on guard for compression of the cauda equina and severe nerve damage. Such problems are usually caused by a massive disc prolapse or a retroperitoneal haemorrhage.

3. What conditions are often missed?

Past experience makes us wise, but it is a human failing to make the same mistakes when we are working under intense pressure or when we become over-familiar with the common dysfunctional problems. For the young woman with upper lumbar pain, the possibility of a urinary tract infection must be considered. The inflammatory disorders must be kept in mind, especially ankylosing spondylitis in the younger patient, and the relatively rare disorders – Reiter's disease, psoriasis, ulcerative colitis and Crohn's disease. The old trap of claudication in the buttocks and legs due to a high arterial obstruction being confused with sciatica must be avoided.

4. Could the patient have one of the masquerades?

Seven important masquerades to consider are listed in Table 21.2. Depressive illness has to be considered in any patient with a chronic pain complaint. This common psychiatric disorder can continue to aggravate and/or maintain the pain even though the provoking problem has disappeared. This is more likely to occur in people who have become anxious about their problem or who are under excessive stress. Many doctors treat such patients with a therapeutic trial of anti-depressant medication – for example, amitryptiline or doxepin taken at night.

5. Is the patient trying to tell me something?

Low back pain following lifting at work is the classic problem that causes considerable anguish to doctors especially in patients whose problem becomes chronic and complex. Such an event may be the 'final straw' for a patient who has been struggling to cope with a personal problem, and their fragile equilibrium is thrown into disarray by their episode of back pain. Many patients who have been dismissed as malingerers turn out to have a genuine problem. The importance of a caring, competent practitioner with an insight into all facets of his or her patient's suffering, organic and functional, becomes obvious. The tests for non-organic back pain are very useful in this context.

The process of diagnosis commences as soon as the patient enters the consulting room. Appearance, movements and responses should be observed carefully at all times. Shoes with laces, for example, should make one cautiously sceptical of the patient who complains of chronic severe low back pain.

The general diagnostic approach is outlined in Chapter 2. It must be emphasised that this process is only one approach and practitioners will necessarily develop their own individual strategy to conform with their knowledge base, training and type of practice.

ACUTE LOW BACK PAIN

The general causes of acute back pain are presented in Figure 2.1. However, the outstanding cause of acute low back pain ('lumbago') is vertebral dysfunction, and the main serious clinical syndromes are secondary to a prolapse of an intervertebral disc, usually L4–L5 or L5–S1.

Table 21.3 *Clinical features and diagnosis of vertebral dysfunction leading to low back and leg pain.*

CLINICAL FEATURES	DIAGNOSIS
Syndrome A (surgical emergency) Saddle anaesthesia (around anus, scrotum, or vaginal) Distal anaesthesia Evidence of UMN or LMN lesion Loss of sphincter control or urinary retention Weakness of legs peripherally	Spinal cord or cauda equina compression
Syndrome B (probable surgical emergency) Anaesthesia or paraesthesia of the leg Foot drop Motor weakness Absence of reflexes	Large disc protrusion, paralysing nerve root
Syndrome C Distal pain with or without paraesthesia Sciatica Positive dural stretch tests	Posterolateral disc protrusion on nerve root or disc disruption
Syndrome D Lumbar pain (unilateral, central or bilateral)	Disc protrusion or apophyseal joint dysfunction

Table 21.3 presents the general clinical features and diagnosis in acute back pain (fractures excluded) following vertebral dysfunction: the symptoms and signs can occur singly or in combination.

Fortunately syndromes A and B are extremely rare but, if encountered, urgent referral to a neurosurgeon or orthopaedic surgeon is mandatory. Syndrome B can follow a bleed in patients taking anticoagulant therapy or be caused by a disc sequestration after inappropriate spinal manipulation.

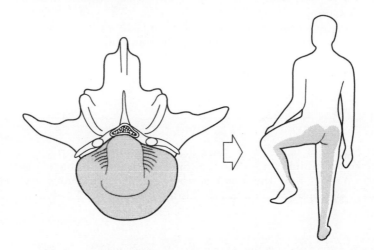

Figure 21.1 Prolapsed intervertebral disc causing a cauda equina syndrome. The distribution of pain, paraesthesia or anaesthesia is illustrated.

Figure 21.1 illustrates the distribution of pain, paraesthesia or anaesthesia with cauda equina lesion which tends to cause features of a lower motor neurone lesion with paralysis of the legs and feet and wasting of the calves.

Radicular pain

Syndromes B and C (Table 21.3) represent nerve root compression problems causing radicular pain which can vary in severity. All these cases reflect a significant disc protrusion and must be handled with care.

Table 21.4 lists the signs and symptoms of a severe disc protrusion such as presenting in syndrome B.

If radicular pain is not severe enough to be treated by surgical removal or chemical destruction of the disc, a protracted course of conservative management lasting at least 6 to 12 weeks can be anticipated. Spinal manipulation is absolutely contra-indicated in these patients.

Treatment

The patient should rest in bed; a firm mattress is essential. Analgesics (ranging from paracetamol to codeine) may be prescribed according to the severity of the pain. Non-steroidal anti-inflammatory drugs (NSAIDs) such as diclofenac, diflunisal, ketoprofen, naproxen or

Table 21.4 *Symptoms and signs of a severe lumbar disc protrusion.*

SYMPTOMS

Latency: pain develops hours or days after the injury
Peripheral (rather than central) pain
Irritability: precipitation of acute pain with simple movements, or activity
Pain or paraesthesia below the knee to foot
Pain present at night, not relieved by lying down
Advancement of symptoms: from pain to paraesthesia to anaesthesia

SIGNS

'Floppy' foot
Weakness in the leg
Marked scoliosis of spine
Muscle spasm
Positive dural stretch signs: straight leg raising and 'slump' test

piroxicam and a tranquilliser or muscle relaxant (such as diazepam) are useful for short-term use.

Swimming and other suitable exercise should be prescribed as the condition improves and the patient should be referred to a therapist skilled in back pain management for mobilisation and traction.

Success rates varying from 30 to 80 per cent have been reported for lumbar and caudal epidural injections and the authors recommend a caudal epidural for severe cases and those not responding to conservative treatment.

Outcome

Most of the problems associated with severe disc protrusion respond to conservative treatment. If they do not, or if the condition deteriorates, early referral to a consultant surgeon is necessary.

Radicular pain (typical profile)

Age:	Any age, usually middle aged.
History of injury:	Yes, lifting or twisting. Can be spontaneous.
Site and radiation:	Unilateral low back, distal radiation along dermatome, tends to have a 'distal' emphasis.
Type of pain:	Deep aching pain (episodic) develops soon after arising in morning. Has a 'travelling' nature.
Aggravation:	Activity, lifting, intercourse, sitting, bending, car travel, coughing, sneezing, straining.
Relief:	Rest, lying, standing.

Associations:	Distal paraesthesia ± numbness, stiffness.
Physical examination: (significant)	Guarded and restricted movement. Loss of lumbar lordosis Lateral deviation (scoliosis) Restricted flexion, extension, lateral flexion SLR and slump test positive ± specific muscle/myotomal weakness ± reduced distal sensation ± reduced ankle jerk (S1) ⎫⎬⎭ Unilateral
Diagnostic confirmation (for special reasons):	CT scan, discogram, radiculogram, MRI or myelogram.

Significance of the level of the prolapsed disc

The clinical patterns for radicular pain can show several variable patterns. Usually only one nerve root is involved, commonly the L5 or S1 nerve root but, unlike discogenic lesions in the cervical spine, more than one nerve root can be involved with a prolapse of the L5–S1 disc: both the L5 and S1 nerve roots. The L4–L5 and L5–S1 disc spaces are the only two lumbo-sacral disc spaces that are regularly crossed closely by nerve roots (Figure 21.2). Significant degenerative disc lesions occur almost exclusively at these two levels.

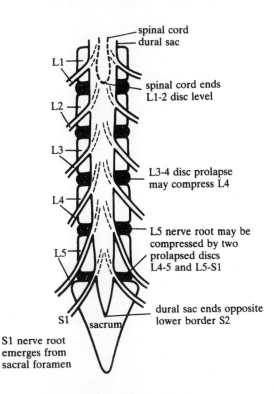

Figure 21.2 Posterior 'window' view of spine illustrating the relationships of the nerve roots to the intervertebral discs (after Cailliet).

When a disc prolapses the direction of the prolapse is either posterolateral or posterior. With the posterolateral prolapses there is low back pain and radicular pain to one leg. The peripheral pain can be more severe than the central pain.

Posterior prolapses tend to be accompanied by intense low back pain with possible radiation into both legs, or the pain may alternate between one side and the other side. This tends to occur with the L4–L5 disc and is usually associated with a significant deformity such as lateral deviation or forward flexion of the spine.

A study of Figure 21.2 explains how the prolapsing disc tends to compress the nerve emerging from the space below rather than at its own level – that is, for a nerve root to be compressed a disc must prolapse *above* its exit through the intervertebral foramen.

In summary

- The S1 nerve root crosses both the L4–L5 and L5–S1 discs.
- An L4 nerve root lesion is usually caused by L3–L4 disc prolapse.
- An L5 nerve root lesion is usually caused by L4–L5 disc prolapse.
- An S1 nerve root lesion is usually caused by L5–S1 disc prolapse.

Non-radicular pain

Syndrome D is the most common clinical presentation in general practice and most cases can be expected to subside within three weeks; spinal manipulation will shorten that period.

A typical patient is a middle-aged person who complains of the sudden onset (after twisting) of right-sided back pain, localised to the fourth or fifth level in the lumbar spine: the dural stretch test is negative.

Treatment

The patient should rest, especially for the first two days following the injury, and then when necessary. Basic analgesics should be taken as required. These patients are usually most suitable for mobilisation and manipulation if they do not settle within three or four days.

A programme of rotation, flexion and extension exercises should be commenced (swimming is best) and the patient should be taught ways to protect the back from further episodes.

CHRONIC LOW BACK PAIN

There are several causes of chronic low back pain but profiles will follow for the most important and common causes. The outstanding common cause is uncomplicated vertebral dysfunction causing non-radicular back pain. This cause is considered to be due mainly to dysfunction of the pain-sensitive apophyseal joint.

Each of the following profiles will depict a typical case for that particular problem, but it must be remembered that individual patients may show variations in presentation.

Vertebral dysfunction with non-radicular pain

Age:	Any age – late teens to old age, usually 30–60.
History of injury:	Yes, lifting or twisting.
Site and radiation:	Unilateral lumbar (maybe central). Refers over sacrum, SIJ areas, buttocks.
Type of pain:	Deep aching pain, episodic.
Aggravation:	Activity, lifting, gardening, housework (vacuuming, making beds, etc.).
Relief:	Rest, warmth.
Associations:	May be stiffness, usually good health.
Physical examination: (significant)	Localised tenderness – unilateral or central L4, L5 or S1 levels May be restricted flexion, extension, lateral flexion.
Diagnosis confirmation:	Investigations usually normal. *Note:* Diagnosis made clinically.

Comment

This case is the most common back problem. The precise pathophysiology is difficult to pinpoint but invariably is dysfunction of one of the spinal joints, most likely an apophyseal joint or the MID as proposed by Maigne.

Malignant disease

Age:	Usually over 50 but the older the patient the greater the risk.
History of injury:	Usually insidious onset.
Site and radiation:	Localised pain anywhere in lumbar spine Radiates into buttocks or legs (if nerve root involved).
Type of pain:	Boring deep ache, can be referred or radicular, unrelenting continuous pain, getting worse.
Aggravation:	Movement Specific activities such as lifting, gardening.
Relief:	Usually none No response to any treatment.
Associations:	Malaise, fatigue, weight loss Muscular weakness Night pain.

Physical examination: Flattened lumbar lordosis
(significant)   Localised tenderness over vertebrae
                               All movements restricted and protective (if
                               advanced)
                               Neurologically   normal   unless   roots
                               involved
                               More than one root may be involved
                               Major neurological signs incompatible with
                               pain level.

Diagnosis confirmation: X-ray (Figure 21.3)
(select from)   Serum alkaline phosphatase
                               Prostatic specific antigen
                               ESR
                               Bone scan.

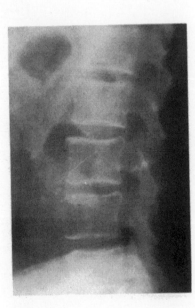

Figure 21.3 Metastatic disease: X-ray of spine showing osteolytic metastasis in the body of L2 from carcinoma of the lung.

Comment

It is most important to identify malignant disease and other space-occupying lesions because of the prognosis and the effect of a delayed diagnosis on treatment. If malignant disease is proved and myeloma is excluded a search should be made for the six primary malignancies that metastasise to the spine (Figure 21.4).

With respect to the neurological features, more than one nerve root may be involved and major neurological signs may be present without severe root pain. The neurological signs will be progressive.

Spondylolisthesis

Age: Any age; young adult if congenital, older
                               person (over 50) if degenerative.

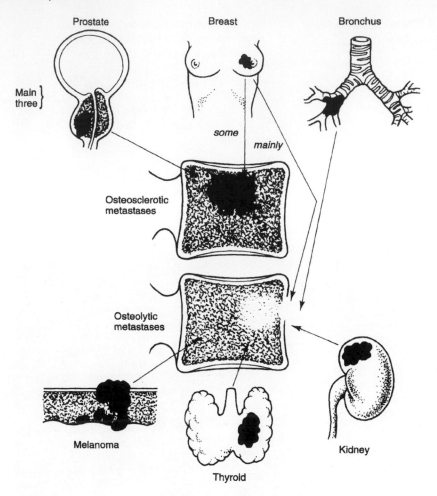

Figure 21.4 Important primary malignancies metastasing to the spine. Note the difference between sclerotic and osteolytic metastases; multiple myeloma also causes osteolytic lesions.

History of injury:	May precipitate problem.
Site and radiation:	Low lumbar Radiates bilaterally or unilaterally into buttocks, hip, thighs and feet.
Type of pain:	Dull ache, episodic depending on activity Onset usually mid-morning after standing.
Associations:	Paraesthesia in legs Stiffness after exercise May be associated discogenic lesion.
Physical examination: (significant)	Stiff waddling gait Increased lumbar lordosis Flexed knee stance Tender prominent SP of 'slipped' vertebra Limited flexion Hamstring tightness or spasm.
Diagnosis confirmation:	Lateral X-ray (standing).

Comment

About 5 per cent of the population have spondylolisthesis but not all are symptomatic. The pain is caused usually be extreme stretching of the interspinous ligaments or of the nerve roots. The onset of back pain in many of these patients is due to a concurrent disc degeneration rather than a mechanical problem.

Ankylosing spondylitis

Age and sex:	Young men 15–30 (rare onset after 40) Women – up to 20 per cent of all cases.
History of injury:	None, unless coincidental Has a slow insidious onset.
Site and radiation:	Low back, may radiate to both buttocks or posterior thighs (rare below knees) Can alternate sides.
Type of pain:	Aching throbbing pain of inflammation Commonly episodic.
Aggravation:	Often worse at night, turning over in bed and arising in the morning.
Relief:	Activity including exercise Patient may walk around during night for relief.
Associations:	Back stiffness especially in morning Pain and stiffness in thoracic or cervical spine. Pain and stiffness in chest cage Peripheral joint pain (up to 50 per cent of cases) Iritis (up to 25 per cent of cases).
Physical examination: (significant)	Absent lumbar lordosis Lateral flexion limited first, then flexion and extension Positive sacro-iliac joint stress tests.
Diagnosis confirmation:	X-ray of pelvis (sacro-iliitis) Bone scans and CT scans ESR usually elevated HLA B27 antigen positive in over 90 per cent of cases.

Comment

Ankylosing spondylitis and other spondyloarthropathies represents an often overlooked cause of low back pain, especially in the younger patient. It is a chronic inflammatory arthropathy of the axial skeleton which usually originates in the sacro-iliac joints; it can also involve the peripheral joints such as the knees and hips, entheses especially around the pelvis, and certain extra-articular structures such as iritis and cardiac lesions. Psoriasis and Reiter's disease have a similar effect on the spine.

The patient's history provides significant clues to differentiate it from other causes of back pain. Five specific features to search for in the diagnosis of this inflammatory disease are:

- insidious onset of low back pain
- morning stiffness (often severe and prolonged)
- onset before the age of 40 (usually before 30)
- pain unrelieved by rest but eased by exercise
- duration of three or more months.

The radiological features are shown in Figure 21.5.

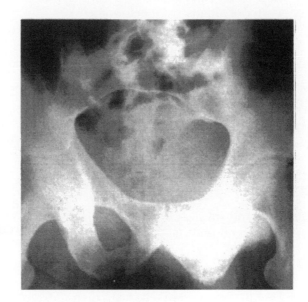

Figure 21.5 Ankylosing spondylitis: X-ray of sacral area showing sclerosis with obliteration of the sacro-iliac joints on the left side and partial fusion on the right side.

The earlier treatment is initiated, the better the outlook for the patient: the prognosis is usually good. The basic objectives of treatment are:

- prevention of spinal fusion in a poor position
- relief of pain and stiffness
- maintenance of optimum spinal mobility.

The basic methods of management are:

- advice on good back care and posture
- exercise programmes to improve the range of movement
- drug therapy, especially tolerated NSAIDs (indomethacin recommended). Sulfasalazine is second line treatment.

Lumbar spondylosis

Age:

Over 50 years
More common with increasing age.

History of injury:

Heavy manual work, trauma to spine – for
example, motor vehicle accident.

Site and radiation:

Low back pain
May radiate to buttocks.

Type of pain:

Dull nagging ache (often constant)
Acute episodes on chronic background.

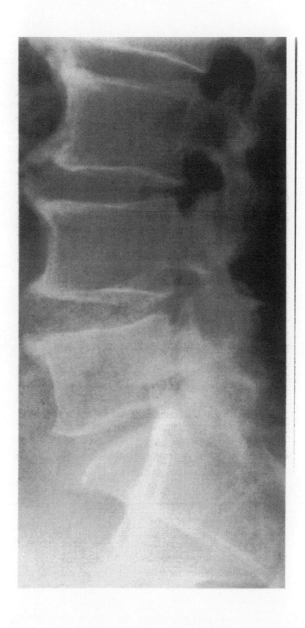

Figure 21.6 Lumbar
spondylosis: X-ray of
lumbosacral spine showing
advanced degenerative
disease.

Aggravation:	Heavy activity, bending Limited tolerance of standing and sitting.
Relief:	Resting by lying straight, gentle exercise, hydrotherapy.
Associations:	Stiffness, especially in mornings Stiffness with immobility Generally good health.
Physical examination:	All movements restricted.
Diagnosis confirmation:	X-ray (Figure 21.6).

Comment

Spondylosis or degenerative arthritis is the term used to describe degenerative or osteoarthritic changes in the spine which cause back pain, although stiffness is the main feature. There are gradual degenerative changes in all aspects of the functional unit – primarily a consequence of intervertebral disc degeneration. With progressive deterioration, subluxation of the apophyseal joints can occur. Subsequent narrowing of the spinal canal and intervertebral foramen (canal) leads to spinal canal stenosis, thus compressing the cauda equina and nerve roots respectively (Figure 21.7).

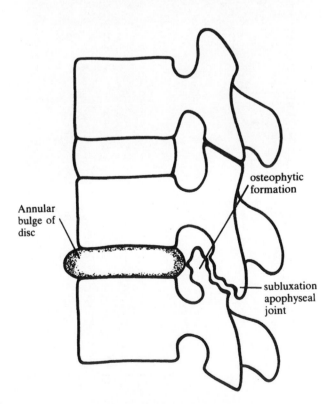

osteophytic formation

Annular bulge of disc

subluxation apophyseal joint

Figure 21.7 Lumbar spondylosis with narrowing of disc space and intervertebral foramen.

Spinal canal stenosis and vascular claudication
(see Chapter 22, p. 342–343)

Degenerative changes in the lumbar spine can result in narrowing of the spinal canal, often at several levels, with cauda equina and nerve root compression, kinking and entrapment (Figure 21.8).

As a rule these patients are free of pain and no abnormalities are found when they are examined at rest.

Depression or other non-organic back pain

Age:	Any age, typical 30–50.
History of injury:	Yes – usually remote in the past; often motor vehicle accident.
Site and radiation:	Low back, central, often bilateral May radiate to leg (may be bizarre pattern).
Type of pain	Variable, usually deep ache or burning Continuous – acute or chronic.
Aggravation:	Work, especially housework, or manual Worse in mornings on waking Stress and worry.

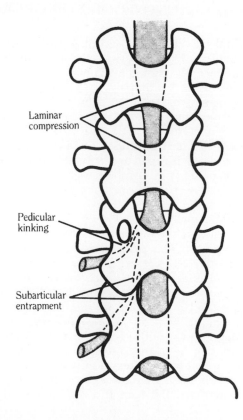

Laminar compression

Pedicular kinking

Subarticular entrapment

Figure 21.8 Illustration of nerve root compression, kinking and entrapment.

Relief:	Better in the evenings and on retiring.
Associations:	Headache Fatigue, exhaustion, tiredness Insomnia, inability to cope Other aches and pains.
Physical examination	Diffuse tenderness to palpation Possible hyperactive reflexes.
Diagnosis confirmed:	Trial of anti-depressants (minimum three weeks).

Comment

Like headache, back pain is a symptom of an underlying functional, organic or psychological disorder. Preoccupation with organic causation of symptoms may lead to serious errors in the assessment of patients with back pain. Any vulnerable aching area of the body is subject to aggravation by emotional factors.

Depressed patients are generally less demonstrative than patients with extreme anxiety and conversion disorders and malingerers, and it is easier to overlook the non-organic basis for their problem.

THE DIAGNOSIS OF NON-ORGANIC BACK PAIN

Failure to consider psychological factors in the assessment of low back pain may lead to serious errors in diagnosis and management. Each instance of back pain poses a stimulating exercise in differential diagnosis. A comparison of organic and non-organic features is presented in Table 21.5.

Assessment of the pain demands a full understanding of the patient. One must be aware of his or her type of work, recreation, successes and failures, and one must relate this information to the degree of incapacity attributed to the back pain.

Patients with psychogenic back pain, especially the very anxious, tend to overemphasise their problem. They are usually demonstrative, the hands being used to point out various painful areas almost without prompting. There is diffuse tenderness even to the slightest touch and the physical disability is out of proportion to the alleged symptoms. The pain distribution is often atypical of any dermatome and the reflexes are almost always hyperactive. It must be remembered that patients with psychogenic back pain – for example, depression and conversion disorders – do certainly experience back pain and do not fall for the traps set for the malingerer.

The problem of malingering with back pain is extremely difficult. Magnuson's method can be very useful. He advises performing the pointing test and seeking areas of tenderness on two occasions separated by an interval of several minutes. He presses randomly over the whole of the lower back, marking the area or areas of specific tenderness. Between the two examinations the patient's attention is

Table 21.5 *Comparison of general clinical features of organic and non-organic based low back pain.*

	ORGANIC DISORDERS	NON-ORGANIC DISORDERS
Symptoms		
Presentation	Appropriate	Often dramatic
Pain	Localised	Bilateral/diffuse Sacrococcygeal
Pain radiation	Appropriate Buttock, specific sites	Inappropriate Front of leg/whole leg
Time pattern	Pain-free times	Constant, acute or chronic
Paraesthesia/ anaesthesia	Dermatomal Points with finger	May be whole leg Shows with hands
Response to treatment	Variable Delayed benefit	Patient often refuses treatment Initial improvement (often dramatic) then deterioration (usually within 24 hours)
Signs		
Observation	Appropriate Guarded	Over-reactive under scrutiny Inconsistent
Tenderness	Localised to appropriate level	Often inappropriate level: Withdraws from probing finger
Spatial tenderness (Magnuson)	Consistent	Inconsistent
Active movements	Specific movements affected	Often all movements affected
Axial loading test	No back pain (usually)	Back pain
SLR 'distraction' test	Consistent	Inconsistent
Sensation	Dermatomal	Non-anatomical: 'sock' or 'stocking'
Motor	Appropriate myotome	Muscle groups, e.g. leg 'collapses'
Reflexes	Appropriate May be depressed	Brisk/hyperactive

diverted from his back by other examinations. The examination of the back is then resumed. In most malingerers the tender areas do not correspond. Various other tests are outlined in Chapter 23.

'A patient who, as a result of a comparatively minor accident, insists that he cannot put on his shoes and socks, but always has this done for him, is seldom genuine.' (Sir Hugh Griffiths)

SUMMARY

Figure 21.9 Chronic back pain: a diagnostic flow chart.

There are several common causes of low back pain, and various manifestations of vertebral joint dysfunction, but familiarisation with

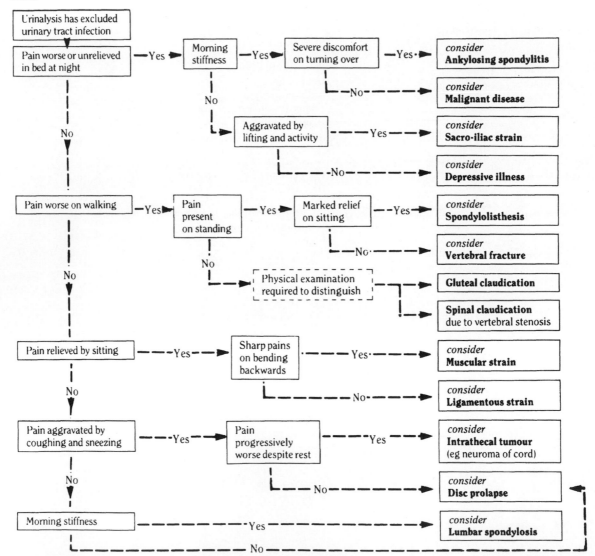

the general clinical features will help the practitioner arrive at the appropriate diagnosis. A diagnostic flow chart for chronic back pain is presented in Figure 21.9.

It is vital to be able to recognise quickly the surgical emergency of spinal cord or cauda equina compression and refer the patient immediately. Distal symptoms and signs and involvement of more than one nerve root should be treated with suspicion since they indicate a serious underlying disorder. It is recommended that the practitioner become familiar with the comparative features of neurogenic and vascular claudication and of organic and non-organic pain.

22
Pain in the buttock, hip and legs

'Which of your hips has the most profound sciatica?'

William Shakespeare (1564–1616)
Measure for Measure

Contents
☐ Key checkpoints
☐ A diagnostic approach
☐ Sacro-iliac pain
☐ Gluteus medius tendinitis and trochanteric bursitis
☐ 'Hip pocket nerve' syndrome
☐ Nerve entrapments
☐ Chronic lower limb ischaemia
☐ Neurogenic versus vascular claudication
☐ Determining the origin of buttock pain
☐ Summary

Pains in the hip, buttock, groin and upper thigh tend to be interrelated. Patients often present complaining of pain in the hip yet are referring to pain in the buttock or lower back.

The spine is the most likely cause of pain in the buttocks in adults.

A major cause of leg pain lies in the source of the nervous network to the lower limb, namely the lumbar and sacral nerve roots of the spine. It is important to recognise radicular pain, especially from L5 and S1 nerve roots, and also the patterns of referred pain such as from apophyseal (facet) joints and sacro-iliac joints.

KEY CHECKPOINTS

● Always consider the lumbosacral spine, the sacro-iliac joints and hip joints as important causes of leg pain.
● Nerve root lesions may cause pain in the lower leg and foot only (without back pain).
● Most pain in the buttock has a lumbosacral origin.
● Pain originating from disorders of the lumbosacral spine (commonly) and the knee (uncommonly) can be referred to

the hip region while pain from the hip joint (L3 innervation) may be referred commonly to the thigh and the knee.

- If a woman, especially one with many children, presents with bilateral buttock or hip pain, consider dysfunction of the sacro-iliac joints as the cause.
- Nerve entrapment is suggested by a radiating burning pain, prominent at night and worse at rest.
- Older people may present with claudication in the leg from spinal canal stenosis or arterial obstruction or both.
- Think of the hip pocket wallet as a cause of sciatica from the buttocks down.
- Acute arterial occlusion to the lower limb requires relief within four hours (absolute limit of six hours).

A DIAGNOSTIC APPROACH

A summary of the diagnostic model is presented in Table 22.1.

Table 22.1 *Pain in the buttock, hip and legs: adult diagnostic strategy model (modified).*

Q. *Probability diagnosis*
A. Lumbosacral spine dysfunction
    referred pain, or
    radicular pain
  Traumatic muscular strains, e.g. hamstring
  Osteoarthritis (hip, knee)

Q. *Serious disorders not to be missed*
A. Cardiovascular
    arterial occlusion (embolism)
    claudication from chronic obstruction
    deep venous thrombosis
  Neoplasia
    metastases, e.g. breast to femur
  Septic infections, e.g. osteomyelitis

Q. *Pitfalls (often missed)*
A. Polymyalgia rheumatica
  Sacro-iliac disorders
  Spinal canal stenosis → claudication
  Herpes zoster (pre-eruption)
  Nerve entrapment
    sciatica 'hip pocket nerve'
    obturator
    lateral cutaneous nerve to thigh
  Bursitis or tendinitis
    gluteus medius tendinitis
    trochanteric bursitis
    ischial bursitis
  Paget's disease

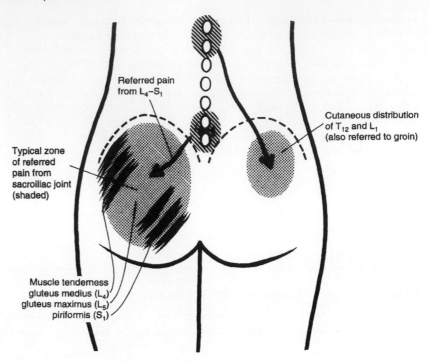

Figure 22.1 Referral patterns of pain from thoracolumbar region, the lumbosacral spine and the sacroiliac joint.

Probability diagnosis

The commonest cause of hip and buttock pain presenting in general practice is referred pain from the lumbosacral spine and the sacro-iliac joints. The pain is invariably referred to the outer buttock and posterior hip area (Fig. 22.1). The origin of the pain can be the facet joints of the lumbar spine (Figure 1.3), intervertebral disc disruption or, less commonly, the sacro-iliac joints.

One of the commonest causes is nerve root pain, invariably single, especially affecting the L5 and S1 nerve roots. Tests of their function and of the lumbosacral spine for evidence of disc disruption or other spinal dysfunction will be necessary. Should multiple nerve roots be involved other causes such as compression from a tumour should be considered. Remember that a spontaneous retroperitoneal haemorrhage in a patient on anti-coagulant therapy can cause nerve root pain and present as intense acute leg pain. The nerve root sensory distribution is presented in Figure 23.34.

Serious disorders not to be missed

Vascular problems

Acute severe ischaemia can be due to thrombosis or embolism of the arteries of the lower limb. Such occlusions cause severe pain in the limb and associated signs of severe ischaemia, especially of the lower leg and foot.

Chronic ischaemia due to arterial occlusion can manifest as intermittent claudication or rest pain in the foot due to small vessel disease.

Aorto-iliac occlusion

Ischaemic muscle pain including buttock claudication secondary to aorto-iliac arterial occlusion is sometimes confused with musculoskeletal pain. An audible bruit over the vessels following exercise is one clue to diagnosis.

Pitfalls

The many disorders of the sacro-iliac joint and hip region can be traps, especially the poorly diagnosed yet common gluteus medius tendinitis. Another more recent phenomenon is the 'hip pocket nerve syndrome', where a heavy wallet crammed with credit cards can cause pressure on the sciatic nerve.

One of the biggest traps, however, is when hip disorders, particularly osteoarthritis, present as leg pain, especially on the medial aspect of the knee.

SACRO-ILIAC PAIN

Pain arising from sacro-iliac joint (SIJ) disorders is normally experienced as a dull ache in the buttock but can be referred to the groin or posterior aspect of the thigh. It may mimic pain from the lumbosacral spine or the hip joint. The pain may be unilateral or bilateral.

There are no accompanying neurological symptoms such as paraesthesia or numbness but it is common for more severe cases to cause a heavy aching feeling in the upper thigh.

Causes and management of sacro-iliac joint pain are outlined in Chapter 25.

GLUTEUS MEDIUS TENDINITIS AND TROCHANTERIC BURSITIS

Pain around the lateral aspect of the hip is a common disorder, and is usually seen as lateral hip pain radiating down the lateral aspect of the thigh in older people engaged in walking exercises, tennis and similar activities. It is analogous in a way to the shoulder girdle, where supraspinatus tendinitis and subacromial bursitis are common wear-and-tear injuries.

The two common causes are tendinitis of the gluteus medius tendon, where it inserts into the lateral surface of the greater trochanter of the femur, and bursitis of one or both of the trochanteric bursae (Figure

28.4). Distinction between these two conditions is difficult, and it is possible that, as with the shoulder, they are related. The pain of bursitis tends to occur at night; that of tendinitis occurs with such activity as long walks and gardening. Treatment is described on page 426.

'HIP POCKET NERVE' SYNDROME

An interesting modern phenomenon is the so-called 'hip pocket nerve' syndrome. If a man presents with 'sciatica', especially confined to the buttock and upper posterior thigh (without local back pain), consider the possibility of pressure on the sciatic nerve from a wallet in the hip pocket. This problem is occasionally encountered in people sitting for long periods in cars (e.g. taxi drivers). It appears to be related to the increased presence of plastic credit cards in wallets (Figure 22.2).

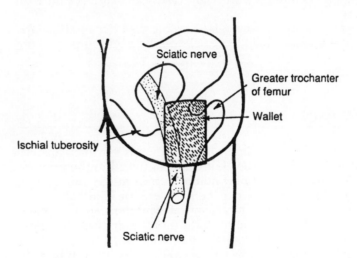

Figure 22.2 'Hip pocket nerve' syndrome: location and relations of sciatic nerve in the buttock.

NERVE ENTRAPMENTS

Nerve entrapments (Figure 22.3) are an interesting cause of leg pain, although not as common as in the upper limb. Some entrapments to consider include:

- lateral cutaneous nerve of thigh, known as meralgia paraesthetica
- common peroneal nerve
- posterior tibial nerve at ankle (the 'tarsal tunnel' syndrome)
- obturator nerve, in obturator canal
- femoral nerve (in inguinal region or pelvis).

Meralgia paraesthetica, which can be easily misdiagnosed, causes pain and paraesthesia over the lateral aspect of the hip.

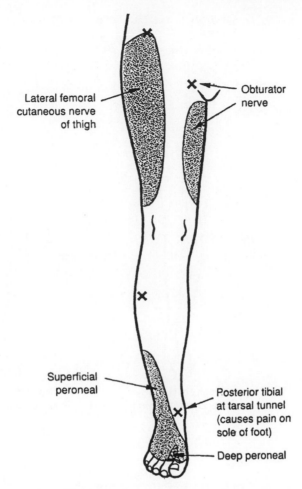

Lateral femoral
cutaneous nerve
of thigh

Obturator
nerve

Superficial
peroneal

Posterior tibial
at tarsal tunnel
(causes pain on
sole of foot)

Deep peroneal

Figure 22.3 Distribution of pain in the leg from various nerve entrapments: the site of entrapment is indicated by an X.

CHRONIC LOWER LIMB ISCHAEMIA

Chronic ischaemia caused by gradual arterial occlusion can manifest as intermittent claudication or rest pain in the foot.

Intermittent claudication

The level of obstruction determines which muscle belly is affected (Figure 22.4).

Proximal obstruction, e.g. aorto-iliac

- Pain in the buttock, thigh and calf, especially when walking up hills and stairs
- Persistent fatigue over whole lower limb
- Impotence is possible (Leriche syndrome).

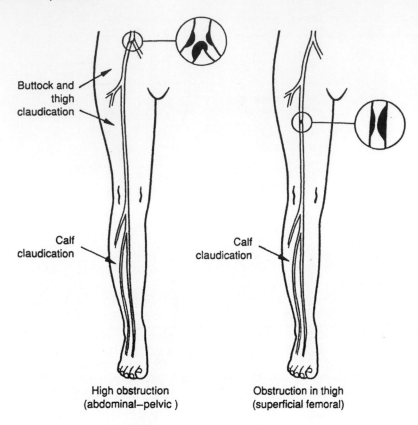

Figure 22.4 Arterial occlusion and related symptoms according to the level of obstruction.

High obstruction (abdominal–pelvic)

Obstruction in thigh (superficial femoral)

Obstruction in the thigh

● Superficial femoral (the commonest) causes pain in the calf, e.g. 200–500 metres
● Profunda femoris → claudication about 100 metres
● Multiple segment involvement → claudication 40–50 metres.

NEUROGENIC VERSUS VASCULAR CLAUDICATION

Patients with spinal canal stenosis are often free of pain at rest but buttock pain and leg pain with weakness are initiated by prolonged standing or walking. These symptoms of neurogenic claudication, which are caused by relative hypoxia of the nerve root trunks of the cauda equina, have to be differentiated from the symptoms of vascular claudication due to obstructive arterial disease (Table 22.2).

The onset of vascular claudication is gradual, with the onset of symptoms following a regular pattern, after walking a similar distance on each occasion. The symptoms of neurogenic claudication vary, often having minimal relationship to the distance walked.

Table 22.2 *Clinical features of neurogenic and vascular claudication.*

	NEUROGENIC CLAUDICATION	VASCULAR CLAUDICATION
Cause	Spinal canal stenosis	Aorto-iliac arterial occlusive disease
Age	Over 50 Long history of back ache	Over 50
Pain site and radiation	Proximal location, initially lumbar, buttocks and legs Radiates distally	Distal location Buttocks, thighs and calves (especially) Radiates proximally
Type of pain	Weakness, burning, numbing or tingling (not cramping)	Cramping, aching, squeezing
Onset	Walking (uphill and downhill) Distance walked varies Prolonged standing Lying with back arched	Walking a set distance each time, especially uphill
Relief	Lying down Flexing spine – e.g. squat position May take 20–30 minutes	Standing still – fast relief Slow walking decreases severity
Associations	Bowel and bladder symptoms	Impotence Rarely, paraesthesia or weakness
Physical examination **Peripheral pulses**	Present	Present (usually) Reduced or absent in some, especially after exercise
Lumbar extension **Neurological**	Aggravates Saddle distribution Ankle jerk may be reduced after exercise	No change
		Note: Abdominal bruits after exercise
Diagnosis confirmation	Radiological studies	Duplex ultrasound Arteriography

The symptoms of vascular claudication cease rapidly when the patient stands still, but with neurogenic claudication it is usually necessary for the patient to lie down to relieve the pain. With the latter problem the patient can continue to walk by leaning forward to reduce the lumbar lordosis and enlarge the spinal and intervertebral canals.

DETERMINING THE ORIGIN OF BUTTOCK PAIN

Clinically it can be very difficult to determine the cause of buttock pain. One practical method is to examine by palpation the tissue layers of the buttock to determine the origin of the tissue pain.

The tissues involved are the skin, muscle and periosteum. At any one region in the buttock these three tissues can have different innervation levels from the spine. It is practical to palpate the skin and muscle.

Method of examination

Skin

Pick up a roll of skin (over the painful area of the buttock) between the thumb and index finger. Using a gentle yet controlled firmness pinching method roll the skin (Figure 22.5). A positive test is if this pinch/roll effect is very painful (it should be compared with the other side) and a skin 'flare' is reproduced.

Interpretation

A positive test indicates that the dermatome is involved. The spine from T10 to L1 on the painful side should be examined to determine a dysfunctional level.

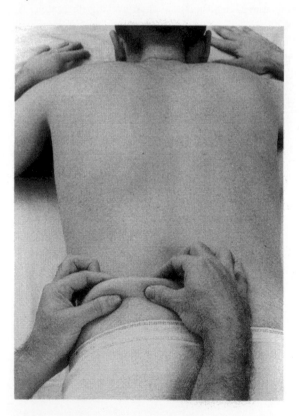

Figure 22.5 The pinch/roll test for increased skin sensitivity at the level of the iliac crest.

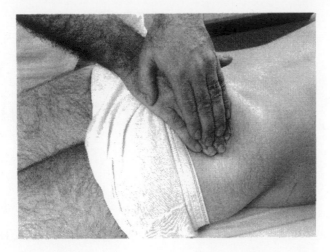

Figure 22.6 Deep palpation over the buttock to detect tender and/or taut muscle bands.

Muscle

In this method palpate deeper to feel for trigger points or, more importantly, taut muscle bands. Use one hand for palpation and an overlying hand for reinforcement and pressure (Figure 22.6).

Interpretation

A positive test indicates myotomal dysfunction with innervation from L4, L5 or S1. The lower lumbar spine should be examined.

Summary

If a patient presents with pain in the buttock or adjacent areas it is likely that the origin of the pain is the lumbosacral spine or even the thoracolumbar region of the spine. The physical examination should cover these areas. Dysfunction or arthritis of the sacroiliac joints which can also refer pain into the buttocks should be considered in grand-multiparous women and young people respectively presenting with pain in this region.

23
Examination of the lumbosacral spine

'A patient who, as a result of a comparatively minor accident, insists that he cannot put on his shoes and socks, but always has to have this done for him, is seldom genuine.'

Sir Hugh Griffiths

Contents
- ☐ Key checkpoints
- ☐ Inspection
- ☐ Movements
- ☐ Provocation tests
- ☐ Palpation
- ☐ Measurements
- ☐ The neurological examination
- ☐ Tests for non-organic back pain
- ☐ Examination of other joints
- ☐ Practice tips
- ☐ Summary

There is a logical progression to the examination of the lumbosacral complex, a procedure which can be performed quickly.

The examiner must follow the time-honoured rule for the examination of any joint: look, feel, move, measure and X-ray. When the back is involved, a neurological examination is important if radicular pain is present; or if pain or paraesthesia extends below the buttock.

Findings may be recorded on a chart such as that shown in Figure 2.8.

The three objectives of the examination are:

- to reproduce the patient's symptoms
- detect the level of the lesion
- determine its cause (if possible).

The physical examination is the foundation on which effective treatment is based. The reasons for the importance of this examination from the viewpoint of manual therapy are summarised in Table 23.1.

It begins from the moment the patient is sighted in the waiting room. A patient who is noted to be standing in preference to sitting is likely to have a significant disc lesion. Considerable information can be obtained

Table 23.1 *Manipulation and the importance of the physical examination.*

OBJECTIVE	REASON
Determine level of lesion	Provide specific mobilisation or manipulation
Determine irritability and nerve root signs	If positive, mobilisation is preferable to manipulation
Determine dural signs	Manipulate or mobilise with care
Determine neurological damage	Manipulation contra-indicated

from the manner in which the patient arises from a chair and moves into the consulting room. The patient who carefully removes slip-on shoes, with the spine straight and knees flexed, is a different picture from the patient who casually bends over with the spine flexed to unlace the shoes. Observing the patient when he or she is unaware of being watched is useful in establishing the nature of the complaint.

KEY CHECKPOINTS

- The key objectives are to reproduce the patient's symptoms and to detect the level of the lesion.
- Knowing the surface anatomy is the key to identifying the correct anatomical level of the lesion.
- The top of the iliac crests lie opposite the L4 spinous process or the L4–L5 intervertebral disc.
- If the pain cannot be reproduced on active movement, apply passive overpressure or a provocative test such as the quadrant test.
- The neurological examination should be performed only if symptoms are present in the lower limbs.
- The L5 and S1 nerve roots are the roots almost exclusively affected by disc lesions of the lumbar spine.
- The examination of the sacro-iliac joints and hips must not be overlooked if pain in the pelvic or buttock area is present.

INSPECTION

The spine must be adequately exposed and inspected in good light. Patients should undress to their underpants; women may retain their brassiere and it is proper to provide them with a gown that opens down the back. Note the general contour and symmetry of the back and legs, including the buttock folds, and look for muscle wasting. Note the lumbar lordosis and any abnormalities such as lateral deviation. If

Table 23.2 *Inspection checklist.*

OBSERVATION	SIGNIFICANCE
Lateral deviation/scoliosis	Congenital/structural Compensatory; unequal leg length Protective: ● ipsilateral or contralateral (most common) ● disc prolapse (if severe, suggests L4–L5 disc) ● apophyseal joint syndrome
Lumbar lordosis ● increased	Sway back Weak anterior abdominal wall Spondylolisthesis
● absent or decreased (flattened spine)	Paravertebral muscle spasm Disc degeneration
Lumbar insufficiency (pelvis moves under trunk)	Segmental instability Hypermobility
Lateral tilt of pelvis	Unequal leg length
Unequal leg length	Congenital variation Stress on hip joint on long side
Movements on and off couch	If incongruous might be non-organic
Muscle wasting and fasciculation	Lower motor neurone lesion Nerve root pressure

lateral deviation (scoliosis) is present it is usually away from the painful side.

An inspection checklist is presented in Table 23.2. Anatomical landmarks should be noted and include the iliac crest, spinous processes, the sacrum, posterior superior iliac spines (PSIS), the erector spinae (Figures 23.1 and 23.2). Note the presence of midline moles, tufts of hair or haemangioma that might indicate an underlying congenital anomaly such as spina bifida occulta.

MOVEMENTS

With all movements, determine the range and quality of active movement, the 'end feel', muscle spasm and any onset or increase in pain. It is most important that the patient actively extends the movements as far as possible. Record each range of movement on the DOM diagram.

The movements to test are:

1. *Extension*: perform first (normal range 20–30 degrees).
2. *Lateral flexion*: left first, then right side (30 degrees each way).
3. *Flexion*: normal range 75–90 degrees (average 80 degrees).
4. *Rotation*: left then right.

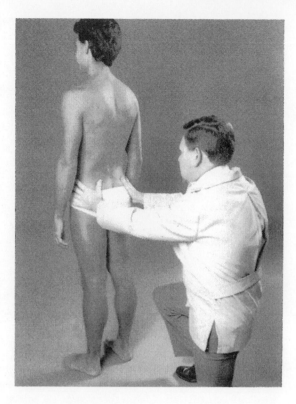

Figure 23.1 Inspection of the lumbar spine.

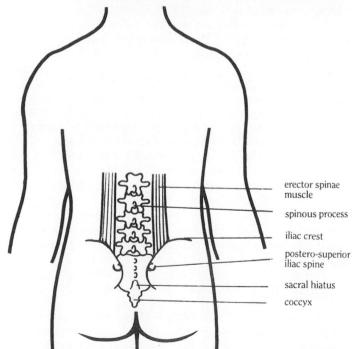

erector spinae
muscle

spinous process

iliac crest

postero-superior
iliac spine

sacral hiatus

coccyx

Figure 23.2 Important landmarks of the lumbosacral spine.

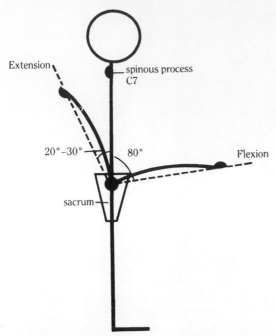

Figure 23.3 Illustration of degrees of movement of the lumbar spine: flexion and extension.

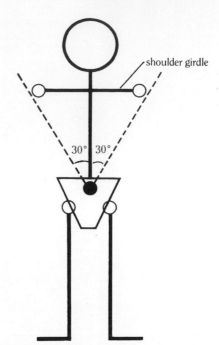

Figure 23.4 Illustration of the degree of lateral flexion of the lumbar spine.

Measurement of the angle of movement can be made by using a line drawn between the sacrum and the large vertebral prominence of C7 (Figures 23.3 and 23.4). If the movement (direction) is pain-free then *gentle* overpressure is applied to test fully that particular direction of movement.

Extension

Perform this first. Kneel behind the patient and observe the point on the spine at which extension originates (Figure 23.5). Note the movement in relation to the painful site. Does the patient extend through the painful area or does the movement originate from above that area? Note any restriction of movement. The usual range of movement is 20–30 degrees. If there is no restriction, apply gentle overpressure to ensure that the patient is not stopping short of pain (Figure 23.6). Extension is often the stiffest and most painful movement with lumbar problems. With discogenic lesions, hyperextension is often more painful than flexion.

Lateral flexion

Lateral flexion or side bending is also a significant movement to test. Test the left side first (Figure 23.7). Ask the patient to slide the fingers down the leg. Note if the movement occurs through the level of the pain.

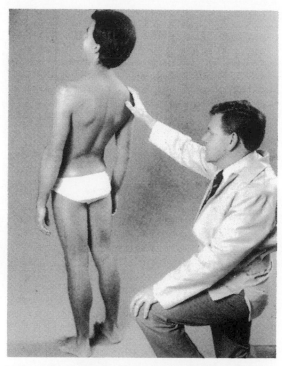

Figure 23.5 Extension of the lumbar spine.

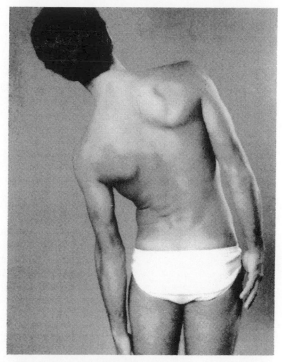

Figure 23.7 Left lateral flexion.

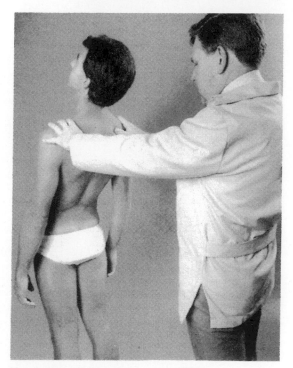

Figure 23.6 Overpressure into extension.

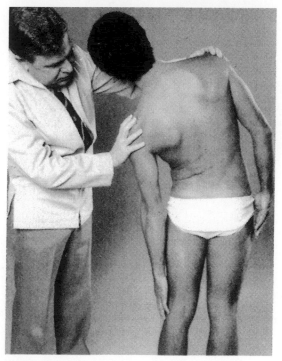

Figure 23.8 Overpressure into left lateral flexion.

When at full active range, apply gentle overpressure (Figure 23.8) to check if the patient is stopping short of pain. The normal range of movement is approximately 30 degrees. All serious diseases of the lumbar spine (such as malignancy and ankylosing spondylitis) result in an equal limitation of left and right lateral movements. With disc lesions it is common to have restriction to one side and normal range in the other side.

Perform the same test for the right side and apply overpressure if necessary.

Flexion

Forward flexion (Figure 23.9) is an important movement and one most likely to be limited by a disc lesion. Ask the patient to bend over slowly; warn the patient not to bend over forcefully to touch the toes. Note the level at which lumbar flexion originates and note its relationship to the painful level. Normally the lumbar area moves and is 'flattened' during flexion. Lack of movement in this area is abnormal.

If there is restriction, record the degree. If pain is not produced, apply gentle overpressure (Figure 23.10) to try and provoke the patient's pain. This is the movement that patients usually complain about as being painful and restricted. It is inevitably reduced if there is

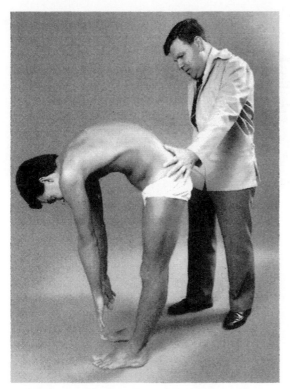

Figure 23.9 Flexion of the lumbar spine.

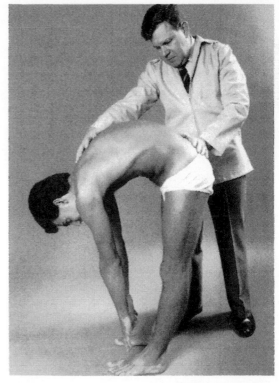

Figure 23.10 Overpressure into flexion.

nerve root compression from a disc prolapse. The normal range varies from 75 to 90 degrees, with an average of 80 degrees.

Rotation

There is no significant rotation of the lumbar spine but it is a useful test for the patient with non-organic back pain (for example, in depression).

While the patient sits on the couch, examine for pain by rotating the trunk to the left and right (Figure 23.11). Patients with marked restriction in other directions can usually demonstrate a good range of rotation. It is a function of the thoracic spine.

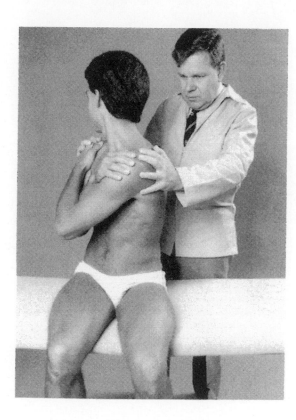

Figure 23.11 Testing for rotation.

PROVOCATION TESTS

The quadrant test

If the preceding active movements fail to reproduce the patient's pain, the quadrant test is a useful compressive provocation test designed to determine if the origin of the pain is truly in the lumbar spine. It places a greater stress on the articular pillar of apophyseal joints, the posterior and lateral wall of the disc and the posterior longitudinal ligament.

The first step in this test is to stand behind the patient, place a hand on each shoulder and extend the lumbar spine to its limit. Ensure that the patient does not bend the knees. Now apply overpressure and add lateral flexion (side bending) towards the painful side.

The next step is to rotate the spine to the same side. When the limit of range is reached (Figure 23.12) hold the position for 20 seconds to allow for a delayed response. This applies especially for peripheral symptoms. The test is positive if pain is reproduced.

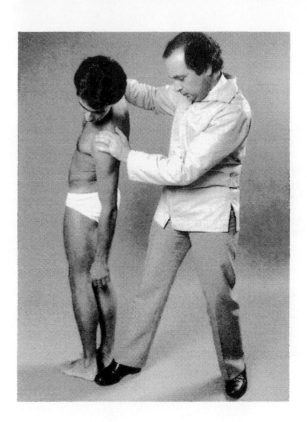

Figure 23.12 The quadrant test: rotation superimposed on extension and lateral flexion.

The slump test

The slump test is a very useful screening test for a disc lesion and dural tethering because it stretches the dura from above and below, via the sciatic nerve. It indirectly stresses the posterior and lateral walls of the spinal canal, including the posterior longitudinal ligament.

It is performed on the patient who has low back pain with or without leg pain, especially if leg pain includes posterior thigh pain.

The slump test is positive if the back or leg pain complained about by the patient is reproduced. At the end of each progressive step (1 to 5 below) any reproduction of pain is noted. As soon as pain is reproduced the hamstring status is evaluated and the test then ceased.

Method

- The patient sits on the couch in a relaxed manner.
- The patient slumps forward without excessively flexing the trunk (Figure 23.13). The test is negated by excessive flexion of the back from the lumbar area.
- The patient now places the chin on the chest (Figure 23.14). Ask the patient if the pain is reproduced.
- The patient now straightens the unaffected leg (the leg on the side opposite the pain) (Figure 23.15).
- The patient is now asked to straighten the affected leg so that both legs are straightened (Figure 23.16). Note how this will provoke hamstring tightness. If no pain is reproduced, hold in this position for 20 seconds to allow for a delayed response.
- Finally, if the pain is not reproduced, added stretching of the dura can be achieved by dorsiflexion of the foot on the affected side (Figure 23.17).

Differential diagnosis

If pain in the thigh is reproduced, particularly during step 4, the problem could be in the lumbosacral spine or the hamstring.

To establish the cause, maintain this position and then ask the patient to extend the head (Figure 23.18). If the pain disappears it is probably of spinal origin. If it persists, it is likely to be due to a hamstring problem.

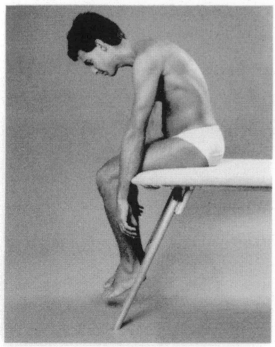

Figure 23.13 The slump test 1: patient slumps forward.

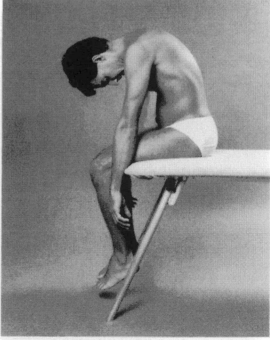

Figure 23.14 The slump test 2: patient places chin on chest.

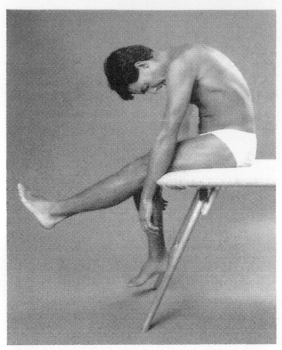

Figure 23.15 The slump test 3: patient straightens unaffected leg.

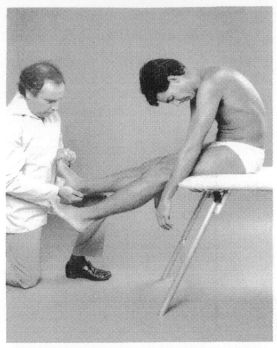

Figure 23.17 The slump test 5: dorsiflexion of foot of affected leg.

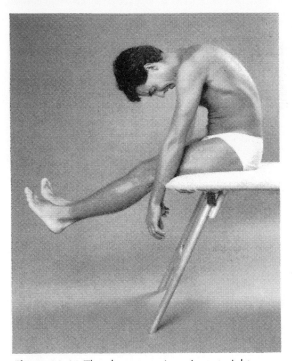

Figure 23.16 The slump test 4: patient straightens both legs.

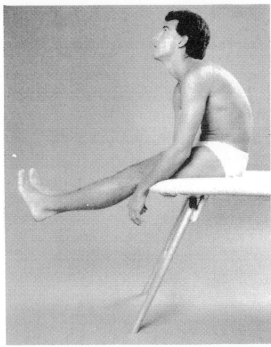

Figure 23.18 The slump test 6: patient extends head to differentiate between pain of dural origin and hamstrings.

Significance of slump test

- It is positive if the back or leg pain is reproduced.
- It is positive for dural pressure if the hamstring accessory test (deflexing the neck) relieves the reproduced pain.
- If positive, one should approach manual therapy with caution.
- If negative, it *may* indicate lack of serious disc pathology or dural tethering.

PALPATION

Palpation is the essential component of the manual medicine examination. A working knowledge of the anatomical structures and surface anatomy of the structure being palpated is a prerequisite for the procedure, which has two objectives:

1. to apply this knowledge to correctly (a) determine the level of the lesion; (b) detect abnormalities in bone structures (such as spina bifida and spondylolisthesis); and
2. to establish the nature of the problem (pain, stiffness or muscle spasm).

Surface anatomy

It is essential to develop a clear picture of exactly what one is feeling or palpating and, using a logical sequence, to build up a picture of the bony landmarks of the lumbosacral region.

1. Determine the L4 and L5 levels

Method

The patient must be relaxed, lying prone, with the head to one side and arms by the sides. Standing behind the patient, place your fingers on the top of the iliac crests and your thumbs at the same level on the midline of the back, at the level of the fourth and fifth lumbar disc interspace (Figure 23.19).

The iliac crests lie at the same level of the fourth and fifth lumbar interspace (Figure 23.20) or slightly higher at the fourth lumbar spinous process. Mark this important reference point and then mark out the spinous processes of the five lumbar vertebrae, especially those of L4 and L5. Remember that most lumbar problems originate from the L4, L5 and S1 levels.

2. Determine the PSIS and S2 level

Palpate (and feel) the posterosuperior iliac spines (PSIS) and the S2 spinous process which lies on the line between the two PSISs (Figures 23.21 and 23.22).

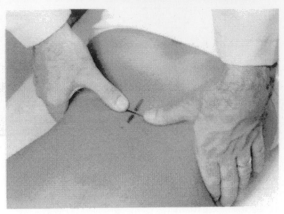

Figure 23.19 Palpation: determining the L4–L5 interspace.

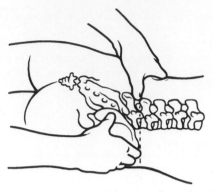

Figure 23.20 Illustration of the main bony landmarks of the lumbosacral area and palpation of the L4–L5 interspace which lies at the same level of the tops of the iliac crests.

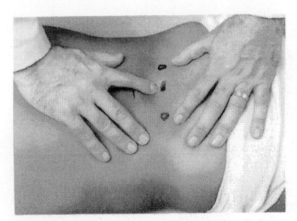

Figure 23.21 Palpation: determining the level of S2 by palpation of the PSISs.

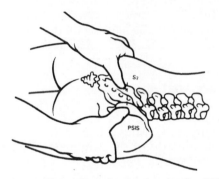

Figure 23.22 Illustration of palpation for the PSISs and the S2 spinous process.

Palpation of the vertebrae

The objectives of palpation are:

● to determine the level of the lesion
● to reproduce the pain.

Hence it is necessary to look for:

● irritability
● provocation of pain (in back or legs)
● maximum tenderness
● a sense of resistance
● muscular spasm.

With practice it is possible to appreciate small differences in ranges of movement, end feel and resistance.

Method

- The palpation of the vertebrae should ideally commence at L1 and systematically proceed distally to L5 and then over the sacrum and coccyx if applicable. By starting superiorly it is possible to obtain an appreciation of movement (joint play) before reaching the symptomatic level (usually L4 and L5).
- There are various techniques of palpation that can be used but the two methods that are recommended are the use of the tips of the thumbs or the pisiform prominence of the wrist as the presenting part of the examiner's hand. Some examiners prefer the pads of the tips of the thumbs or the tips of the index and middle fingers, but the preferred method of these two is the use of the thumbs either side by side (preferably) (Figure 23.23), or with one thumb on top of the other.
- Since the thumbs tend to slide off the tips of the spinous processes, some examiners prefer to use the pisiform using the grip as illustrated in Figure 23.24. The authors recommend the use of the pisiform palpatory method for central palpation over the spinous processes and the application of the thumbs for interspinous central, unilateral and transverse palpation.

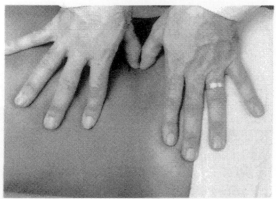

Figure 23.23 Palpating the spinous processes centrally. The thumbs move the vertebrae ventrally in a postero-anterior gliding movement.

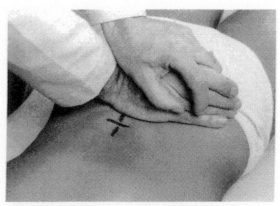

Figure 23.24 Palpating the spinous processes using the pisiform prominence of the hand.

- If the continued use of the pisiform method is uncomfortable, the presenting part can be shifted slightly (about 1 to 2 cm) so that the softer base of the hypothenar eminence over the base of the fifth metacarpal is applied to the spinous processes. However, it is important not to lose sensitivity of touch for palpation.
- Always use light or gentle pressure initially. Firmer pressure is used if the lighter pressure does not reproduce the patient's symptoms.

Golden rule: The harder one presses, the less one feels.

Talk to the patient

Explain to the patient that you want to 'find out where the pain is coming from' and that you want him or her to indicate if and when you reach the level that brings on the pain.

The three main sites for palpation

1. *Central palpation.* With central palpation, the thumbs or pisiform are firmly applied to the spinous processes which are then gently moved with a rocking movement into a postero-anterior glide (Figure 23.23). The initial movement therefore is to push the vertebra forwards (anteriorly) in relation to the others. After this, palpate in the interspinous spaces with the tips of the thumbs.

2. *Unilateral palpation.* After palpating the spinous processes, move laterally a thumb's breadth (from where the thumb lies adjacent to the spinous processes) and gently palpate, systematically and on both sides at each corresponding level (to the spinous processes) (Figure 23.25). The same postero-anterior glide is imparted and any reproduction of pain in the underlying soft tissue is noted. Although it is claimed that one is exerting pressure over the transverse process, it does appear that the pain is more likely to be reproduced by compressing a myofascial trigger zone in the adjacent segment of the muscle (erector spinae). This is a consequence of a stiff and tender spinal segment. Furthermore, pressure is being imparted over the apophyseal joints and disorders of these joints may be indirectly detected by this unilateral method.

3. *Transverse pressure to the spinous processes.* With this technique, pressure is applied to the side of the spinous process, which produces a degree of rotation of the vertebrae. This appears to be a very sensitive movement for detecting pain in a restricted segment; it quickly localises the problem and for many practitioners is the preferred method of palpation.

   The thumbs or fingers are placed firmly against the side of each spinous process and a gentle rhythmic pressure applied (Figure 23.26)

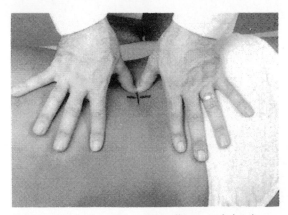

Figure 23.25 Palpating unilaterally at each lumbar level.

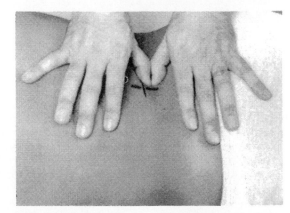

Figure 23.26 Palpation by transverse pressure to the side of the spinous process of a lumbar vertebra.

with the direction angulated downwards towards the opposite side. This method is illustrated in Figure 16.15.

The process is repeated on each side (right and left) of the spine.

Note: The transverse pressure method will often indicate which is the symptomatic side of the pain, even in the presence of central pain.

If this method produces pain, the painful lesion is on the side from which the palpation is performed. For example, if palpation on the left side of the L4 spinous process produced pain, the problem lies on that side (the left side).

MEASUREMENT

Thigh and calf circumference

Sometimes it is necessary to test for muscle atrophy in the thighs and calves by measuring the circumference at a fixed reference point in both limbs.

To measure the circumference of the thighs, measure 15 cm from the superior pole of the patella of both legs and then place the tape measure around the thighs and compare the measurements.

For the leg, use the tibial plateau as a reference point and measure 15 to 16 cm distally with the tape measure. Compare both sides.

Leg length

Observation of the patient may indicate inequality of leg length. Apparent and real leg length should be measured. Invariably the real leg lengths are found to be equal – a fact which can be very reassuring to the patient, who may have been informed otherwise.

THE NEUROLOGICAL EXAMINATION

A neurological examination is performed only when the patient's symptoms, such as pain, paraesthesia, anaesthesia and weakness, extend into the leg.

The importance of the neurological examination is to ensure that there is no compression of the spinal nerves from a prolapsed disc or from a tumour. This is normally tested by examining those functions that the respective spinal nerves serve, namely skin sensation, muscle power and reflex activity.

The examination is not daunting but can be performed quickly and efficiently in two to three minutes by a methodical technique that improves with continued use.

The neurological examination consists of:

1. Quick tests
   - walking on heels (L5)
   - walking on toes (S1)
2. Dural stretch tests
   - slump test
   - straight leg raising (SLR)

3. Specific nerve root tests (L4, L5, S1)
   - sensation
   - power
   - reflexes.

Table 23.3 summarises important clinical signs that can be elicited during the examination, giving the typical responsible nerve root and the disc level where the disc lesion usually originates.

Table 23.3 *Typical nerve root and responsible disc lesion for various clinical signs.*

SIGN	NERVE ROOT	TYPICAL DISC LEVEL
Femoral nerve stretch test (positive)	L3	L2–L3
Marked lateral deviation of spine	L5	L4–L5
Crossover sign	L5	L4–L5
Weakness walking on heels	L5	L4–L5
Weakness walking on toes	S1	L5–S1

Sensory changes usually follow the dermatomes but if a 'glove and stocking' type sensory loss is found, causes such as peripheral neuropathy (caused by alcohol, diabetes and other disorders) and non-organic disorders have to be considered. The lower sacral nerve roots mainly supply the perineum.

Quick tests

These two tests will quickly help estimate whether the patient has a serious motor disorder of L5 or S1 or both.

Walking on the heels

A good screening test for the integrity of the L5 nerve root is to request the patient to walk a reasonable distance (for example, twice or three times the length of a consulting room of reasonable size) on his or her heels (Figure 23.27). Note dorsiflexion of the great toe. If this can be managed normally without fatigue, then a major weakness of L5 can be excluded. If foot drop is present, the patient cannot walk on the heels.

Walking on the toes

Similarly, assessing the ability of the patient to walk on the toes will test the integrity of the S1 nerve root (Figure 23.28). A flopping foot indicates weakness of the nerve root.

The straight leg raising (SLR) test

The SLR test is a passive test performed by the practitioner up to 75 degrees. The straight leg raising, which should be performed slowly,

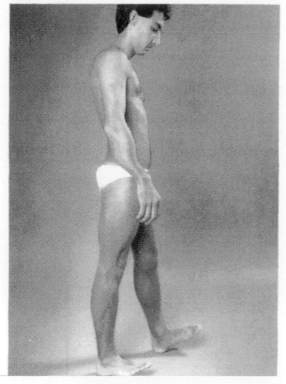

Figure 23.27 Walking on the heels test for L5 motor power.

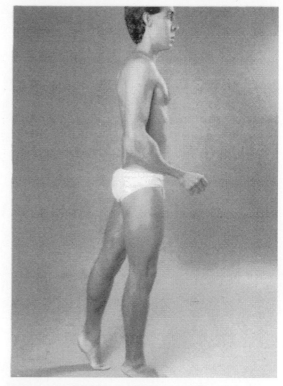

Figure 23.28 Walking on the toes test for S1 motor power.

pulls the nerve root downwards, which, if the nerve root is under tension, will provoke leg pain.

If the test reproduces pain in the back and causes radiation of pain down the leg along the course of the sciatic nerve, it is positive and indicates nerve root tension in the lumbosacral spine.

Method

- First lift the leg and slightly internally rotate it.
- Then raise the leg passively and slowly with the knee extended (Figure 23.29).
- Test for limitation by pain, on both sides (Figure 23.30).
- If forced dorsiflexion of foot increases pain, dural involvement is confirmed (Figures 23.31 and 23.32).
- If neck flexion increases pain, dural involvement is again confirmed (stretches dura upwards by 3 cm).
- The contralateral SLR test is performed by raising the 'good leg' (Figure 23.33). It may reproduce pain (sciatic radiation) in the opposite leg in the presence of a large central disc protrusion (usually L4) when the dura is stretched to the extent that a contralateral lesion can be 'triggered'. This is called the 'crossover' sign. It is recommended that SLR is performed on the pain-free leg first.

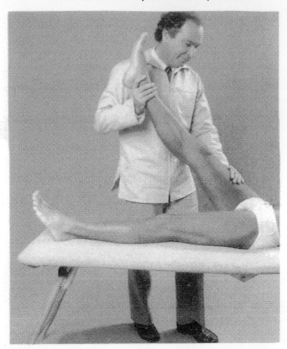

Figure 23.29 The straight leg raising test: raise the leg to the point of discomfort (maximum to 75°).

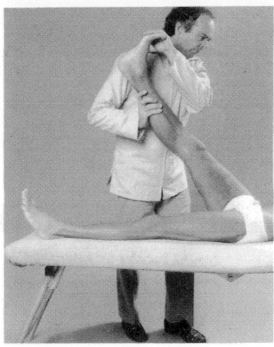

Figure 23.31 The straight leg raising test – forced ankle dorsiflexion: this causes further painful sciatic stretching.

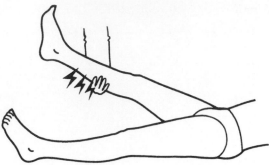

Figure 23.30 Diagrammatic representation of how the SLR reproduces pain that is more severe in the leg than in the back in the presence of nerve root entrapment.

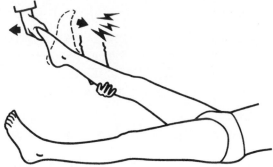

Figure 23.32 Diagrammatic representation of how forced dorsiflexion of the ankle increases the pain due to further sciatic stretching; plantar flexion relieves the pain.

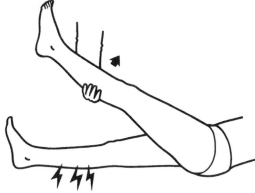

Figure 23.33 The contralateral SLR. Raising the 'good' leg can cause sciatic radiation of pain in the opposite 'painful' leg by stretching the dura sufficiently to 'trigger' contralateral pain. It usually signifies a large L4–L5 disc prolapse.

Significance of the SLR test

- It is an excellent sign of dural irritation by a lumbar disc protrusion.
- It places a varying degree of tension on each of the lumbosacral roots in their dural sleeves from L4 to S2 but especially S1.
- The test is positive if it reproduces the patient's back pain or, especially, pain in the sciatic nerve.
- The test is negative if pain is not produced before 75 degrees of hip flexion, since further flexion may rotate the back and cause pain.
- If limited to 30 degrees or less, entrapment of nerve roots by disc pathology is indicated.
- A negative test is rare in the presence of a lumbar disc protrusion but is possible.

Individual nerve roots

The main nerve roots to test are L4, L5 and S1. When testing muscle power and reflexes, it is important to look for unusual fatigue. Elicit the reflex six times, to test for fatigue, and always compare both sides.

The dermatomes for the lower limb are presented in Figure 23.34 and this should provide a ready reference for the practitioner.

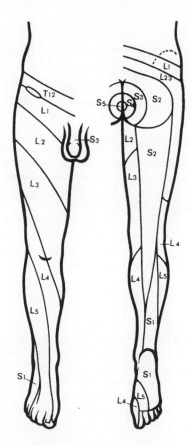

Figure 23.34 Dermatomes of the lower limb representing approximate cutaneous distribution of the nerve roots.

Table 23.4 *Nerve root syndromes.*

NERVE ROOT	PAIN DISTRIBUTION	SENSORY LOSS	MOTOR WEAKNESS CHANGES	REFLEX
L3	Front of thigh, inner aspect of thigh, knee and leg	Anterior aspect of thigh	Extension of knee	Knee jerk
L4	Anterior thigh to front of knee	Lower inner aspect of thigh and knee, inner great toe	Flexion, adduction of knee	Knee jerk
L5	Lateral aspect of leg, dorsum of foot and great toe	Dorsum of foot, great toe, 2nd and 3rd toes, anterolateral aspect of lower leg	Dorsiflexion of great toe	Tibialis posterior (clinically impractical)
S1	Buttock to back of thigh and leg, lateral aspect of ankle and foot	Lateral aspect of ankle, foot (4th and 5th toes)	Plantar flexion of ankle and toes, eversion of foot	Ankle jerk

A summary of the main clinical features of the lumbosacral nerve root syndromes is presented in Table 23.4.

Fourth lumbar

Test the strength of the tibialis anterior by resisting inversion of the foot while it is held in dorsiflexion and inversion (Figure 23.35).

Test the knee jerk to assess whether it is normal, diminished or absent (Figure 23.36).

Test for sensory loss over the inner ankle and medial side of the forefoot (Figure 23.37) down to the outside of the big toe. The L4 root supplies the skin over the medial aspect of the lower leg extending over the ankle and sometimes extends to the inner aspect of the big toe.

Fifth lumbar

Test the strength of the extensor hallucis longus by resisting extension of the great toe with the thumb pressed against the nail of the toe (Figure 23.38). Both sides should be compared, so it is necessary to perform this test on both big toes simultaneously.

Test for sensory loss over the dorsum of the foot, especially the second and third toes.

Ask the patient to walk on the heels of the feet (Figure 23.27). Inability to perform this normally represents weakness of this nerve root.

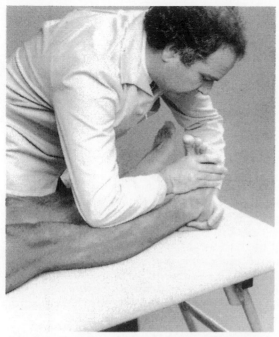

Figure 23.35 Motor testing L4: testing the strength of tibialis anterior by resisting inversion of the foot.

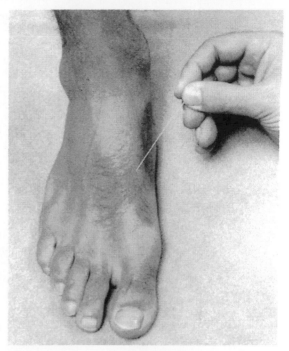

Figure 23.37 Sensory testing L4: test for sensation by pin prick over the medial ankle and forefoot.

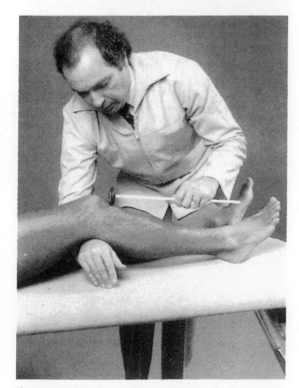

Figure 23.36 Reflex testing L4: testing the knee jerk.

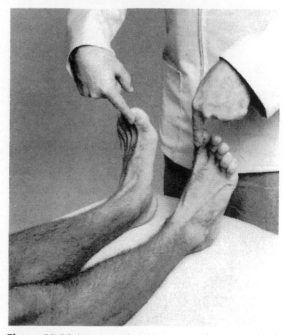

Figure 23.38 Motor testing L5: testing the strength of extensor hallux with the thumb or index finger against the nails bilateral. Compare the strength and look for fatigue.

Testing a suitable reflex for the L5 nerve root is not an easy clinical task as it is difficult to elicit. The tibialis posterior provides an L5 reflex but it is very slight and inconsistent. However, if there is some doubt about the presence of the L5 nerve root, the tibialis reflex should be elicited. The method is to hold the ankle in eversion and tap the tendon of tibialis posterior just behind the medial malleolus (or just before it inserts into the navicular bone of the foot). A positive response (which is slight) indicates inversion of the ankle.

First sacral

Test the strength of the peroneus longus and brevis by opposing eversion of the foot while it is plantar flexed and everted (Figure 23.39).

Test the Achilles tendon reflex (ankle jerk) by asking the patient to kneel on a chair and grasp the back of it firmly (Figure 23.40). Test for sensory loss over the lateral malleolus, the fourth and fifth toes, especially the fifth toe and the sole of the foot (if necessary). Patients with an S1 lesion may complain that it hurts to walk on the feet.

Note whether the finding of the walking on the toes test (Figure 23.28) matches these tests.

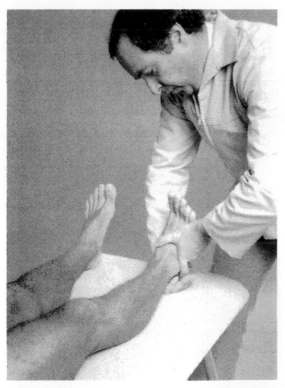

Figure 23.39 Motor testing S1: testing the strength of peroneus longus and brevis by resisting eversion.

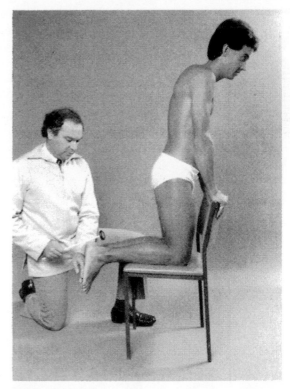

Figure 23.40 Reflex testing S1: testing the ankle jerk.

The femoral nerve stretch

With the knee flexed to 90 degrees, passively extend the hip. This places tension on the femoral nerve roots, especially the lumbar third, and will reproduce the patient's pain (Figure 23.41).

Plantar reflex test

With the patient's leg extended, use a blunt instrument to stimulate the lateral border of the sole of the foot, moving from the heel towards the little toe (Figure 23.42).

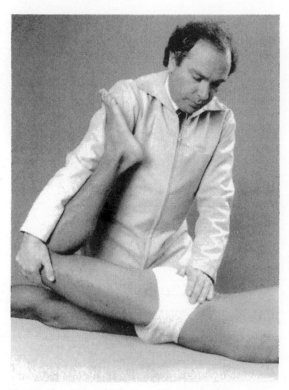

Figure 23.41 The femoral nerve stretch test.

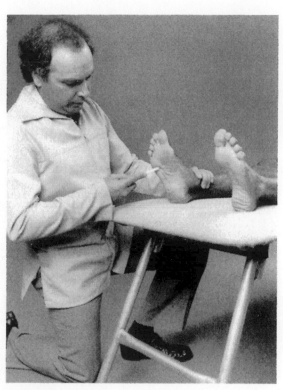

Figure 23.42 The plantar reflex test.

Plantar flexion is a normal response but dorsiflexion (a positive 'Babinski' response) is pathological and indicates spinal cord injury (upper motor neurone lesion).

TESTS FOR NON-ORGANIC BACK PAIN

A series of tests is useful in the differentiation of organic and non-organic back pain (for example, that in the depressed or malingering patient).

Magnuson's method (the 'migratory pointing' test)

Request the patient to point to the painful sites. Palpate these areas of tenderness on two occasions separated by an interval of several minutes and compare the sites. (Between the two tests divert the patient's attention from his or her back by another examination.)

Axial loading

Place your hands over the patient's head and press firmly downward. Few patients whose lumbar pain is organic will suffer discomfort (Figure 23.43).

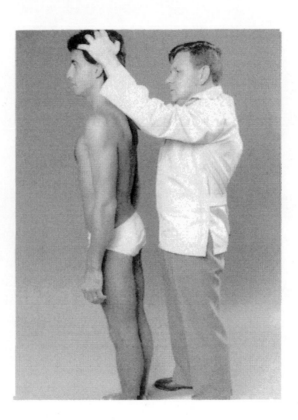

Figure 23.43 The axial loading test.

Hip and shoulder rotation

Examine for pain by rotating the patient's hips and shoulders while the feet are kept in place on the floor. The manoeuvre usually is painless for patients with an organic back disorder (Figure 23.11).

Kneeling on a stool

Ask the patient to kneel on a low stool, lean over and try to touch the floor (Figure 23.44). Even with a severely herniated disc, most patients

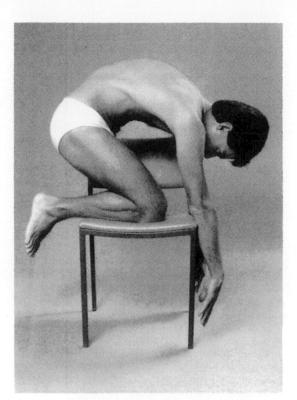

Figure 23.44 Kneeling on stool test: normal test attempt.

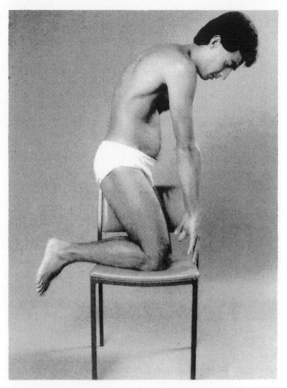

Figure 23.45 Kneeling on stool test: abnormal attempt.

will attempt the task to some degree. Persons with non-organic back pain will usually refuse on the grounds that it would cause great pain or they would overbalance in the attempt (Figure 23.45).

Paradoxical straight leg raising

Perform the usual straight leg raising test (Figure 23.29). The patient might manage a limited elevation, for example 30 degrees (Figure 23.46). Keep the degree in mind. Ask the patient to sit up and swing the legs over the end of the couch. Distract attention with another test or some questions (Figure 23.47), then attempt to lift the straight legs to the same level achieved on the first occasion (Figure 23.48). If it is possible, then the patient's response is inconsistent. A variation is to lift the straight legs while the patient is supine (Figure 23.49).

EXAMINATION OF OTHER JOINTS

It is necessary to assess other joints which can cause pain similar to that which originates from the lumbosacral spine. In particular the hip and sacro-iliac joints should be assessed.

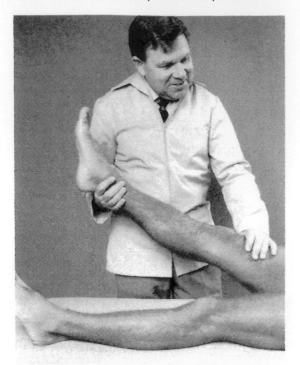

Figure 23.46 Leg raising test: stage 1.

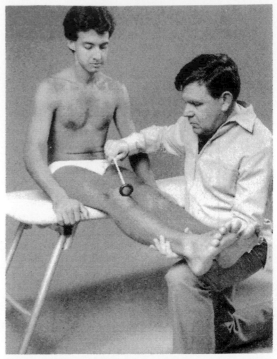

Figure 23.48 Leg raising test: stage 3.

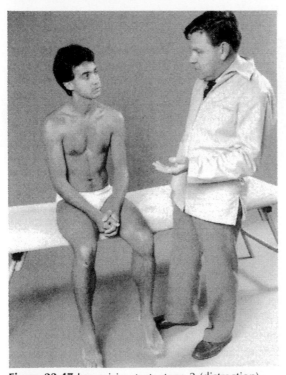

Figure 23.47 Leg raising test: stage 2 (distraction).

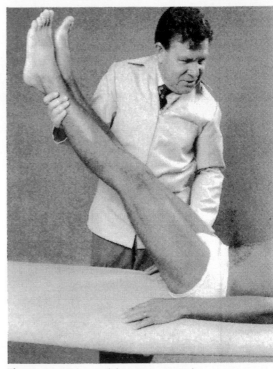

Figure 23.49 Leg raising test: stage 4.

Hip joint

First ask the patient to squat for several seconds. If there is any pathological condition, the stress on the hip and knee joints will cause pain and discomfort (Figure 23.50). The examiner can apply over-pressure by pushing down on the shoulders to stress the joint.

Perform a routine examination on the hip. Remember that the first movements to be affected with osteoarthritis of the hip are internal rotation, extension and abduction.

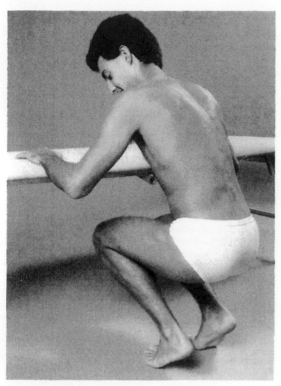

Figure 23.50 The squat test.

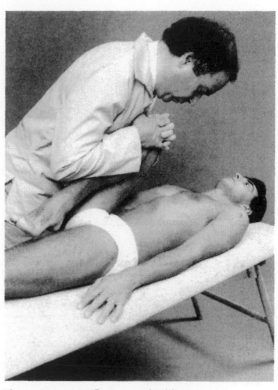

Figure 23.51 Hip flexion and adduction compression test.

The passive hip flexion and adduction test stresses the hip joint considerably. The knee and hip are fully flexed as the examiner compresses the hip joint (Figure 23.51).

Sacro-iliac joints

The SIJs are difficult to palpate and examine but there are several tests that provoke the SIJs. These tests are described in Chapter 25.

An example of the significance of these tests is given in Table 23.5.

Table 23.5 *Pain reproduction in joints.*

	KNEE	HIP	SACRO-ILIAC JOINT	LUMBAR SPINE
Squat test	X	X	X	X
Flexion and adduction test	X	XX	XX	
'Patrick' test		X	X	
Winged compression test			X	
Lateral compression test			X	
Postero-anterior pressure over sacrum			X	
Postero-anterior pressure over lumbar spine				X
Unequal sacral 'rise' test			X	

Table 23.6 *Physical examination of the lumbar spine (a summary).*

Objectives

1. Reproduce the patient's symptoms
2. Detect the level of the lesion
3. Determine its cause (if possible)

Key Points

Surface anatomy:
The tops of the iliac crest lie at the level of the L4–L5 interspace (or L4 spinous process) while the PSISs lie opposite S2. Use tips of opposed thumbs for palpation of spinous processes, interspinous spaces and 2 cm lateral to midline.

Main Components (check list)

1. Inspection
2. Palpation
    centrally
        •• spinous processes L1
            to coccyx
        •• interspinous spaces
    unilateral (R & L sides)
        2 cm from midline
    transverse pressure to sides
        of spinous processes
        (R & L)
3. Movements
    extension (20°–30°)
    lateral flexion, L & R (30°)
    flexion 75°–90°
4. Provocation Tests
    quadrant test
    slump test
5. Other Joints
    sacroiliac
    hip

6. Neurological
    if radicular pain present, or pain or
    paraesthesia below buttocks
    1. Quick tests
        walking on heels (L5)
        walking on toes (S1)
    2. Dural stretch tests
        slump test
        straight leg raising (SLR)
    3. Specific nerve root tests
        (L4, L5, S1)
        sensation
        power
        reflexes
    Main nerve roots
        L3 – femoral stretch test (prone, flex
            knee, extend hip)
            – motor-extension of knee
            – sensation-anterior thigh
            – reflex-knee jerk (L3, L4)
        L4 – motor–resisted inversion foot
            – sensation–inner border of foot to
                great toe
            – reflex – knee jerk
        L5 – motor–walking on heels
                –resisted extension great toe
            – sensation–middle three toes
                (dorsum)
            – reflex–nil
        S1 – motor–walking on toes
                –resisted eversion foot
            – sensation–little toe, most of sole
            – reflex–ankle jerk

PRACTICE TIPS

- The T12–L1 and L1–L2 discs are the groin pain discs.
- The L4–L5 disc is the back pain disc.
- The L5–S1 disc is the leg pain disc.
- Severe limitation of SLR (especially to less than 30 degrees) indicates lumbar disc prolapse.

SUMMARY

The physical examination is the key to the diagnostic process and for decision-making about the selection of the most appropriate manual technique. The preceding tests will help the examiner determine the severity of the back pain, the level of the lesion, the presence of nerve root pressure and the authenticity of the patient's pain. A summary is presented in Table 23.6.

24
Mobilisation of the lumbar spine

'Force is never more operative than when it is known to exist but is not brandished.'

Alfred Thayer Mahan

Contents
☐ Key checkpoints
☐ Classification of techniques
☐ Lumbar mobilisation techniques
    1. Accessory rotation
    2. Anterior directed central gliding
    3. Anterior directed unilateral gliding
    4. Transverse directed rotational gliding
    5. Longitudinal distraction gliding (traction)
☐ Practice tips
☐ Summary

The advantage of lumbar mobilisation is that it generally permits the practitioner to commence treating the lumbar spine immediately when manipulation may be inappropriate. This applies particularly to acute low back pain where a high degree of irritability with or without muscle spasm makes manipulation impossible or, if attempted, liable to aggravate the patient's condition.

By means of carefully applied oscillatory movements, mobilisation can begin gently to decrease muscle spasm, increase mobility and thus lessen pain. Mobilisation can be used either as a treatment technique per se or as a pre-manipulation procedure. This choice depends upon the patient's condition and the practitioner's management strategy.

One of the great advantages of mobilisation is that there are a number of techniques from which to choose. This is in contrast to manipulation, where a higher degree of skill is required and there is a narrower margin of error for the technique to be successful. Furthermore, many patients find mobilisation a relatively pleasant hands-on procedure and not as threatening as manipulation. The practitioner can never take for granted his or her clinical right to launch straight into a forceful manual technique on the patient. It is important to offer the patient an explanation of the planned treatment and the right to refuse.

KEY CHECKPOINTS

- Mobilisation is the treatment of choice for acute low back pain.
- Stage 1 to 2 accessory rotational mobilisation is a very useful method for the patient with very acute unilateral low back pain.
- Mobilisation in rotation and anterior directed central gliding has three separate stages (or grades) ranging from the gentler initial range, the wide amplitude mid range to the short amplitude end range.
- Mobilisation is safe and can be given over a relatively long period in one treatment session, for example 30 to 60 seconds, which can be repeated two or three times.
- Mobilisation of the lumbar spine can be very useful during the last trimester of pregnancy.
- The pisiform method of hand application is the most comfortable for anterior directed gliding.

CLASSIFICATION OF TECHNIQUES

Mobilisation techniques can be divided into direct and indirect according to whether a body lever is used. Direct techniques are those where a direct pressure or force is applied to the affected area and hence are generally quite specific for that area. Indirect techniques, on the other hand, use body levers to produce the effect and are non-specific, producing movement not only at the affected level but also over wider areas of the spine.

Table 24.1 *Mobilisation techniques for the lumbar spine.*

TECHNIQUE	TYPE	INDICATIONS

1. Accessory rotation
  a. Initial range
  b. Mid range
  c. End range
	Indirect	Unilateral pain (one or both sides)
		Acute severe pain at one or several levels

2. Anterior directed central gliding	Direct	Midline pain radiating bilaterally
3. Anterior directed unilateral pain	Direct	Unilateral pain
4. Transverse directed rotational gliding	Direct	Unilateral pain
5. Longitudinal distraction gliding (= traction) a. Both legs	Indirect	Bilateral (central) pain Unilateral pain
b. One leg	Indirect	Unilateral pain

It is appropriate to use the less effective indirect techniques when the affected part is too painful to withstand direct pressure and the indirect method can mobilise the area without direct touching. Indirect techniques are also appropriate where a wide region is affected rather than one level, thus enabling all involved levels to be treated simultaneously.

The site of the pain has to be considered, since some techniques are better for unilateral pain and others for central or bilateral pain. The indications for various mobilisation techniques are outlined in Table 24.1.

LUMBAR MOBILISATION TECHNIQUES

1. ACCESSORY ROTATION

This technique is effective over a wide range of rotation and is considered over three aspects (or arcs) of the range of movement, namely the initial, mid and end ranges. Its versatility is such that it can be used for either acute or chronic conditions with equal effect. Generally the initial rotatory range is used for acutely painful backs, including the so-called hyperacute lumbago, and the range is increased as the severity of the problem decreases.

A. Initial range

This method is ideal for the acutely painful lower back or the very irritable back where the patient cannot tolerate much movement yet where some movement is desirable.

Position of the patient

- The patient lies on the pain-free side.
- The body lies in a 'neutral' position; that is, with the spine not rotated.
- The head is supported by a pillow and the shoulders and body are at right angles to the couch.
- The legs are slightly flexed at the hips and knees.

Position of the therapist

- The therapist stands behind the patient opposite the pelvis.
- Both hands are placed over the pelvis – from the antero-superior iliac spine to the greater trochanter.

Method

- A gentle small amplitude oscillatory movement is applied to the pelvis (Figure 24.1).
- The rotation is such that the patient is allowed to roll back to the starting position, using the hands to guide this movement. It is a gentle 'push and pull' method with the emphasis being on the push with a gentler guiding pull in the posterior direction.

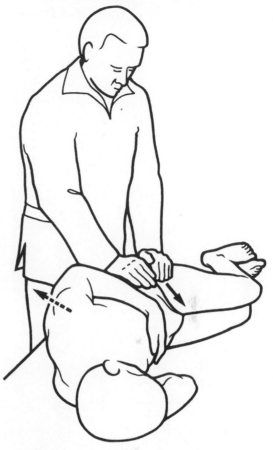

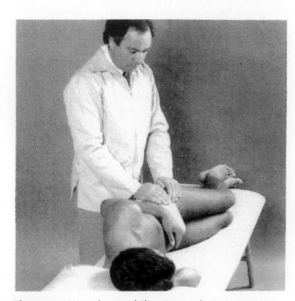

Figure 24.1 Lumbar mobilisation technique 1: accessory rotation – initial range (stage 1).

Figure 24.2 Diagrammatic illustration of the effective forces for initial range accessory rotation shown in Figure 24.1.

Comment

It will be noted that there is a gentle rocking movement along the entire length of the spine with the shoulder oscillating about one-half an amplitude out of phase from the pelvis (Figure 24.2).

This mobilisation produces a gentle, small but effective oscillation in the mobile segment and although the movement appears minimal, it is capable of producing a significant therapeutic effect – sufficient to break the cycle of painful muscle spasm that restricts movement.

Time span

- The procedure occupies about 30 to 60 seconds and may be repeated one, two or three times during the first treatment session or later that day. It may be repeated two or three days later, depending on the assessment at the next consultation.

B. Mid range

This wider arc mobilisation can be used as a first-up technique or following a satisfactory response to the preceding technique when the patient's low back pain has improved.

Position of the patient

- The patient lies on the pain-free side.
- The lower shoulder is pulled forward by grasping the arm at the elbow and gently but firmly rotating the spine (Figure 24.3).

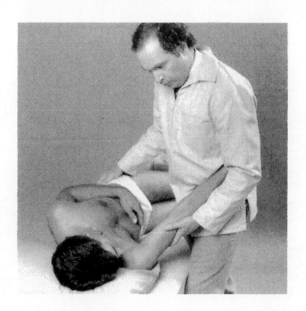

Figure 24.3 Lumbar mobilisation technique 1: method of rotating the trunk by gripping the arm at or just above the elbow.

- The uppermost arm rests on the lateral wall of the chest.
- The uppermost leg is flexed at the hip (to about 50 to 60 degrees) and the knee flexed to a right angle (Figure 24.4).
- The foot rests behind the knee of the lower leg.
- The patient places the palm of the lowermost hand under the head.

Method

- Adopting the same position as for the initial movement, the therapist's hands rest on the pelvis and a large range oscillatory movement with an amplitude of about 40 degrees is produced (Figure 24.5).

Comment

It is evident that the uppermost trunk is about half a rotatory movement behind the pelvis. Note that the patient's uppermost arm helps to promote a counter movement and thus reinforce the leverage.

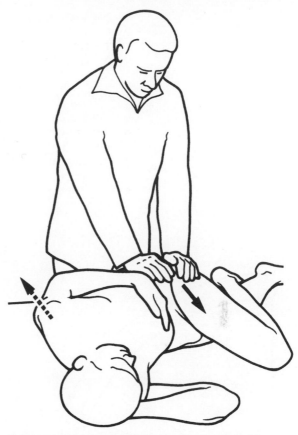

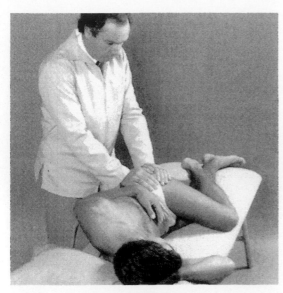

Figure 24.4 Lumbar mobilisation technique 1: accessory rotation – mid range (stage 2). A larger amplitude of movement is achieved. Note that the upper knee is more flexed and the trunk further rotated.

Figure 24.5 Diagrammatic illustration for the mid range of accessory rotation shown in Figure 24.4.

The net effect is the production of a large accessory oscillatory movement in the mobile segment of the lumbar spine. The key strategy here is to produce the appropriate degree of rotation whereby it falls just short of reproducing the patient's pain. To achieve this, the patient is asked to state if he or she starts to feel their back pain. If this occurs the amplitude of rotation is reduced or the patient's degree of rotation slightly reversed.

Time span

● This method occupies 30 to 60 seconds and can be repeated two or three times at any one treatment session.

C. End range

This technique is very effective when painful symptoms are present only at the end range, whether produced by an active movement or upon palpation. Since the amount of force used at the end range can be controlled, there are several variations of this technique ranging from gentle oscillations to firm stretching at the end range.

The range of movements for the accessory rotation techniques are summarised in Figure 24.6.

Position of the patient

- The patient lies on the pain-free side.
- The uppermost leg is flexed at the hip to a right angle and the knee rests over the side of the couch
- The patient's trunk is rotated (Figure 24.3) until the hip begins to lift off the table (this signifies full rotation).
- The uppermost hand rests on the chest wall (Figure 24.7).

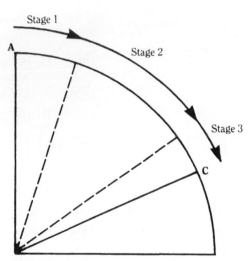

Figure 24.6 Illustrating the various ranges (termed 'stages') of accessory rotation mobilisations.

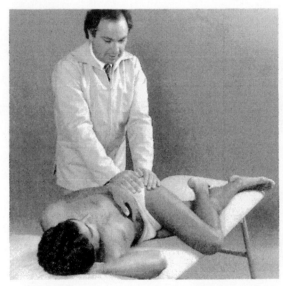

Figure 24.7 Lumbar mobilisation technique 1: accessory rotation – end range (stage 3). Note the increased rotation of the pelvis and of the trunk.

Method

- The therapist, who places the hands on the hip and pelvis as for previous methods, finds that only a slight forward movement is now required to rotate the lower lumbar spine to the end range (elastic limit).
- A rotatory force in the form of short amplitude oscillations is applied and the required movement tends to generate freely, without much applied force. The contra-oscillatory but synergistic movement between the pelvis and shoulder is again noted.
- The therapist should always be alert for signs of discomfort and should adjust the movement, if necessary, to fall just short of any painful 'nipping'.

Time span

● The end range technique is applied for a shorter period of time, perhaps 30 seconds, with two or three repeats in a treatment session.

Variations of this technique

If the patient's problem is not severe, three variations, all relying on the application of more stretch at the end range, can be utilised and all tend to be more effective than previous methods.

The shoulder lock

The uppermost shoulder is grasped gently and locked in a fixed position by pulling towards the therapist. At this position of increased stretch on the trunk the other hand is used to apply rotatory mobilisation of the pelvis at the end range (Figure 24.8).

The free falling leg

The leg is now extended at the knee and dropped over the edge of the table. This permits a slight increase in the end range force with the help of the added weight of the leg. The same mobilisation technique with short amplitude oscillations is applied (Figure 24.9).

The end range stretch

The third variation (which is not a true mobilisation) is the technique of simply stretching the lumbar spine to the elastic limit by stretching

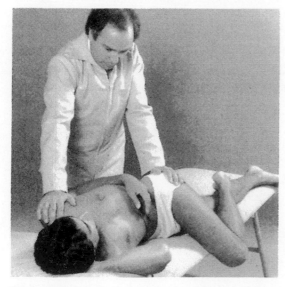

Figure 24.8 End range mobilisation technique with the shoulder 'fixed'.

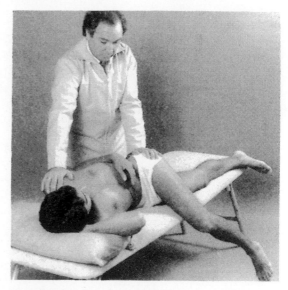

Figure 24.9 End range mobilisation (or stretching only) with the upper leg falling freely over the couch.

and locking the shoulder above and applying a firm controlled stretch to the pelvis. Figure 24.9 shows the position for this method. This is usually held, according to patient comfort, for 5 to 15 seconds and gently released. This technique, which must provide full stretch at end range, is very effective.

2. ANTERIOR DIRECTED CENTRAL GLIDING

This technique is most effective at the mid or end range and, unlike the previous treatment, involves direct pressure to the affected vertebral level. The transmitted force, which produces a gliding effect in the vertebrae, is directed with the thumbs or hands from posterior to anterior and can be applied in three stages.

Position of the patient

The position of the patient remains unaltered for all stages of this technique of anterior directed central gliding.

- The patient lies prone (as for palpation) with no pillow on the head of the couch.
- A small pillow or cushion can be placed under the pelvis to achieve a slight degree of forward flexion of the lumbar spine and aid patient comfort.

Position of the therapist

- The main consideration for the therapist is the position of the hand for this technique. There are two main but very different positions, which are the same as that for palpation – the thumbs or the pisiform applied to the spinous process.

The thumb method

In this method both thumbs are closely aligned and pressure is exerted by the tips of the thumbs directly over the spinous processes (Figure 24.10 and 24.11).

The advantage of this technique is that it is very sensitive to tissue change. However, only a limited amount of force can be employed before it becomes uncomfortable for the therapist or the thumbs fatigue and begin to extend at the interphalangeal joint. This technique is best used for early stage 1.

The pisiform method

For this technique the pisiform area of the hand at the back of the hypothenar eminence acts as the specific point for the application of thrust to the back (Figure 24.12).

Although this method may seem relatively insensitive when compared with finger tip methods, skilled therapists find this presenting part better because a firmer, more controlled application can be achieved and it can be used for all three stages of mobilisation.

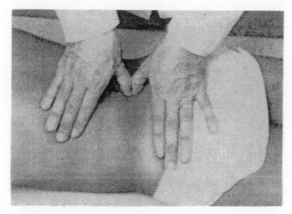

Figure 24.10 Lumbar mobilisation technique 2: the thumb position for anterior directed central gliding mobilisation techniques.

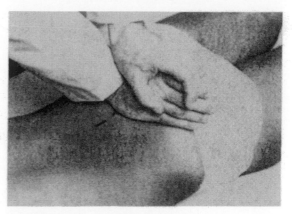

Figure 24.12 The pisiform position for anterior directed central gliding mobilisation techniques.

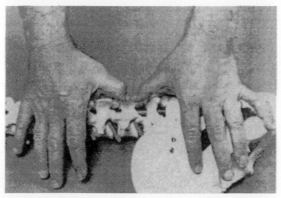

Figure 24.11 Illustrating the position of the thumbs over the spinous process of L4 on the spinal model.

How to adopt the '*pisiform*' position

1. Stretch the palpating hand out in front of you (consider the right hand in this case) and extend the wrist (Figure 24.13). This presenting hand should be your normal working hand.
2. Grip this hand with the other hand (left in this case) with the wrist comfortably extended. The gripping or reinforcing hand should grip comfortably over the top of the index finger of the lower hand with the lowermost three or four fingers embracing the palm of this right hand. The grip is similar to a golfer's grip (Figure 24.14).
3. Laterally rotate and extend the wrist so that the pisiform becomes the lowest prominent presenting part (Figure 24.15).
4. Place the pisiform on the spinous process of the vertebrae at the painful level.

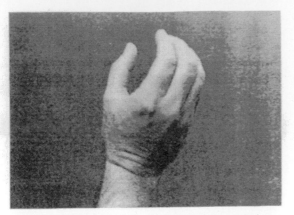

Figure 24.13 The pisiform grip, step 1: the initial position of the presenting mobilising hand.

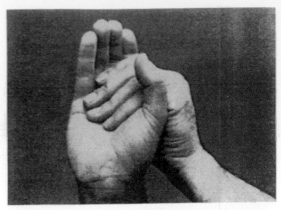

Figure 24.15 The pisiform grip, step 3: a close up view of the grip. The presenting part is indicated with a mark.

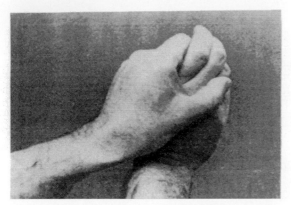

Figure 24.14 The pisiform grip, step 2: the interlocking hand grip of the reinforcing upper hand.

Variation of this method

Some therapists find it more comfortable to apply the padded proximal end of the fifth metacarpal (adjacent to the pisiform) to the spine. This is quite acceptable and should achieve the same results although the prominent pisiform can obtain more localised pressure per unit area.

The mobilising technique

Initial range (stage 1)

The therapist stands at the patient's side and places the thumbs or (preferably) pisiform over the appropriate spinous process. It is important to lean over the patient with the arms perfectly straight and the head and shoulders over the spine. For this reason the couch should be low or the therapist standing on a stool.

The oscillatory movement is obtained by gently rocking the upper trunk up and down with pressure being transmitted by the shoulders and the arms to the spinous process (Figure 24.12).

Mid range (stage 2)

This is a deeper movement with a wider range. The oscillations should be rhythmic and of a constant depth. This constant range is very important. The stretching pressure on the spine should not be completely released at any stage.

End range (stage 3)

For this technique the presenting part (the pisiform) should take up the slack with very firm, but not painful, pressure being applied to reach the end range. A small amplitude well controlled oscillation is produced at this end range. It should be employed for less painful problems.

Figure 24.16 illustrates the three stages of mobilisation for anterior gliding.

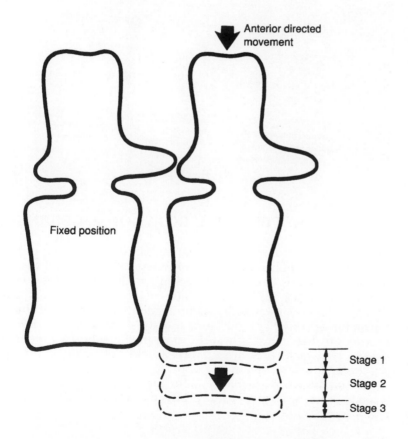

Figure 24.16 Anterior directed central gliding mobilisation, illustrating the three stages of mobilisation.

Time span

● The mobilisation should be applied for approximately 30 to 60 seconds with two or three repeats in one treatment session.

3. ANTERIOR DIRECTED UNILATERAL GLIDING

This technique is similar to the central method but it is used for unilateral pain where the painful lesion is localised, lateral to the spinous process.

The pressure is primarily directed at the transverse process of the symptomatic level and thus is transmitted through the erector spinal musculature and associated fascia.

The method is similar to that of the central pressure method and either the thumbs or pisiform can be used to transmit the pressure. Most therapists prefer to use the thumbs (Figure 24.17), but others consider that the pisiform method gives better results. The unilateral method is most effective as a mid range (stage 2) or end range (stage 3) technique.

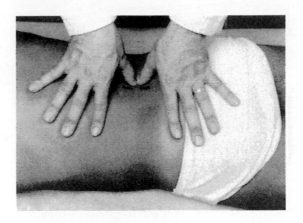

Figure 24.17 Lumbar mobilisation technique 3: anterior directed unilateral gliding mobilisation using the thumbs to transmit pressure to the painful site lateral to the midline.

4. TRANSVERSE DIRECTED ROTATIONAL GLIDING

This technique achieves a rotational mobilisation by means of localised direct pressure applied to the side of the spinous process of the affected vertebral level. It is an end range technique, since there is minimal joint play in this direction. The direction of the pressure is critical and should always be towards the painful side. For example, if the pain is unilateral on the right side and transverse pressure to the spinous process on that side aggravates the pain, then the treatment should involve transverse pressure applied to the left side of the spinous process at that level (Figure 17.5, p. 262).

This method is particularly useful for unilateral pain in the upper lumbar spine, where it is more effective than in the lower lumbar region.

Position of the patient

- The patient lies prone with the head facing towards the painful side.
- The arms should be by the side or relaxed over the sides of the couch.

Position of the therapist

- The therapist stands on the pain-free side.
- The thumbs are applied against the side of the spinous process at the painful level (Figure 24.18).

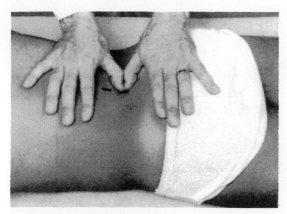

Figure 24.18 Lumbar mobilisation technique 4: transverse directed rotational gliding using the thumbs.

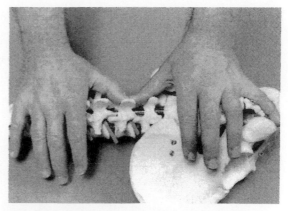

Figure 24.19 Lumbar mobilisation technique 4: position of the thumbs on the spinous process for transverse gliding.

Method

- Allow the thumbs to fit deeply into the groove beside the spine in a relaxed manner.
- Exert pressure from the side of the spinous process – not from near the tip of the process because this can be uncomfortable or painful for the patient.
- The thumbs apply a rhythmic oscillatory force directed towards the painful side (the pisiform can also be used for this technique).
- As this technique requires some degree of force it is useful to overlap the thumbs to generate reinforcement. Figure 24.19 shows the appropriate position of the thumbs on the spinous process.

Time span

- Mobilise for approximately 30 to 60 seconds with two or three repetitions.

5. LONGITUDINAL DISTRACTION GLIDING (TRACTION)

It is often overlooked that traction is another form of mobilisation except that it is in a longitudinal direction. Although it can be, and usually is, administered by machines, it can also be performed manually, often with great benefit.

Indication

Low back pain (central or unilateral), with or without sciatica, where the pain is acute and uncomfortable with the preceding techniques is suitable for traction. Traction is particularly useful for sciatica radiating to the foot.

Determining pelvic tilt

Although several structures can be palpated it is convenient to palpate the ischial tuberosities and note their level. If one is higher (Figure 24.20) it is called an 'upslip' and may represent a hypomobile lesion on that side (in this patient on the right side) which is then the side subjected to traction.

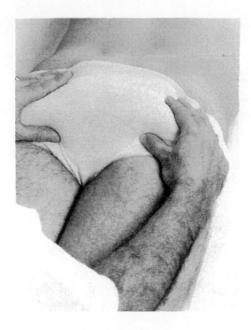

Figure 24.20
Determination of any pelvic 'upslip': determining position of the ischial tuberosities by palpation. Illustration of pelvic 'upslip' where the ischial tuberosity on the right side is at a higher level.

Rules

- Traction can be used on both legs simultaneously or just one leg (on the side on which there is upward pelvic tilt).
- If there is a pelvic tilt apply traction to the one leg first.
- Follow this with traction to both legs.

Position of the patient

- The patient lies prone and can grasp the end of the table for support. This provides suitable counterpressure. Alternatively an assistant can provide countertraction at the axilla.

Position of the therapist

- The therapist stands at the feet of the patient.
- The therapist should use a belt since it allows the body weight to supply the force, thus making a smooth, gentle and well controlled traction.
- Although the hands can be used, the arms tire quickly and cannot sustain the traction if prolonged traction is desired.

Method

A: Using hands only

Unilateral

- One hand grips the foot and the other grips the heel of the affected leg (that is the one on the side with the upslip)
- Ask the patient to relax especially at the knee (Figure 24.21).
- Apply firm traction along the line of the leg with sufficient force that the patient experiences stretching in the lumbosacral area.

Bilateral

- Grasp both feet as shown (Figure 24.22) and apply steady traction.

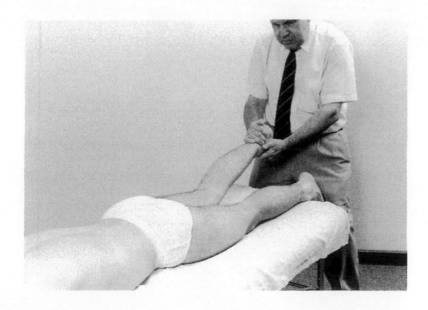

Figure 24.21 Lumbar mobilisation technique 5: manual traction applied to the affected leg using a hand grip on the foot and pulling in the line of the leg.

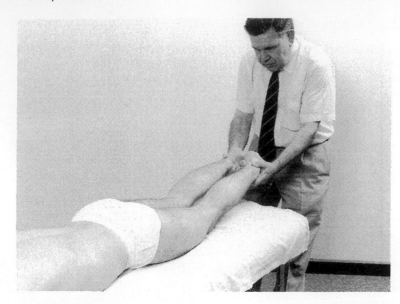

Figure 24.22 Lumbar mobilisation technique 5: manual traction to both legs for a bilateral problem.

B: Using a belt

- The belt (such as a car seat belt or packing belt from a camping store) is applied to the affected leg (Figure 24.23) and the application of body weight achieved by leaning backwards. This action provides the traction force.
- The traction is applied gently until any symptoms begin to ease and then maintained at this level for about two minutes. A gentle oscillatory force can be applied if this proves to be effective.
- A key point is to keep talking to the patient so as to determine what is happening as the traction is applied.

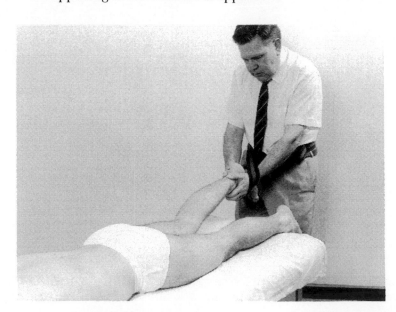

Figure 24.23 Lumbar mobilisation technique 5: traction applied to one leg using the belt which allows the body weight to provide stretch simply leaning back.

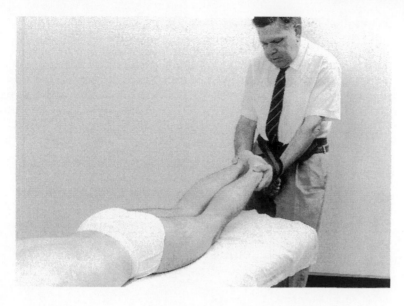

Figure 24.24 Lumbar mobilisation technique 5: traction applied to both legs simultaneously.

- If the pain increases – stop (ease off gently).
- If the pain decreases – maintain or increase traction.
- If the pain is unchanged – apply stronger traction.
- Apply the traction to one leg initially and conclude by applying traction to both legs simultaneously (Figure 24.24).

Time span

- Duration is between two and three minutes.

PRACTICE TIPS

- Lumbar mobilisation permits a wide range of techniques.
- Stage 1 accessory rotation mobilisation is a very useful method for the patient with very acute unilateral low back pain.
- Mobilisation of the lumbar spine can be very useful during the last trimester of pregnancy.
- Maintain mobilisation treatment for about 30 to 60 seconds with each treatment and repeat twice or three times in one treatment session.
- The pisiform method is the most comfortable for anterior directed gliding.

SUMMARY

Mobilisation is an effective mode of treatment for lumbar pain but its effectiveness depends on patient assessment and the correct selection of technique. If in doubt, commence with an early (initial) range technique. The progression through the stages is dependent on the patient's response to therapy.

This chapter has emphasised that, for a technique to be effective, it must be competently performed. The oscillatory movements should be maintained at a constant depth and rhythm. A beginner's mistake is that the arc or range becomes wider and the depth deeper. Throughout the technique it is recommended that the therapist communicate effectively with the patient to assess the effect of the technique.

25
Sacro-iliac joints: clinical features, examination and treatment

Contents
- ☐ Key checkpoints
- ☐ Pain in the sacral area
- ☐ Sacro-iliac pain
- ☐ Physical examination
- ☐ Mobilisation techniques
    - 1. Direct oscillation
    - 2. Direct central pressure with hyperextension
- ☐ Muscle energy therapy
    - Technique 1
    - Technique 2
- ☐ Manipulation techniques
    - 1. Sacral thrust in sitting position
    - 2. Sacral thrust in side lying
    - 3. Ileal thrust in side lying
    - 4. High velocity leg traction

KEY CHECKPOINTS

- A frequently misdiagnosed sacro-iliac problem is an inflammatory disorder such as ankylosing spondylitis. Such disorders require anti-inflammatory medication – not physical therapy.
- Mechanical dysfunction is commonly seen in multiparous women.
- Hypomobile problems of the SIJ can be diagnosed by the unequal rise of the sacrum during forward flexion. This is determined by placing the thumbs over the PSIS. The problem is on the side where the PSIS moves first and furthest.
- Physical therapy includes mobilisation, muscle energy therapy and manipulation.

PAIN IN THE SACRAL AREA

The dilemma

Pain presenting in the sacral area is a difficult and controversial area. Although it certainly can arise from dysfunction of the sacro-iliac joints, pain experienced in the sacral area is commonly referred from the lumbar spine and not necessarily originating from the SIJ.

Some therapists perceive pain over the region of the posterior superior iliac spines as due to SIJ disorders but this pain may be referred from several levels higher in the lumbar spine via sensory nerves (posterior rami of nerve roots) or possibly distal insertions of either the multifides or the erector spinae muscle.

It can be a useful concept to consider the sacrum as an extra vertebra. Where there is dysfunction there is a rotational and side bending torsion of the sacrum.

SACRO-ILIAC PAIN

Pain arising from sacro-iliac joint (SIJ) disorders is normally experienced as a dull ache in the buttock but can be referred to the groin or posterior aspect of the thigh. It may mimic pain from the lumbosacral spine or the hip joint. The pain may be unilateral or bilateral.

There are no accompanying neurological symptoms such as paraesthesia or numbness but it is more common for more severe cases to cause a heavy aching feeling in the groin and upper thigh.

Causes of sacro-iliac joint disorders

- Inflammatory (the spondyloarthropathies)
- Infections – for example, TB, *Staphylococcus aureus* (rare)
- Osteitis condensans ilii
- Degenerative changes
- Mechanical disorders (dysfunction of the SIJ)
- Post-traumatic, after sacro-iliac disruption or fracture.

Dysfunction of the SIJ

These problems are more common than appreciated and can be caused by hypomobile or hypermobile joints.

Hypomobile SIJ disorders are usually encountered in young people after some traumatic event, especially women following childbirth (notably multiple or difficult childbirth), and those with structural problems – for example, shortened leg. Pain tends to follow rotational stresses of the SIJ – for example, tennis, dancing. Excellent results are obtained by passive mobilisation or manipulation.

Hypermobile SIJ disorders are sometimes seen in athletes with instability of the symphysis pubis, in women after childbirth and in those with a history of severe trauma to the pelvis – for example, motor vehicle accidents, horse riders with foot caught in stirrups after a fall. The patient presents typically with severe aching pain in the lower back, buttocks or upper thigh. Such problems are difficult to treat and manual therapy usually exacerbates the symptoms. Treatment consists of relative rest, analgesics and a sacro-iliac supportive belt.

PHYSICAL EXAMINATION

The SIJs are difficult to palpate and examine but there are several tests that provoke the SIJs and diagnose SIJ dysfunction. The following tests are a useful guide to dysfunction.

Direct pressure

With the patient lying prone a firm direct springing pressure is applied directly downwards over the sacrum (Figure 25.1). If there is no (or any equivocal response) the sacral pressure can be varied by concentrating

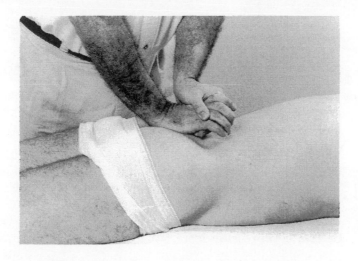

Figure 25.1 Direct pressure is applied over the sacrum with the heel of the hand, producing a firm downward springing pressure.

the pressure either above or below the central axis (of rotation). The sacrum can thus be rotated or counter-rotated by exerting downward pressure over the proximal part (base) of the sacrum or applying the pressure to the distal part of the sacrum, near the coccyx.

Patrick or Fabere test

This method can provoke the hip as well as the SIJ. The patient lies supine on the table and the foot of the involved side and extremity is placed on the opposite knee (the hip joint is now flexed, externally rotated and abducted). The knee and opposite ASIS are gently pressed downwards simultaneously (Figure 25.2). If low back or buttock pain is reproduced the cause is likely to be a disorder of the SIJ.

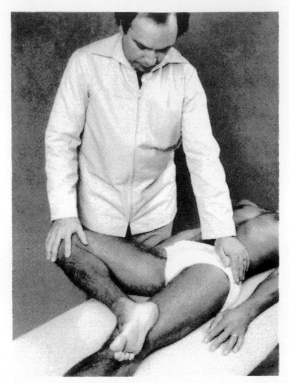

Figure 25.2 The Patrick (Fabere) test.

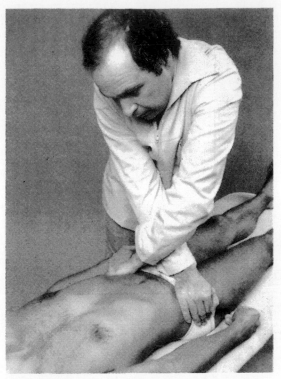

Figure 25.3 The 'winged' compression test for the sacro-iliac joint.

Winged compression test

With the patient lying supine with the examiner's arms crossed, 'separate' the iliac crests with a downwards and outwards pressure. This compresses the SIJs (Figure 25.3).

Lateral compression test

With hands placed on the iliac crests, thumbs on the ASISs and heels of hand on the rim of the pelvis, compress the pelvis. This distracts the SIJs (Figure 25.4).

Unequal sacral 'rise' (Piédallu) test

Method

- Squat behind the standing patient and place your thumbs under but on the posterior superior iliac spines. Ask the patient to bend slowly forwards and observe for symmetry. If one side moves higher relative to the other a problem may exist in the SIJs, invariably a hypomobile lesion in the painful side if that side's PSIS moves higher.
- This test can be performed with a patient sitting over the edge of the couch.

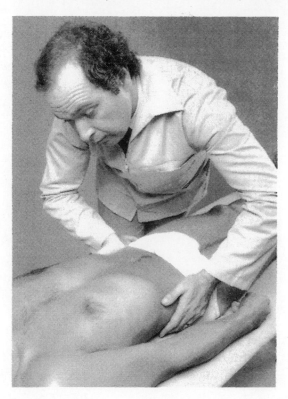

Figure 25.4 The lateral pelvic compression test for the sacro-iliac joints.

Unequal sacral 'rise' in sitting position

● Examination of the PSIS in forward flexion is best performed in the sitting position with feet well supported since this tends to eliminate leg muscle imbalance and pelvic muscle distortion as a factor. The thumbs are placed on the PSISs (Figure 25.5). If one PSIS moves first

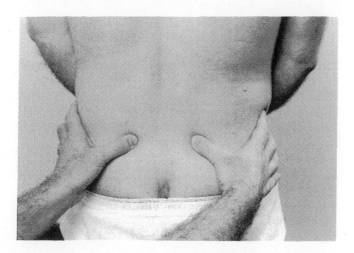

Figure 25.5 Testing sacral 'rise': step 1 – The thumbs are placed over the PSISs.

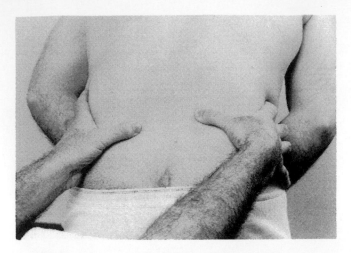

Figure 25.6 Testing sacral 'rise': step 2 – the patient flexes forward. The unequal rise shown here indicates pathology (hypomobility) on the right side where the thumb moves first and higher.

and higher during forward flexion (Figure 25.6) this is a more reliable guide to restriction of SIJ movement on that side.

● This test can be performed with a patient sitting over the edge of the couch.

Treatment

Before treating dysfunction of the SIJ:

● check for unequal leg length (upslip) and treat if present;
● correct any associated lumbar dysfunction;

then focus treatment on the SIJs.

MOBILISATION TECHNIQUES

1. Direct oscillation

Position of the patient and therapist

● The patient lies prone and the therapist stands to one side as shown in Figure 25.1.

Method

● Using the pisiform process or metacarpal border of the leading hand apply firm downward pressure over the sacrum (position as in Figure 25.1) and using an oscillatory movement mobilise at the limit of pain.
● The pressure can be applied at three levels:
  1. Over the axis (S2–S3 level): this achieves general depression of the sacrum, with no rotation.
  2. Proximally (above the axis): this achieves rotation of the proximal sacrum (if this is desired – should it be the painful movement).

3. Distally (lower sacrum): this achieves counter-rotation of the proximal sacrum.

2. Direct central pressure with hyperextension

The use of extension often proves to be effective in treating sacro-iliac problems, especially resistant cases. This technique combines the use of anterior directed central pressure and extension of the spine via hyperextension of the leg at the hip. Thus greater extension is achieved by using the thigh as a lever.

Indications

Sacro-iliac dysfunction manifests as low central back pain, especially with bilateral radiation into the buttocks and with loss of flexion. It should not be used as a first line technique but reserved for conditions not responding to conventional techniques.

Position of the patient

- The patient lies prone, with the head turned to the painful side and the arms relaxed over the side of the couch.

Position of the therapist

- The therapist stands level with the patient's hips on the side opposite the painful side (if pain is unilateral).

Method

- Grasp the patient's furthermost thigh just above the knee with the hand and wrist under the thigh in a cradling manner.
- Place the heel of the other hand over the sacrum centrally at its affected level.
- Elevate the thigh thus extending the hip joint and increasing the extension of the lumbar spine (Figure 25.7). If this position increases the patient's pain, lower the leg until a pain-free position is reached.

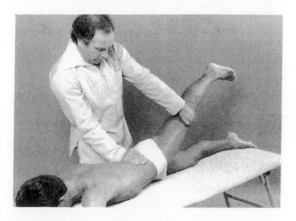

Figure 25.7 Sacral mobilisation technique 2: direct central pressure with hyperextension.

Two variations of this technique can be used

1. The leg can be held at a constant level and a mobilising anterior directed force applied with the pisiform of the other hand to the spine.
2. The pisiform of the hand on the spine applies a constant anterior directed pressure while the leg can be oscillated into extension, keeping just short of any discomfort.

MUSCLE ENERGY THERAPY

Muscle energy therapy can be used for sacro-iliac dysfunction. Two basic techniques are described.

Technique 1

Note

- This technique is for right-sided dysfunction.
- Sitting forward flexion is positive on the right.
- There is posterior torsion on the right.
- The springing test is positive.

Position of the patient and therapist

- The patient lies on the left side (affected side uppermost).
- The therapist stands in front of the patient and extends the spine by rotating the pelvis forwards.
- The right hand palpates the lumbosacral area to ensure the L5–S1 joint is not locked by overextension (extension should achieve tautness down to L5).
- With the left hand extend the left hip by easing the left leg backwards to the point where the sacrum just begins to move (without movement of L5).
- Ask the patient to grasp the table with the right hand – ensure sufficient rotation has occurred so that the tension does not extend beyond L5.
- Steady the patient's trunk with the right forearm on the trunk and monitor tension at the lumbosacral area with the right hand.
- Use the left hand to control movement of the upper leg.

Method

- Ask the patient to lift their upper (right) leg against your hand.
- Resist this upward movement in an isometric hold for five seconds (Figure 25.8).
- Ask the patient to relax. It should be possible to feel the right sacral bone move forwards away from the palpating fingers.
- Repeat so that the slack is taken up to the new barrier.
- Repeat three to four times.

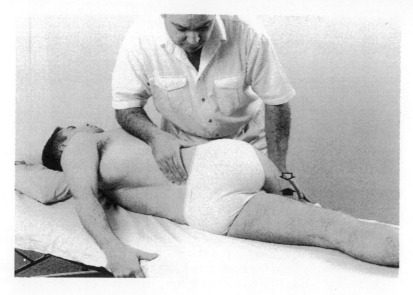

Figure 25.8 Muscle energy technique 1 (right-sided SIJ dysfunction): upward lift of the right leg is resisted by the therapist.

Technique 2

Note

- This technique is for right-sided dysfunction.

Position of the patient and therapist

- The patient lies prone with the right shoulder close to the side of the table and with the right arm hanging over the edge.
- The therapist manoeuvres the legs so that the patient adopts the flexed position as shown (Figure 25.9). The hip flexion must be

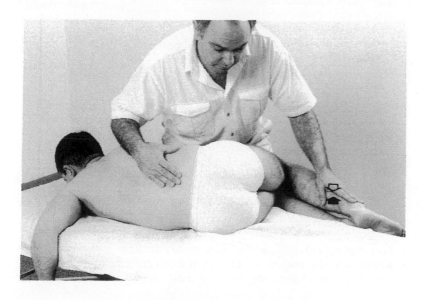

Figure 25.9 Muscle energy technique 2 (right-sided SIJ dysfunction): upward lift of the leg is resisted in an isometric hold.

stopped just before the sacrum begins to move. The sacral movement is monitored by the fingers of the right hand.

- A small cushion can be placed under the thigh to protect it from the edge of the table.

Method

- The patient breathes deeply and slowly while reaching out for the floor with the right hand.
- The therapist's palpating right hand monitors lumbosacral movement and stops the patient movement when L5 just begins to move.
- The exhalation and reaching for the floor is repeated until the point of tension is reached.
- The necessary left side-bend is achieved by dropping the patient's feet over the edge of the table (the cushion under the thigh makes this more comfortable).
- The patient is then instructed to 'lift the lower legs or feet towards the ceiling' while this is resisted with a equal and opposite force with your left hand.
- Maintain this isometric hold for five seconds, then relax by asking the patient to drop the feet.
- It should be possible to feel the right sacral base move back during this process.
- The slack is taken up to the new point of tension as palpated with the fingers. This can be achieved by dropping the feet and adjusting the degree of flexion of the hips.
- The process of isometric contraction is repeated two or more times.

MANIPULATION TECHNIQUES

1. Sacral thrust in sitting position

Note

- This technique demonstrates left-sided SIJ dysfunction.

Position of the patient and therapist

- The patient sits astride the examination table with the left arm crossing the right so that the left hand holds the right shoulder.
- The therapist stands behind and to the right and places the left hand (the pisiform bone can be the point of contact) over the left sacral base at the level of the PSIS (Figure 25.10).

Method

- The right arm grasps the patient's left arm or shoulder (while supporting the patient's right shoulder), flexes the trunk then locks the spine into right side bending and right rotation, including the

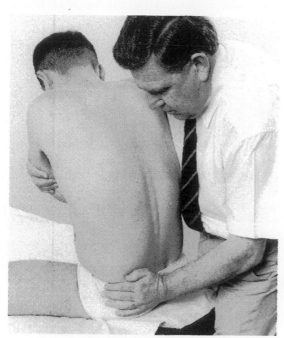

Figure 25.10 Manipulation technique 1 for SIJ dysfunction (left side) sacral thrust in sitting position: step 1 – the hand is placed firmly over the left sacral place.

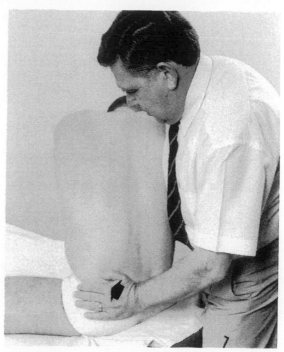

Figure 25.11 Manipulation technique 1 (for SIJ dysfunction (left side) sacral thrust in sitting position: step 2 – a direct forward thrust is applied with the hand as the patient is rotated in the end range.

sacrum. This will cause the left sacral base to move forwards which can be felt with the left hand.

- As the patient's trunk is taken into further rotation with the right hand and the slack is taken up, a low amplitude high velocity thrust is applied with the left hand in an anterior direction (Figure 25.11). The small arc of movement must be applied at full stretch.

2. Sacral thrust in side lying

Note

- This technique demonstrates left-sided SIJ dysfunction.
- It moves the sacrum on the ileum.

Position of the patient and therapist

- The patient lies on the left side with the right shoulder elevated.
- The therapist stands in front, flexes the right hip to a right angle.
- The left hand (usually the pisiform bone) is then placed over the left side of the sacrum, that is, the lower side. The elbow is bent so that the forearm is aligned for the required thrust.
- By placing the right hand on top of the shoulder the therapist rotates the shoulder backwards to lock the spine down to L5.

- The slack is taken up by means of the lower hand exerting firm sacral pressure in the direction of the right shoulder.
- At this point a low amplitude, high velocity thrust is applied by a scooping movement of the left hand in the direction of the right shoulder (Figure 25.12).

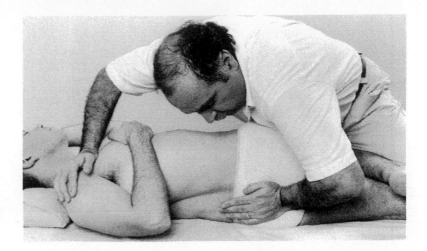

Figure 25.12 Manipulation technique 2 for SIJ dysfunction (left side). The therapist's left side thrusts with a scooping movement towards the patient's right shoulder.

3. Ileal thrust in side lying

Note

- This technique demonstrates a left-sided SIJ dysfunction.
- It moves the ileum on the sacrum.
- It can be used as a rotational mobilisation technique as well as a manipulation technique.
- It is similar in principle and process to the specific rotational manipulation technique for the lumbar spine.

Position of the patient and therapist

- The patient lies on the unaffected side so that the restricted joint is uppermost.
- The therapist faces the patient.
- The uppermost leg is flexed until tightening can be felt in the lower sacrum.
- The trunk is rotated until the spine is locked down to the L5–S1 level. This is monitored with the left hand.

Method

- The therapist applies tangential pressure over the ileum (usually the iliac crests) with the forearm. This achieves gapping of the posterior SIJ.
- A rhythmic pressure is applied with this forearm – this achieves mobilisation with limited gapping of the stiff joint.

Manipulation

- While the left arm steadies the trunk by exerting a counterforce on the upper trunk and axillary area the right arm applies full stretch to the ileum.
- At this full stretch a low amplitude high velocity thrust is applied with the forearm. This produces rotation of the ileum on the sacrum (Figure 25.13).

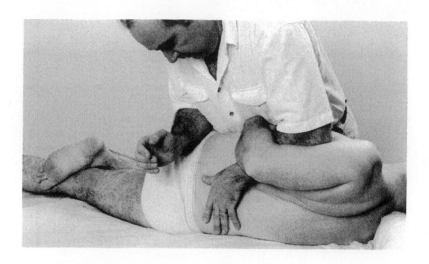

Figure 25.13 Manipulation technique 3 for SIJ dysfunction (left side). The forearm applies a rotational thrust to the ileum.

4. High velocity leg traction

This technique is a modification of the mobilisation techniques for sciatica as described in Chapter 24.

Note

- The technique here is for a left-sided dysfunction characterised by a higher ischial tuberosity on that side.
- It should not be used if there is disease of the knee, hip or ankle joints on that side.
- The patient should be warned that there may be increased discomfort for a few days.

Position of the patient and therapist

- The patient can lie supine as shown but can also lie prone (Figure 24.21). The feet should be just over the end of the table.
- The therapist stands at the foot of the table and lifts the leg (on the affected side) off the table gripping either just above the ankle or with one hand at this level and the other grasping the foot (Figure 24.21).
- Downward movement of the right leg can be blocked by pressing the left thigh against it or using an assistant to block it.

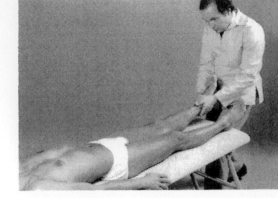

Figure 25.14
Demonstration of the position for leg traction with the patient lying supine (the belt is not usually used).

- The therapist applies traction with slight abduction and internal rotation applied to the hip (Figure 25.14 shows the position).
- The therapist then flexes the hip and knee three times to achieve relaxation of the leg and at the end of the third movement a sharp high velocity tug is applied to the leg, in the plane of the SIJ.

26
Muscle energy techniques for the lumbar spine

Contents
☐ Key checkpoints
☐ Indications for the use of MET in lumbar
   disorders
☐ Examination in flexion and extension
☐ General interpretation
☐ Joint signs
  ● Techniques
     1: MET for restricted flexion – method A
     2: MET for restricted flexion – method B
     3: MET for restricted extension
☐ Summary

KEY CHECKPOINTS

● Muscle energy therapy (MET) is ideal for lumbar disorders with
  excessive pain, muscle spasm and irritability.
● Patients have to be examined carefully in extension and flexion
  by a method called positional analysis.
● Separate techniques are used for restriction into flexion or
  extension.

INDICATIONS FOR THE USE OF MET FOR LUMBAR DISORDERS

MET is indicated when at the barrier

● there is an inability to engage the end range
● there is excessive pain
● there is excessive muscle spasm
● the condition is too irritable.

MET can also be used as a pre-manipulative technique.

Objective

The post isometric muscle relaxation from MET results in recession of the barrier of pain and movement.

EXAMINATION IN FLEXION AND EXTENSION

Techniques

There are two main techniques but one is chosen on the basis of the examination of the patient which is performed in flexion and extension of the lumbar spine using a method called positional diagnosis. The aim of this method is to assess the degree of rotation of the vertebrae by noting the relative posteriorisation of the transverse processes and comparing the vertebrae.

Examination in flexion

Method

- The patient sits across a low couch or stool but can stand.
- The examiner's thumbs are placed on either side of the same vertebra (can use T11 to L5). The thumbs lie on the transverse processes which may be felt in the lateral gutter (between longissimus and iliocostalis lumborum muscles).
- The patient flexes into a forward-bent position as the examiner determines which transverse process is most posterior (Figure 26.1).
- The sequence is repeated rapidly and individually at each level of the lumbar spine.

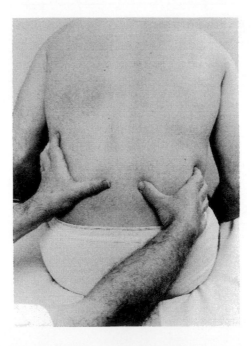

Figure 26.1 Positional analysis for lumbar diagnosis in flexion. The thumbs lie on the transverse processes. Note the different levels of the thumbs, the right being more posterior indicating a blocked joint on the right.

Interpretation

If there is restriction into flexion one of the transverse processes indicated by the thumb level will become posterior relative to the other. If there is no restriction the levels of the thumbs are equal.

Examination in extension

This is performed in two positions: one with the patient prone (standing position is acceptable) and the other propped up on elbows. The prone position whereby the patient lies in a 'neutral' position is shown in Figure 26.2 and the extended position in Figure 26.3. Each level is examined using the thumbs as for the previous method and noting, for each segmental level, whether the thumbs are symmetrical or asymmetrical.

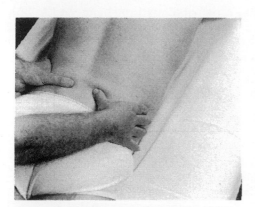

Figure 26.2 Positional analysis for lumbar diagnosis in a neutral position with the patient lying prone.

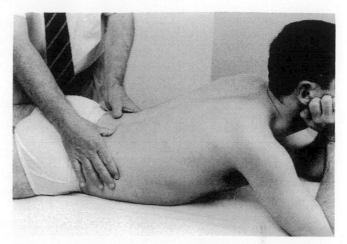

Figure 26.3 Positional analysis in extension.

GENERAL INTERPRETATION

1. Consider restriction of L4 relative to L5 when painful on forward flexion

In neutral: The transverse processes of L4 are at the same level and thumbs are symmetrical.

In flexion: The R transverse process a therefore R thumb becomes more posterior and prominent.

In extension: The asymmetry disappears.

Implication: The R L4–L5 facet joint is blocked and will not open or flex leading to loss of L rotation of L4 and associated lateral flexion (side bending).

Rule: In flexion, the side of the most posterior transverse process is the side of the blocked joint.

2. Consider restriction of L4–L5 on extension

In extension: The R transverse process or thumb becomes more prominent.

In flexion: The asymmetry disappears.

Implication: Restriction is under extension.
The joint cannot fully extend (close).
The L L4–L5 facet joint will not extend and there is a loss of L rotation and side bending.

Rule: In extension the blocked joint is on the opposite side to the most posteriorly placed thumb.

JOINT SIGNS

Another sign of joint dysfunction is palpable texture change at L4–L5 particularly over the R L4–L5 facet joint. As one palpates in the paravertebral gutter the increased muscle tone can be felt due to spasm in the posterior motor unit (multifidus and rotatores).

Technique 1: MET for restricted flexion (lesion uppermost) – method A

Note

- The posterior transverse process is uppermost.
- The example used is a blocked R L4–L5 facet joint.

Position of the patient and therapist

- Place the patient in Sims position with L side down, the left arm hanging over the couch behind the patient and the right shoulder close to the edge of the couch.
- Place the palpating hand at the level of restriction (L4–L5).
- The patient's knees are supported on the therapist's knees – either from the front or from behind whereby the therapist sits on the couch (Figure 26.4).
- The patient drops the feet towards the floor as far as they will go.

Method

- Ask the patient to raise the feet (ankles) towards the ceiling.
- The therapist resists this by an equal and opposite downward force.
- This isometric position is held for five seconds (Figure 26.4).
- Ask the patient to relax and then 'stretch' the legs down until you feel the new point of tension with the palpating fingers at L4–L5.
- Repeat this step two to three times more.
- Recheck to determine if the alignment is now equal.

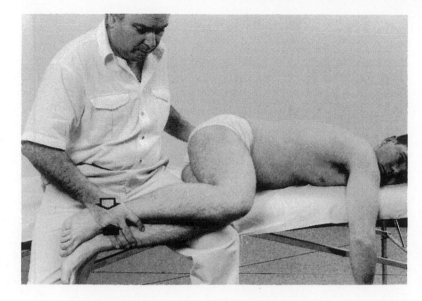

Figure 26.4 Technique 1: MET for restricted flexion – method A (right sided L4–L5 facet joint blockage): the therapist resists the patient raising the leg in an isometric hold. *Note*: Patient's force shown by filled arrow; therapist's force shown by 'open' arrow.

Technique 2: MET for restricted flexion (lesion lowermost) – method B

Note

- The posterior transverse process is placed down
- The example used is a blocked R L4–L5 facet joint.

Position of the patient and therapist

- Place the patient on the right side.
- The patient's trunk is rotated to their left so the left shoulder moves posteriorly towards the table.
- The patient's thighs are flexed to approximately 75 degrees.

Method

- Palpate the affected level – for example, R L4–L5.
- Raise the patient's feet towards the ceiling until side bending is localised to the restrictive segment, i.e. when movement is felt at L4–L5 (Figure 26.5).
- Ask the patient to attempt to pull their feet down against your resistance.
- Hold for five seconds in an isometric hold then relax.
- Take to the new barrier by a further lift of the patient's feet.
- Repeat about three times.
- Retest.

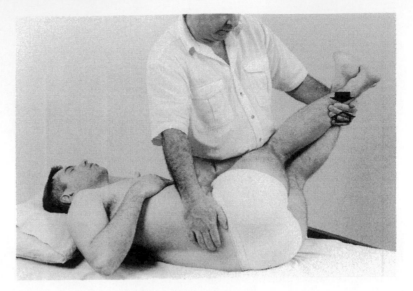

Figure 26.5 Technique 2: MET for restricted flexion – method B (right sided lesion lowermost): the therapist resists elevation of the legs towards the ceiling. *Note:* Patient's force shown by filled arrow; therapist's force shown by 'open' arrow.

Technique 3: MET for restricted extension

Note

- The posterior process is asymmetrical into extension.
- The example used is a blocked L L4–L5 facet joint.

Position of the patient and therapist

- The patient lies on the left side and the therapist brings the pelvis forwards and then pushes the shoulders back to extend the lumbar spine.
- The lower leg is fully extended.
- The patient's right hand grasps the far side of the table thus introducing some rotation and side bending (Figure 26.6).

Method

- The palpating hand is placed over the level of the upper L4–L5 facet joint to feel for tissue and positional change (Figure 26.6).
- The patient's right ankle is gripped and lifted to a position above the other knee until tension is felt with the monitoring hand.
- The patient is asked to contract the upper leg by putting the ankle down onto the medial aspect of the knee.
- When contraction is felt at L4–L5 an isometric hold is performed (Figure 26.7).
- This position is held for five seconds.
- The slack is then taken up into the new barrier by lifting the right foot.
- Repeat about three times.
- Retest.

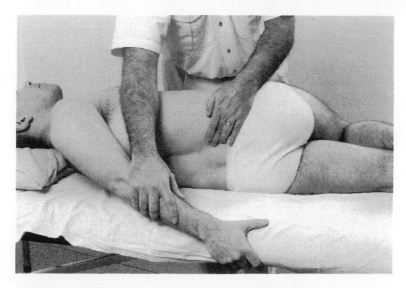

Figure 26.6 Technique 3: MET for restricted extension: showing position of the patient and therapist for treatment for a blocked left L4–L5 facet joint.

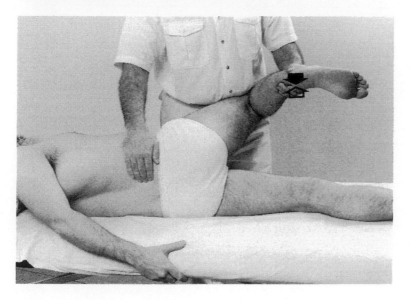

Figure 26.7 Technique 3: the therapist resists adduction of the leg as the patient brings the ankle towards the medial aspect of the knee. *Note*: Patient's force shown by filled arrow; therapist's force shown by 'open' arrow.

SUMMARY

Muscle energy therapy can be a very useful method for acute conditions of the lumbar spine that are very painful, especially those with muscle spasm. The method used depends on whether there is restriction into flexion and extension and preliminary examination is necessary.

27
Manipulation of the lumbar spine

'The secret of successful spinal manipulation is first to select the correct technique for the correct reason and second to be at absolute full stretch (elastic end range) for the final thrust so that the resultant arc of movement will be almost imperceptible.'

Experienced teacher of physical therapy

Contents
☐ Key checkpoints
☐ Classification of techniques
☐ Guidelines for manipulation: dos and don'ts
☐ Lumbar manipulation techniques
    1. Non-specific rotation: method A
    2. Non-specific rotation: method B
    3. Rotation into flexion
    4. Rotation into extension
    5. Specific rotation
    6. Rotation in the sitting position
☐ Lumbar manipulation under general anaesthesia
    7. Trunk rotation with fixed pelvis (for general anaesthesia)
☐ Dangers of manipulating the lumbar spine
☐ Reassessment of manipulation
☐ The best back to manipulate
☐ Practice tips
☐ Cautionary advice

Manipulation of the lumbar spine has a long and colourful history that has been recorded since ancient times. It must be emphasised that there are myriads of techniques practised on the lumbar spine thoughout the world.

Almost everyone has heard of the 'lumbar roll'. This so-called lumbar manipulation can be performed in several ways but the particular method chosen should depend on the nature of the individual patient's problem and the clinical signs. It is useful to be able to learn and perform several variations of lumbar manipulation, since any one type may be unsuitable for a particular patient.

This chapter will describe a few basic methods which are considered important to master. It is better to know a small but broadly selected group of techniques well, rather than to be poorly acquainted with a larger number. Although some therapists claim that their particular method is the 'one and only' technique, the end result achieved by different therapists, each employing their own particular technique, is generally similar. What is important is to know when to apply manipulative therapy and to choose the appropriate methods for the individual patient.

KEY CHECKPOINTS

- Explain to the patient what you intend to do.
- Always attempt to use the most specific technique.
- Manipulation should always be executed at absolute full stretch.
- Take care not to make an asymptomatic degenerative joint symptomatic.

CLASSIFICATION OF TECHNIQUES

Six different lumbar manipulations are described in this chapter. As stated in Chapter 4, manipulation is a high velocity thrust of small amplitude performed at the end range. Manipulations can be classified according to their degree of *directness* or according to their *specificity* (see Table 27.1).

Table 27.1 *Classification of techniques for manipulation of the lumbar spine.*

TECHNIQUE	DIRECTNESS	SPECIFICITY
1. Rotation method A	Indirect	Non-specific
2. Rotation method B	Indirect	Non-specific
3. Rotation with flexion	Semi-direct	Semi-specific
4. Rotation with extension	Semi-direct	Semi-specific
5. Specific rotation	Semi-direct	Specific
6. Rotation in sitting	Semi-direct	Semi-specific

Indirect techniques are those that mainly involve the use of body levers – usually the leg, although the trunk is also used as a lever. Strictly speaking, no really direct methods are described here, but *semi-direct* methods which involve not only the use of body levers but also the application of a localised force over the affected level or segment. Thus the semi-direct techniques tend to be more specific in localisation, compared with the non-specific indirect techniques.

GUIDELINES FOR MANIPULATION: DOs AND DON'Ts

There are several important guidelines to help achieve optimal conditions for lumbar manipulation. Of course, it is essential that organic disease has been ruled out. Never forget to check whether the patient is taking anti-coagulants – permanent nerve damage can occur in such patients, in whom the risk of spontaneous retroperitoneal haemorrhage is greatly increased with spinal manipulation.

These guidelines are presented as a series of DOS and DON'TS.

Dos

- Be relaxed and positive in your approach to the patient.
- Talk to the patient and explain what is going to happen.
- Remember that warmth and massage to the affected part aids treatment.
- Position the patient with the painful side **up** for rotation methods.
- Ensure that the sharp thrust is smooth and decisive, never jerky.
- Ensure that you gap the joint or joints which you assess as responsible for the problem.
- Carry out immediate assessment of the effect of treatment.
- Use a low couch, or a stable platform if the couch is too high. Ideally, the couch should be slightly above your knees.
- Coordinate the manipulative thrust with the patient's breathing to time it towards the end of expiration, since this is the point of maximal patient relaxation. Ask the patient to breathe in and then out. Take up the slack and time your thrust just before full expiration.

Don'ts

- Never manipulate through protective spasm.
- Avoid manipulating the 'irritable' spine.
- Don't manipulate if cord signs or root signs (weakness) are present.
- Don't manipulate if the patient has sciatica with fixed lateral deviation.
- Don't manipulate if peripheral symptoms (such as pain in the foot) are reproduced while taking up the slack at the end range.
- Don't manipulate if movement is greatly reduced in more than three directions.

LUMBAR MANIPULATION TECHNIQUES

1. Non-specific rotation: method A

This method is a logical extension of the stage 3 rotational mobilisation illustrated in Figure 24.7. It is an indirect method using the principle of the lever. It cannot be performed satisfactorily on a high couch.

Position of the patient

- The patient lies on the pain-free side.
- The body should be in a straight line, with the lower leg extended.
- The patient should lie reasonably square on the lower shoulder.
- The lower arm should lie comfortably in front of the body.
- The hand of the lower arm can be placed under the head.
- The upper leg can be either falling freely over the side of the couch (Figure 27.1) or flexed (Figure 27.2).

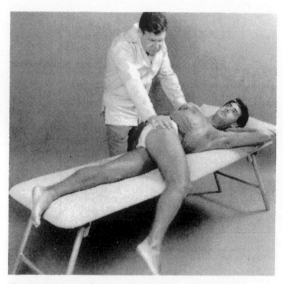

Figure 27.1 Lumbar manipulation technique 1: non-specific rotation, with the lower leg straight and the upper leg falling freely over the couch.

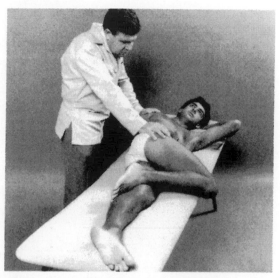

Figure 27.2 Lumbar manipulation technique 1: with the upper knee flexed to about 90 degrees.

Position of the therapist

- The therapist stands behind the patient at the waist level.
- One hand is used to push the trochanteric area of the hip forwards and the other to force the front of the shoulder downwards so that the patient's trunk is rotated in the opposite direction.
- It is best to keep hands in contact with the skin (avoid grasping clothing).

Method

- Now apply a steady rotational movement until a full stretch is applied to both shoulder and hip.
- Don't force the shoulder down too hard – take care to keep it firm and steady during the final thrust.
- Ensure that the thrusting arm is straight and that the line of thrust is tangential along the axis of the femur rather than down into the pelvis.

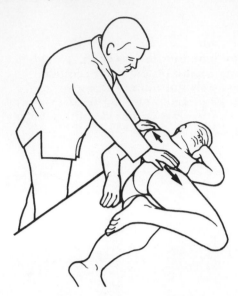

Figure 27.3 Lumbar manipulation technique 1: illustrating the direction of applied forces.

• Maintain sustained pressure for one to two seconds at the end range and then apply a sharp rotational thrust to the hip. The thrust should come from the shoulder and the elbows should be as straight as possible (Figure 27.3).

Post-manipulation

• Immediately after this manipulation re-examine the patient and assess the benefit.

2. Non-specific rotation: method B

This time-honoured method, which some people facetiously call the 'million dollar roll', is the most non-specific of all the lumbar techniques. Although not recommended generally for the lumbar spine it can be an effective technique for a problem at the thoraco-lumbar junction. It has only limited application and should be avoided in the elderly and in those with osteoarthritis of the hip. One spin-off of this method is the occasional ability to detect early osteoarthritis of the hip, as stiffness and loss of movement become apparent during the procedure.

This method is often performed on both sides if the pain is central or bilateral.

Position of the patient

• The patient lies supine, facing upwards with head on a pillow and with arms by the side.
• The patient lies in the centre of the couch.

Position of the therapist

- Stand on the pain-free side.
- Position yourself at about the level of the patient's waist.
- Use your thigh to steady the patient on the couch, if necessary.
- The patient's furthermost shoulder should be firmly 'pinned' to the couch, although it may be necessary to allow some shoulder lift to relieve excessive pressure.

Method

- Grasp the leg of the painful side around or just near the knee and flex the hip to approximately a right angle (Figure 27.4). The degree of flexion of the hip should be determined by patient comfort. Alternatively, if you wish to keep this leg straight, grasp the posterolateral aspect of the patient's calf.
- Steadily and smoothly rotate the patient's pelvis and stretch the lower spine by further rotating the flexed leg across the body and down towards the floor to eventually achieve a maximal lever effect (Figures 27.5 and 27.6).
- With your other hand, keep the patient's shoulder fixed to the couch during this movement.
- Use a gentle oscillatory rotational movement with each hand until you feel absolute full stretch.
  Note: Absolute full stretch is most important – the knee should be quite low at this point.
- At this point apply a sudden sharp amplitude thrust to the leg while maintaining counter pressure on the shoulder (Figure 27.7).
- Always assess the effect of the manipulation.

Common mistakes with non-specific rotation methods

- The patient is not relaxed.
- The couch is too high (one of the biggest drawbacks in general practice).

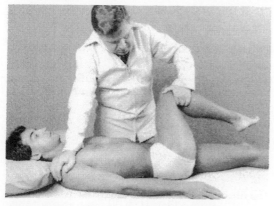

Figure 27.4 Lumbar manipulation technique 2: non-specific rotation – the initial movement.

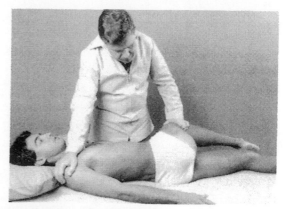

Figure 27.5 Lumbar manipulation technique 2: further rotation of the trunk.

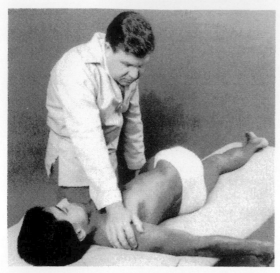

Figure 27.6 Lumbar manipulation technique 2: at the point of full stretch for the manipulative thrust.

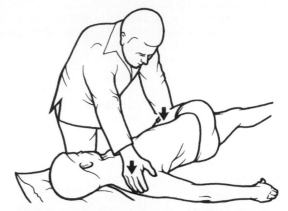

Figure 27.7 Lumbar manipulation technique 2: illustrating the direction of applied forces.

- Insufficient lever action.
- Hurting the patient's shoulder.
- Thrust is not given at absolute elastic limit (novices tend to thrust with some laxity remaining).
- Thrust is directed into the pelvis rather than along the axis of the femur (towards corner of floor and wall!) and there is therefore not a true rotation.
- The leg is adducted rather than the pelvis rotated.
- Manipulation is not abandoned when pain shoots down the leg with the stretch prior to thrusting, or where there is excessive back pain at this limit of stretch.
- Failure to coordinate the patient's breathing with the final thrust.

3. Rotation with flexion

This is an effective pelvic thrust technique that is semi-specific for manipulation of the flexed lumbar spine. The aim of the technique is to increase the lumbar kyphosis (flexion). The appropriate criteria for its use are low back pain with *pain into extension* on examination but freedom from pain into flexion. Thus manipulation is achieved in the correct direction.

Position of the patient
- The patient lies on the pain-free side with the head on a pillow facing the therapist.
- The uppermost leg of the painful side is flexed to 90 degrees with the foot tucked into the popliteal fossa of the lower leg.

Position of the therapist

- Stand in front of the patient at his or her waist level.
- Grasp the patient's lower arm just above the elbow and gently pull the patient into 20 degrees of flexion by applying a force parallel to the ground (Figure 27.8). Then, maintaining the same grip, rotate the thorax to make an angle of approximately 50 degrees with the table by gently pulling upwards (Figure 27.9).
- Now place your hand on the patient's upper shoulder to fix it firmly. *Note*: It is important that this shoulder is maintained at this fixed point by the opposing hand (Figure 27.10).
- Rest the 'thrusting' forearm of your arm against the patient's ischium.

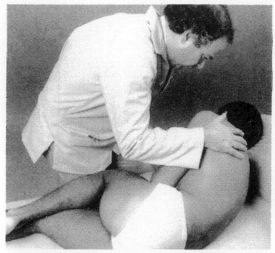

Figure 27.8 Lumbar manipulation technique 3: positioning the patient into flexion.

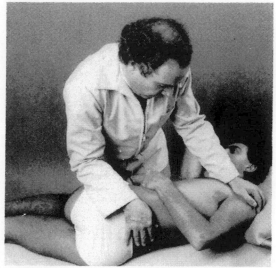

Figure 27.10 Lumbar manipulation technique 3: fixing the upper shoulder.

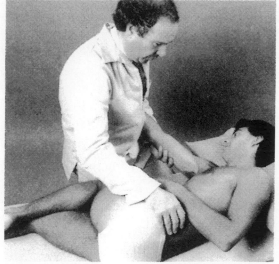

Figure 27.9 Lumbar manipulation technique 3: positioning the patient into rotation.

Method

- With your forearm rotating the patient's pelvis towards yourself take up the slack until the end range is reached (Figure 27.11).
- At this end point manipulation is achieved by imparting the rapid low amplitude thrust to the pelvis with the forearm while the fixed point (upper shoulder) remains unaltered (Figures 27.11 and 27.12).
- Assess the effect of the manipulation.

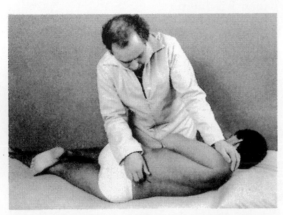

Figure 27.11 Lumbar manipulation technique 3: the position for manipulation.

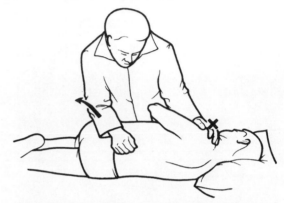

Figure 27.12 Lumbar manipulation technique 3: illustrating the direction of applied forces.

4. Rotation with extension

The aim of this technique is to increase the lumbar lordosis for the purpose of the appropriate manipulative direction. It is indicated where the patient's pain is reproduced into flexion but does not occur into extension.

Position of the patient

- The patient lies on the pain-free side with the head on a pillow facing the therapist.
- The patient's lower leg is fully extended and the upper leg flexed.
- Lordosis of the lumbar spine is achieved by rotating the patient into extension from above while extending the lower leg (Figure 27.13).

Position of the therapist

- The therapist stands level with the patient's pelvis.
- The patient's shoulder is fixed by placing your hand firmly on the shoulder, which should be kept at right angles to the table.
- Your hand is placed on the ilium over the iliac crest.

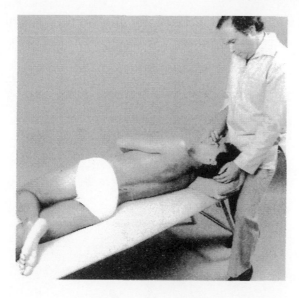

Figure 27.13 Lumbar manipulation technique 4: rotation with extension.

Method

- Adopting the position shown in Figure 27.14, take up the slack by rotating the pelvis firmly with the active hand, while keeping the upper shoulder fixed.
- At full stretch apply a short sharp thrust to the pelvis (Figures 27.14 and 27.15).
- Assess the effect of the manipulation.

5. Specific rotation

This technique has the great advantage of manipulating a specific level without affecting those segments in close proximity. This is particularly useful when it is desirable to manipulate at the painful area yet not

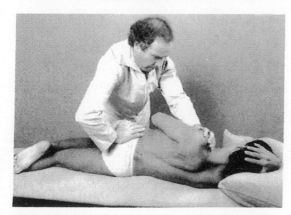

Figure 27.14 Lumbar manipulation technique 4: the position for manipulation.

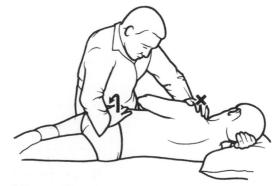

Figure 27.15 Lumbar manipulation technique 4: illustrating the direction of applied forces.

desirable to force a manipulative thrust through another level that may have degenerative changes which are not symptomatic.

This is the ideal manipulative technique for the lumbar spine and is the procedure of first choice for lumbar problems. The importance of being able to identify the specific level of the back problem by careful palpation is thus obvious. This site should be marked with a pen.

Position of the patient

- The patient lies on the pain-free side in a relaxed position with the head on a pillow facing the therapist.
- The upper knee and hip is flexed to about 45 degrees (Figure 27.16).
- The trunk is systematically moved into various positions as outlined in the following notes.

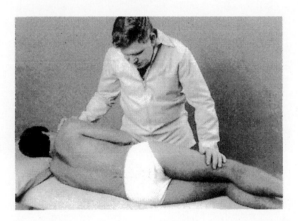

Figure 27.16 Lumbar manipulation technique 5: specific rotation – the starting position.

Position of the therapist

- The therapist faces the patient and stands at waist level.

Method

STEP 1: Position the leg to 'fix' the lower level (Figure 27.17)

- Palpate to indentify the level of the lesion (consider it to be the L4–L5 level in this case).
- Gently press the pad of the index finger of your proximal hand over the interspinous ligament at the affected level.
- Using the other hand on the leg, gradually flex the hip until you feel stretch or tension under the finger as the interspinous gap widens (Figure 27.18).
- As soon as this is felt, fix the leg in that position by tucking the foot in the popliteal fossa.
  Note: It may be necessary to slightly deflex the hip to ensure that this level is not overstretched.

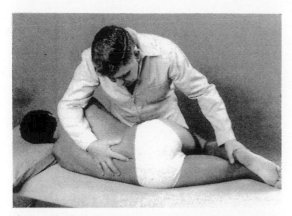

Figure 27.17 Lumbar manipulation technique 5: setting the lower level by positioning the leg.

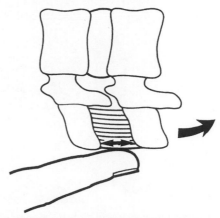

Figure 27.18 Lumbar manipulation technique 5: illustrating the position of the palpating finger over the interspinous ligament between the adjacent spinous processes L4 and L5. It will detect widening (with increased tension) in the gap as the leg is flexed.

STEP 2: Setting the upper level by positioning the trunk (Figure 27.19)

- Ask the patient to turn his or her head and look up at the ceiling.
- Carefully rotate the trunk by grasping the patient's lower arm just above or around the elbow and gently pulling the arm outwards (Figure 27.20). A lower grip may lose control and cause discomfort.
- Maintain smooth slow rotation of the trunk until the palpating finger, which is positioned just under the spinous process of L4 (proximal to the interspinous space), detects a downward movement of this spinous process (Figure 27.21).
- Cease rotating the trunk the instant this movement is detected.
- Now slightly extend the spine by pulling this arm upwards (avoid further rotation).
- Fix the trunk by asking the patient to place the hand of this arm under the head.

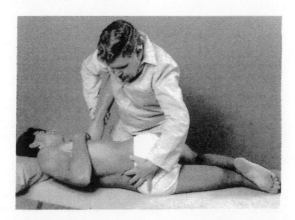

Figure 27.19 Lumbar manipulation technique 5: setting the upper level by positioning the trunk.

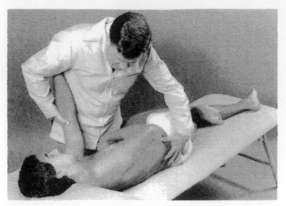

Figure 27.20 Lumbar manipulation technique 5: the arm grip, just above the elbow. Pull through to rotate the trunk.

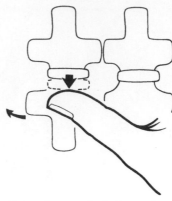

Figure 27.21 Lumbar manipulation technique 5: illustrating the position of the palpating finger just under the proximal spinous process so that it can detect its downward movement.

Note: Excessive friction on the couch can render this movement so jerky that the end point which relies on sensitive palpation can be missed.

STEP 3: The manoeuvre (Figure 27.22)

● Rest the upper forearm against the shoulder and upper chest via the axilla, and the other forearm over the ischium, just below the iliac crest.
● Ensure that you are properly balanced.
● Apply a distracting force, gradually rocking back and forth with the forearms as you move towards maximal rotating stretch.
● The thumb of your proximal hand is placed on the upper side of the spinous process of the upper vertebra (L4) and steadies it by pressing downwards (Figures 27.23 and 27.24).

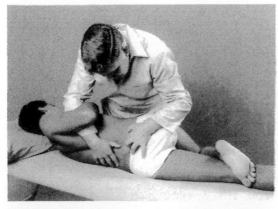

Figure 27.22 Lumbar manipulation technique 5: the end position for manipulation.

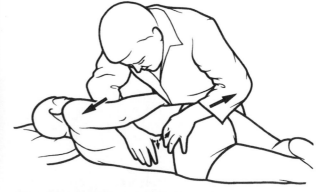

Figure 27.23 Lumbar manipulation technique 5: illustrating the direction of applied forces.

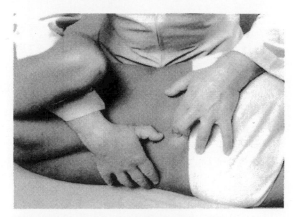

Figure 27.24 Lumbar manipulation technique 5: a close up view of the technique.

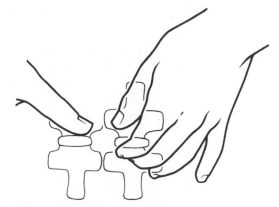

Figure 27.25 Lumbar manipulation technique 5: illustrating the reinforcing position of the hands over the spinous process at the level to be gapped.

- The fingers of your lower hand can be kept free but an appropriate variation is to hook the index and middle fingers beneath the lower spinous process and at the point of thrust with the forearm apply an upward pull on that vertebra (Figure 27.25).
- When all the slack is taken up by your forearms, ask the patient to take a deep breath and exhale. Towards the end of the exhalation execute a sharp increase of rotatory pressure through both forearms, especially through the short lever to the pelvis.
- After this specific manipulation the patient should be reassessed and the manipulation repeated if necessary.

Note: It is important not to dig the elbow of the proximal arm into the patient's body, since this can be painful. Especially in a large patient, this may present a problem; in such a case, it is better to use the proximal forearm to steady and stretch rather than thrust, thus leaving most of the thrust to the forearm on the pelvis. Likewise it is important to find a position for the distal forearm which is comfortable for the patient, and to avoid using the point of the elbow for thrusting, as the buttock area is very sensitive to sharp pressure.

6. Rotation in the sitting position

This very effective technique is different from the preceding methods in that the pelvis is fixed while the trunk is rotated. The patient fixes the pelvis by straddling a low couch or a chair, but the couch provides the better position, because it allows greater flexibility of the trunk.

The main indication is unilateral pain at the thoraco-lumbar junction. The method can be used also for pain (unilateral and bilateral) of the lumbar spine and the lower thoracic spine, especially when other methods prove stubborn or ineffective.

The usual rules for indications and contra-indications apply to this method.

Position of the patient

- The patient straddles the end of the couch as shown in Figure 27.26 and sits firm and erect.
- The patient crosses the arms over the chest so that the hands rest on the opposite shoulders.
- The patient should be comfortable throughout the procedure and proper padding should rest against the inner thighs.

Position of the therapist

- Stand directly behind the patient.
- Adopt a firm wide based stance behind the patient.
- Grasp the patient's shoulders or arm just above the elbow with your hands.

Method

- After grasping the shoulders, rotate the patient's trunk steadily and firmly, away from the painful side, to the limit of rotation.
- Before rotation is attempted the patient must be at the absolute limit of stretch. If any sharp pain is reproduced at this end range the manipulation is abandoned.
- Manipulation consists of a sharp, well controlled rotation. The stretch should be so effective that the final arc of movement of the patient's trunk is almost imperceptible (Figure 27.26).

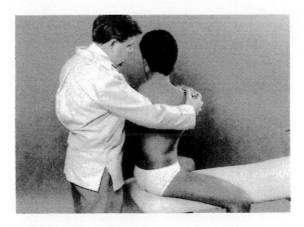

Figure 27.26 Lumbar manipulation technique 6: rotating the trunk to the left because pain was reproduced on rotation of the spine to the right. This method uses the shoulder grip to achieve rotation.

Variations of the sitting technique

An alternative strategy is to 'hug' the patient's trunk using the arm that embraces the trunk to grasp the shoulder or arm on the side to be rotated. The thrusting hand can be applied to the shoulder or to a specific area of the back corresponding to the level of pain. Thus a type of 'push-pull' manoeuvre can be achieved with the embracing arm pulling into rotation and the other hand pushing to achieve a complementary smooth rotation of the trunk (Figures 27.27 and 27.28). Thus some degree of specificity can be achieved by using the thrusting hand over the affected level of the spine and imparting the impulse here during rotation.

Figure 27.27 demonstrates the technique for a problem at the thoraco-lumbar junction, while Figure 27.29 demonstrates the technique for low lumbar pain and Figure 27.30 shows the direction of the applied forces.

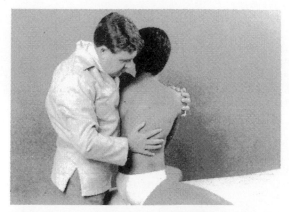

Figure 27.27 Lumbar manipulation technique 6: this variation shows rotatory manipulation of the thoraco-lumbar junction for pain produced on the right side.

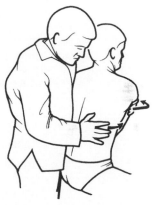

Figure 27.28 Lumbar manipulation technique 6: illustrating the direction of the applied forces for Figure 27.27.

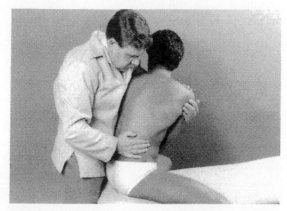

Figure 27.29 Lumbar manipulation technique 6: this variation shows rotatory manipulation for the low lumbar area with the patient being placed in some degree of forward flexion.

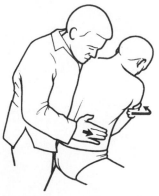

Figure 27.30 Lumbar manipulation technique 6: illustrating the direction of the applied forces for Figure 27.29.

LUMBAR MANIPULATION UNDER GENERAL ANAESTHESIA

Manipulation under general anaesthetic is rarely necessary and should be used as a last resort within the context of manipulation of the lumbar spine. However, the procedure can be dramatically effective, provided the standard guidelines of manipulation are followed.

Indications

● The patient is unable to relax for routine manipulation of the lumbar spine.
● There is persistent stiffness, tightness or a sensation of a deeply locked joint that is not responsive to routine treatment.

The anaesthetic

The simplest and safest method is for an experienced anaesthetist to administer a hypnotic dose of intravenous sodium thiopentone or similar agent. Diazepam can be used for the procedure. The minimum dose to induce sleep and the sensation of relaxation is all that is required and the procedure should take three to five minutes until the patient is awake. Specific muscle relaxants such as suxamethonium are not necessary.

The methods

Three lumbar rotational techniques can be used. They are all non-specific methods: the usual routine is to combine technique 1 or 2 with technique 7.

Lumbar manipulative techniques 1 and 2: under general anaesthetic

The patient is placed on the pain-free side and the manipulation performed as previously outlined (Figure 27.2). This method is preferred to technique 2 (Figure 27.6), where the patient lies supine. However, technique 2 is easier for the anaesthetist to control (see Figures 27.31 and 27.32).

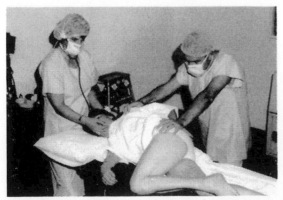

Figure 27.31 Lumbar manipulation technique 1: under general anaesthetic.

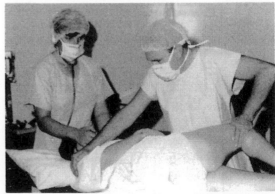

Figure 27.32 Lumbar manipulation technique 2: under general anaesthetic.

7. Trunk rotation with fixed pelvis (for general anaesthesia)

This is another non-specific rotation which mobilises all the lumbar spine, using the principle of a longer lever: the trunk is used to achieve the rotatory force. An assistant is needed to keep the pelvis fixed, and the anaesthetist has to carefully control the head throughout the manoeuvre.

The procedure is commonly performed bilaterally. It is arguably the most effective method to use under general anaesthetic.

Method

- Stand opposite the side to be rotated (the painful side).
- Firmly grasp the patient's arm above the wrist.
- Steadily rotate the trunk towards you until the end range is reached (Figure 27.33). (This should be tested prior to anaesthesia to ensure no reproduction of sharp pain.)
- At the end range give a short rotatory pull (Figure 27.34).

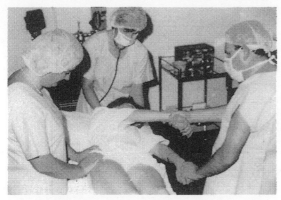

Figure 27.33 Lumbar manipulation technique 7: the initial movement of trunk rotation for pain on the side opposite the therapist.

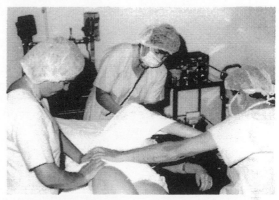

Figure 27.34 Lumbar manipulation technique 7: showing the final position of trunk rotation.

During this procedure the theatre assistant holds the pelvis firm while the anaesthetist controls the patient's head. You can use your spare hand to help the assistant keep the pelvis fixed.

DANGERS OF MANIPULATING THE LUMBAR SPINE

There are many documented cases of manipulation causing sequestration of a prolapsed disc with subsequent damage to nerve roots and the surgical emergency of cauda equina compression.

The danger symptoms and signs contra-indicating manipulation include:

- sciatica to the foot, especially with associated paraesthesia and anaesthesia

- an 'irritable' back when the pain is aggravated by minor trauma, sitting and 'simple' rises in intrathecal pressure such as coughing, laughing, and straining at stool
- protective spasm with lateral scoliosis
- neurological signs, especially weakness
- positive dural signs – positive slump test
  – positive SLR (especially < 30 degrees)
- pain with contralateral SLR.

A good indicator of a problematical potential manipulation is the reproduction of sharp pain when the spine is placed at full stretch immediately prior to manipulation.

One of the worst mistakes is to manipulate a diseased spine or a fractured spine. A proper history and examination and appropriate investigations should lead to the correct diagnosis, especially if the patient has a tumour or metastases in the spine.

Extension thrust techniques can cause cauda equina damage in the presence of a disc prolapse, so assess carefully beforehand.

The rule is 'if in doubt – DON'T manipulate'. Remember that time heals and that mobilisation is a safe technique.

The problem of extension manipulation

The use of forcible postero-anterior central thrusting techniques is fraught with danger, and of all the lumbar manipulation techniques, these are the ones most likely to lead to sequestration of the disc and cause cauda equina damage in the presence of a pre-existing disc protrusion. The method shown in Figure 24.22 is best used, and other mobilisation techniques (as outlined in Chapter 24). Sharp thrusting is to be avoided.

These extension manipulation techniques are described in authoritative literature and have a small place in manual medicine, but should be left to the real experts.

REASSESSMENT OF MANIPULATION

The efficacy of the treatment should be assessed immediately at the end of each treatment.

Methods of assessment

Subjective

- Patient's awareness – relief of pain? increased mobility?
- Response to sitting in and rising out of a chair.

Objective

- Effect on range of a movement, especially flexion or extension.
- Effect on SLR (often an unreliable indicator) and the slump test.
- Response to palpation – less spasm or tenderness?

THE BEST BACK TO MANIPULATE

History

- Pain confined to back
- Sudden onset
- Recent onset.

Examination

- All movements present
- Extension decreased more than flexion if any limitation
- SLR at least 60 degrees
- Slump test negative
- No neurological signs.

PRACTICE TIPS

- A low couch is necessary for optimal lumbar manipulation.
- Don't manipulate through protective spasm.
- Beware of manipulating the patient who has a slow onset of pain and has fixed lateral deviation.
- Never manipulate against the wishes of the patient – talk to the patient and work co-operatively.
- Apply your manipulative thrust just before the end of expiration after requesting the patient to take a deep breath in and out.
- If in doubt, don't manipulate – mobilise or give no manual therapy.

CAUTIONARY ADVICE

Make sure that organic disease is not present in the spine that you are manipulating, especially malignant disease.

Take care not to turn a small disc prolapse into a major sequestration causing nerve root damage or even cauda equina damage. This can occur by manipulating in the presence of neurological signs or by using a forcible postero-anterior direct thrust. Always heed the precautions.

28
Treatment plans, exercises and injection techniques for the lumbosacral spine and hip girdle

Contents
- [ ] Management guidelines for lumbosacral disorders
  - Low back pain (only) due to vertebral dysfunction
  - Acute low back pain (only) with spasm
  - Sciatica with or without low back pain
  - Chronic low back pain
- [ ] Low back pain (LBP) exercises
  - General advice to patients
  - Guidelines
  - Advice and comments
  - Starting the exercises
  - Isometric exercises
  - Extension exercises
  - Flexion exercises
  - Flexion and rotation exercises
  - Flexion and extension exercises
- [ ] Injection techniques
  - Injection of painful myofascial trigger points
  - Injections for gluteus medius tendinitis and trochanteric bursitis
  - Lateral femoral cutaneous nerve of the thigh
  - Epidural injections

MANAGEMENT GUIDELINES FOR LUMBOSACRAL DISORDERS

The management of back pain depends on the cause. Since most of the problems are mechanical and there is a tendency to natural resolution, conservative management is quite appropriate. Practitioners should have a clear-cut management plan with a firm, precise, reassuring and conservative clinical approach.

The problems can be categorised into general conditions for which the summarised treatment protocols are outlined.

Acute pain   = pain less than 2 weeks
Subacute pain = 2–6 weeks
Chronic pain   = greater than 6 weeks

Low back pain (only) due to vertebral dysfunction

The common problem of low back pain caused by facet joint dysfunction and/or limited disc disruption usually responds well to the following treatment:

● back education programme
● encouragement of normal activities according to degree of comfort
● regular simple analgesics – for example, paracetamol
● exercise programme (when exercises do not aggravate), swimming (if feasible)
● spinal mobilisation or manipulation (if no contra-indication on first visit)
● review in about five days (probably best time for physical therapy).

Most of these patients can expect to be relatively pain free in 14 days and can return to work early (some may not miss work).

Acute low back pain (only) with spasm

● back education programme
● strict rest lying on a firm surface for 2–3 days (keep the spine as straight as possible)
● regular simple analgesics with review as the patient mobilises
● cold or hot compresses to the painful area
● simple mobilisation exercises as tolerated
● muscle energy therapy
● relaxant – for example, diazepam (if appropriate) for 4–5 days
● review in 4–5 days.

When the acute phase settles, treat as for uncomplicated low back pain.

Sciatica with or without low back pain

Sciatica is a more complex and protracted problem to treat, but most cases will gradually settle within 12 weeks if the following approach is used:

Acute

● Strict bed rest for three days (keep the spine straight – avoid sitting in soft chairs and for long periods)

- regular simple analgesics with review as the patient mobilises
- NSAIDs for 7 to 10 days
- back education programme
- exercises – straight leg raising exercises to pain tolerance
- swimming
- traction (intermittent only will suffice).

Chronic

- Continue traction
- reassurance that problem will subside (assuming no neurological defects)
- consider epidural anaesthesia (if slow response).

Chronic low back pain

The basic management of the patient with uncomplicated chronic back pain should follow the following guidelines:

- back education programme and ongoing support
- encourage activity
- exercise programme
- swimming
- analgesics – paracetamol
- NSAIDs for 7–10 days (only if inflammation, i.e. pain at rest – relieved by activity); trial of mobilisation or manipulation.

LOW BACK PAIN (LBP) EXERCISES

General advice to patients

Back exercises are extremely important because the muscles of the spine and abdomen support the spine better than any brace or corset. If you have chronic, nagging back pain, it is likely that performing these exercises religiously for three months will greatly reduce your back pain.

The purpose of these exercises is to strengthen the various muscles that support the spine, especially the abdominal muscles and the extensor muscles of the spine.

Guidelines

- Do these exercises on a padded or well carpeted floor.
- Do them at least twice a day for no less than five minutes at a time; once a day is better than not at all.
- Rest between each exercise.
- Avoid jerky movements.
- Do not strain.
- The exercises may be uncomfortable at first, and initially each one should be repeated only two or three times.
- Swimming as an activity is probably the best exercise of all.

Advice and comments

Do not continue with any of these exercises if your symptoms are much worse immediately after exercising or if they remain worse the next day. If any exercise produces or increases leg pain below the knee you should stop doing it. In either case consult your therapist.

It is normal to feel some flare-up of your pain or new pains or aches when starting any new exercises. These new pains are often felt in the arms, along the back, around the shoulders or between the shoulder blades. They simply mean that the body is getting accustomed to new activities. The aching should wear off in a few days.

Starting the exercises

It is very difficult to carry out exercises when you have acute pain so you must not start until you can comfortably lie face down. If you have sciatica, it is a good idea to start straight leg raising exercises as soon as possible, and keep them going. You should always keep up your exercises. At the first signs of a return of low back pain you should immediately start the exercises which previously led to your recovery.

ISOMETRIC EXERCISES: 'SPLINTING' THE LUMBAR SPINE

It is a good idea to learn how to keep the lumbar spine in a fixed position by using the abdominal muscles and the muscles around the spine. These are static (isometric) exercises which can teach you to use the abdominal, low back and pelvic muscles. You can actually feel them tightening and relaxing as you keep the lumbar spine immobile.

Exercise 1: the pelvic tilt

Lie on the floor with your feet flat on the floor, arms at your sides and your knees bent. Draw in your stomach (abdomen) firmly and press your lumbar region (back of waist) against the floor by tightening and slightly raising your buttocks. This will tilt your pelvis upwards. Hold – count to seven – relax; repeat five to ten times.

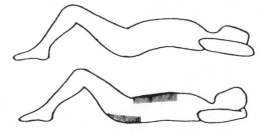

Exercise 2: body flattener

Adopt the same starting position for exercise 2 and then stretch (extend) your legs by sliding your heels forwards while keeping your lumbar spine flat on the floor. You should feel your abdominal and back muscles tighten. Hold – count to seven – relax; repeat five to ten times.

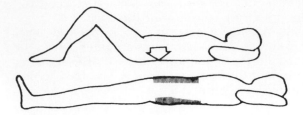

EXTENSION EXERCISES

These exercises are used to strengthen the back muscles and are often used for a disc bulge. They have to be used gently and carefully.

Exercise 3: buttock tightener

Lie on your stomach. Let your head rest comfortably on your folded hands. Tighten your buttock muscles. Hold that position for three seconds, then relax. Repeat five to ten times.

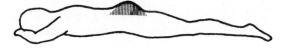

Exercise 4: back leg lift

Keeping your legs straight, lift one as far as possible. Hold for three seconds, drop, and repeat with the other leg. Repeat five to ten times.

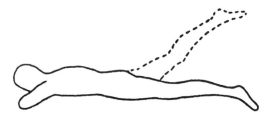

Exercise 5: trunk lift

Lie on your stomach. Place your hands on the floor (as for a lift up) and by straightening your elbows push up as far as possible – keep your pelvis and legs limp – allow your low back to sag. Hold for three seconds, then lower yourself. Repeat five to ten times.

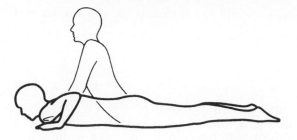

Exercise 6: the back arch (standing extension)

Stand up straight, feet pointing directly forwards and kept apart as wide as your shoulders, hands placed on the small of your back – fingers pointing backwards. Breathe in and breathe out slowly – as you breathe out bend backwards as far as you can while supporting your back with your hands and keeping your knees straight. Hold your lower back arched for three seconds then return to the neutral position. Repeat ten times.

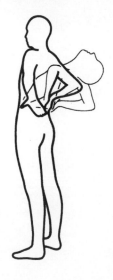

Exercise 7: the horizontal raise

Lie face down with your lower abdomen and pelvis supported across a firm chair or table with suitable padding. Ensure that you are well balanced. Now raise your head, shoulders and legs until your body is horizontal. (Do not raise your shoulders or legs above the horizontal level.) Hold for three seconds – relax; repeat five to ten times.

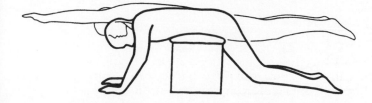

FLEXION EXERCISES

Some of these exercises are very effective for strengthening abdominal muscles.

Exercise 8: the chair exercise

Sit on a chair, feet apart on the floor. Let your neck slowly drop, then drop your shoulders and arms, and bend down between your knees, as far as you can. Return to an upright position, straighten up, and relax. Do not force your downward bend. Repeat five to ten times.

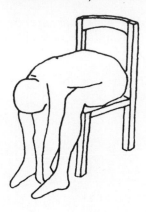

Exercise 9: half sit up

Lie on the floor with your knees bent and your arms relaxed at your sides. Raise your head and shoulders off the floor, hold three seconds, bring them down slowly, and relax. Repeat five to ten times.

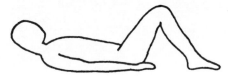

Exercise 10: knee to chest raise

Lie flat on your back, bend one leg up, grasping it with your hand just below the knee, and bend your head forward so that your forehead approaches your knee. Hold three seconds. Repeat on the other side.

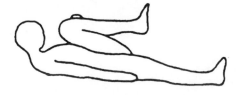

Exercise 11: full sit up

Keeping your arms out straight or folded across the chest, bend your knees slightly, then lift your head and shoulders. You will feel your stomach muscle tighten. Hold three seconds. Repeat five to ten times. Don't do sit ups with your legs straight, unless you are very fit.

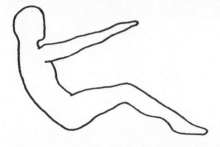

Exercise 12: full sit up with feet locked

This exercise is a variation of exercise 11. Lie on your back with your hands clasped behind your head, knees bent. Fix your feet under a heavy object that won't topple over (a chest of drawers, bed, or heavy chair). Sit up, then lower yourself slowly to a lying position. You should sit up gradually, starting by raising your head, then your shoulders, and then your chest and lower end of the spine. Hold for three seconds. Repeat five to ten times. If you cannot do this exercise with your hands behind your neck, try to do it with your hands at your sides.

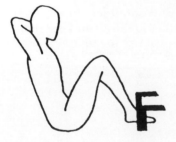

Exercise 13: straight leg raise

With your leg perfectly straight, raise it as high as you can just short of the point of pain. Repeat with the other leg. Take this to the limit of pain. Hold for three seconds. Repeat five to ten times.

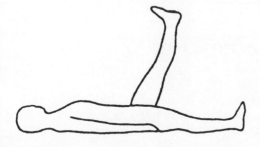

FLEXION AND ROTATION EXERCISES

Exercise 14: straight leg swing

With your arms spread out on either side, raise one leg as high as possible, keeping it straight. Swing the leg in an arc from one side to the other. It is more important to swing the leg on the side of your back that you feel pain (if you have any). Hold for three seconds. Repeat five to ten times.

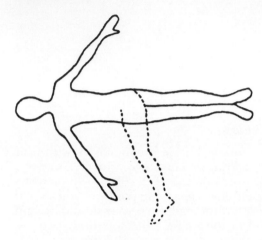

Exercise 15: pelvic roll

You can get better results if someone pins your shoulders to the floor while you do this exercise. Lift your legs together in the air and roll them from side to side. Hold for three seconds. Repeat five to ten times.

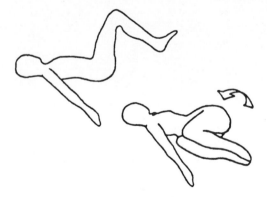

FLEXION AND EXTENSION EXERCISES

Exercise 16: the cat back

Assume a kneeling position, resting on your hands and knees. Arch (hunch) your back like a cat and drop your head at the same time. Hold this position for about seven seconds.

Then reverse the arch by bringing up your head and letting your back sag, as you form a 'U' with your spine. Take a deep breath as you reverse the arch of your back. Arch and sag your back alternately several times.

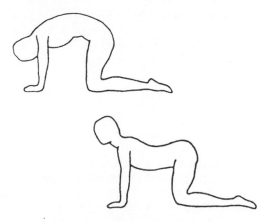

INJECTION TECHNIQUES

Injections have a valuable place in the diagnosis and treatment of specific problems of the spine, the myofascial compartments of the paraspinal regions and the shoulder. It must be emphasised that injection therapy of the soft tissues of the back and neck has a limited place in the overall management of spinal conditions and that there appears to be no proper rationale for the injection of corticosteroid preparations into most of these areas.

A most valuable injection for lumbosacral disorders is the caudal epidural, which is well within the technical capabilities of all practising doctors. This injection is most applicable for those patients with intractable low back pain and sciatica, particularly those confronted with possible surgical intervention.

The one area of the musculoskeletal system that does respond remarkably well to corticosteroid injections is the upper limb, especially the painful disorders of the components of the rotator cuff, and subacromial bursitis.

Rules of procedure for injection therapy

- Accurate diagnosis of the lesion.
- Pinpoint localisation of the painful lesion.
- The injection site should be marked.
- Use a sterile technique.
- For tender trigger points use the needle as a probe.
- Select the shortest needle that will reach the lesion and insert the needle to the minimum effective depth.
- Never inject into a tendon – only into the tendon sheath.

- Always aspirate for blood.
- Use 1% local anaesthetic (or its equivalent) without a vasopressor (adrenaline/epinephrine).
- Avoid corticosteroids in myofascial trigger points.
- Use relatively small volumes of local anaesthetic.
- If the patient is allergic to local anaesthetic, try normal saline as a substitute.
- Do not attempt an ambitious technique or inject blind – for example, apophyseal joint injections or sinuvertebral nerve blocks.

Injection of painful myofascial trigger points

Injection of trigger points in the myofascial tissues of the back and other parts is relatively easy and excellent results are possible.

Identification of these trigger points may be achieved by systematic palpation of paraspinal areas (Figure 28.2). Various alternative terms exist, including 'tender points', 'myalgic points', 'fibrositis', 'myofasciitis' and 'Travell's trigger points'.

Travell (1949, 1952), who has published charts of pain patterns associated with tender trigger points, has defined a trigger point as one characterised by:

- circumscribed local tenderness
- localised twitching or fasciculation with stimulation of juxtaposed muscle
- pain referred elsewhere when subjected to pressure.

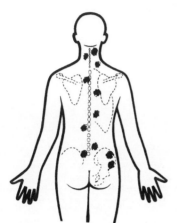

Figure 28.2 Typical distribution of trigger points and areas of pain referral.

The points would also correspond to the MID hypothesis of Maigne with the reflex skin activity. Interestingly, they tend to correspond to the acupuncture points used for pain relief.

An explanation of the pain relief following injection of these trigger points with local anaesthetic has been proposed by Mooney and Cairns (1978), who suggest that these areas of focal irritability represent areas of referred pain and autonomic nerve dysfunction and, 'by a poorly understood mechanism, local injection with anaesthetic can provide pain relief at a distant location for far longer than can be explained by the pharmacological action of the drug. Probably the most simplistic explanation of this phenomenon is the break-up of a cycle of neurological action and response'.

The authors believe that some of these trigger points actually represent the site of emergence of the posterior primary rami through the fascia to supply the skin. These points tend to lie three vertebral levels below the origin of the nerve root. (Refer to Chapter 15, Figures 15.3, 15.5 and 15.7).

Successful injection therapy has been described by many renowned therapists including Wilkinson (1971), for pain and spasm associated with cervical spondylosis; Mehta (1973), for temporary pain relief from chronic pain, muscle strains and spasms, lumbago and acute torticollis; Sheon et al. (1978) for a wide range of back disorders; and Stoddard (1969).

Bourdillon (1973), who also describes occasions of dramatic pain relief from trigger spot injections (especially into muscle), uses 1%

lignocaine in preference to the often used mixture of 2% lignocaine and hydrocortisone.

Principles of injection into trigger points

- Use local anaesthetic (LA) only.
- Corticosteroids irritate trigger points (Mennell, 1986).
- Use a moderate volume of LA.
- Large volumes of solution irritate by local stretching of tissue.
- Avoid bleeding, because blood irritates the points.

Anaesthetic

- Lignocaine/lidocaine, procaine or bupivacaine (1% or 0.5%) can be used.
- Travell prefers the use of 5% procaine in normal (physiological) saline.
- If the patient is allergic to local anaesthetic, use normal saline.
- The volume is 5 to 8 ml.

Method

- Ask the patient to mark the stated area of pain on a blank body chart and note if it compares with a Travell trigger point.
- Identify and mark the trigger point, which must be the maximal point of pain.
- Select a 21, 22 or 23 G needle of a length compatible with the injection site. This may vary from 25 mm in parts of the neck, low lumbar and sacral area, and the thoracic spine to 90 mm in deeper areas such as the upper lumbar spine. A 38 mm needle will cover most areas of the back and neck.
- Insert the needle into the point until the patient complains of reproduction of pain which may be referred distally.
- At this point introduce 5 to 8 ml of local anaesthetic of your choice (Figure 28.3).
- Post-injection stretching exercises to the affected segment are recommended.

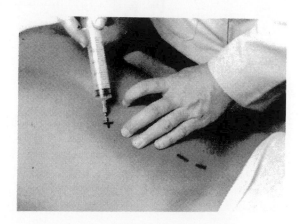

Figure 28.3 Trigger point injection for thoracic back pain at the T9 level.

Injections for gluteus maximus tendinitis and trochanteric bursitis

Pain around the greater trochanter

Pain around the lateral aspect of the hip is a common disorder, and is usually seen as lateral hip pain radiating down the lateral aspect of the thigh in middle aged and older people engaged in walking exercises, tennis and similar activities. It is analogous in a way to the shoulder girdle, where supraspinatus tendinitis and subacromial bursitis are significant wear-and-tear injuries.

The two common causes are tendinitis of the gluteus medius tendon, where it inserts into the lateral surface of the greater trochanter of the femur, and bursitis of one or both of the trochanteric bursae. Distinction between these two conditions is difficult, and it is possible that, as with the shoulder, both are related. The pain of bursitis tends to occur at night; that of tendinitis occurs with such activity as long walks and gardening.

Method

Treatment of both is similar.

- Determine the points of maximal tenderness over the trochanteric region and mark them. (For tendinitis, this point is immediately above the superior aspect of the greater trochanter; Figure 28.4.)
- Inject aliquots of a mixture of 1 ml of long acting corticosteroid with 5 ml of LA into the tender area, which usually occupies an area similar to that of a standard marble.

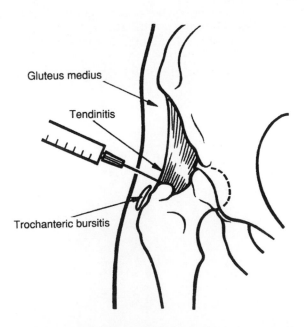

Gluteus medius

Tendinitis

Trochanteric bursitis

Figure 28.4 Injection technique for gluteus medius tendinitis and trochanteric bursitis (into area of maximal tenderness).

The injection is invariably very effective. Follow-up management includes sleeping with a small pillow under the involved buttock and stretching the gluteal muscles with knee–chest exercises. One or two repeat injections over 6 or 12 months may be required. Surgical intervention is rarely necessary.

Lateral femoral cutaneous nerve of the thigh

Meralgia paraesthetica

This is the commonest lower limb nerve entrapment and is due to the lateral femoral cutaneous nerve of the thigh being trapped under the lateral end of the inguinal ligament, about 1 cm medial to the anterior superior iliac spine.

The nerve is a sensory nerve from L2 and L3. Entrapment occurs mostly in middle-aged people, due mainly to thickening of the fibrous tunnel beneath the inguinal ligament, and is associated with obesity, pregnancy, ascites or local trauma such as belts, trusses, corsets. Its entrapment causes a burning pain with associated numbness and tingling (Figure 28.5).

The distribution of pain is confined to a localised area of the lateral thigh and does not cross the midline of the thigh.

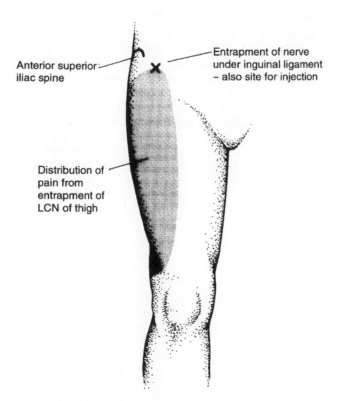

Anterior superior iliac spine

Entrapment of nerve under inguinal ligament – also site for injection

Distribution of pain from entrapment of LCN of thigh

Figure 28.5

Differential diagnosis

- L2 or L3 nerve root pain (L2 causes buttock pain also).
- Femoral neuropathy (extends medial to midline).

Treatment options

- Injection of corticosteroid medial to the ASIS, under the inguinal ligament.
- Surgical release (neurolysis) if refractory.

Note: Meralgia paraesthetica often resolves spontaneously.

Injection treatment

Mix 1 ml of LA corticosteroid with 3 ml of plain local anaesthetic and using an inferior approach inject it under the inguinal ligament at a site 1 to 1.5 cm medial to the anterior superior iliac space.

Epidural injections

Epidural injections have been considered for many years to be a very effective treatment for severe back pain and sciatica. Success rates of between 35 per cent and 86 per cent have been reported, with the average success rate being around 60 per cent after three to six months (Bogduk and Cherry, 1985).

There are two anatomically based epidural injections – lumbar and caudal. Anaesthetists tend to favour the lumbar route because the anaesthetic agent is introduced closer to the target area and a smaller volume is required. In the lumbar technique, the patient lies on the side with the spine, hips and knees flexed, and the injection is introduced at either the L3–L4 or L4–L5 level in a manner similar to a lumbar puncture except that it is strictly extradural. The needle must not puncture the dura; should this occur the procedure should be abandoned. A small amount of local anaesthetic or long-acting corticosteroid, or both, is introduced at this level.

In Australia the Australian Drug Evaluation Committee and Medical Defence Organisations advise against the use of long-acting corticosteroid preparations for epidural injections because of claims of there being no convincing evidence of their efficacy and that they are of doubtful safety.

Cyriax claims that the caudal epidural injection is the nerve block *par excellence* and produces very good results when indicated. He claims that it is an easier procedure and avoids the danger of thecal puncture. However, larger volumes must be injected to reach the affected level. The caudal epidural injection is presented because

- it is technically easier
- it is safer
- it can be performed in the outpatient department of hospitals or in the office treatment room provided resuscitation facilities are available

- the patient can go home after resting for half an hour (lumbar epidural injections usually require hospital admission for 24 hours.)
- it has diagnostic value. (It will relieve, albeit temporarily, the pain from disc compression on dura mater and on nerve roots as well as inflammation of nerve roots, but will not relieve the pain from problems such as ischaemic claudication to the lower limb, ankylosing spondylitis, and invasive lesions including osteomyelitis, neuroma and malignancy.)

The caudal (trans-sacral) injection

Caussade and Chauffard used the caudal epidural technique for the treatment of sciatica as long ago as 1909. Evans (1930) employed an epidural block for the treatment of low back pain with sciatic radiation. He injected an enormous volume (60–145 ml) of 1% novocaine and saline with immediate or complete relief in over 60 per cent of patients.

In 1961 Coomes investigated two groups of 20 patients with severe sciatica. After full clinical and radiological assessment one group was treated by caudal epidurals and the other by bed rest. The groups were matched in terms of symptomatology and duration of pain (average 34 days). He injected 50 ml of a solution of 0.5% procaine into the patients of the test group. The average time for recovery of the control group having bed rest was 31 days and for the injection group 11 days. The injected group also demonstrated a greater improvement in neurological signs.

Harley (1984), in treating 50 successive patients using one or two injections, achieved complete relief in 20 patients, improvement in 13 and no change in 17.

Two debatable issues are the volume of anaesthetic agent and the addition of a corticosteroid to the injection. Cyriax and others use up to 50 ml of solution per injection while others consider that in excess of 40 ml is dangerous. Mehta (1973) observed that the mechanical stretching of nerve roots, by the physical mass of fluid volumes greater than 40 ml is unnecessary and potentially dangerous.

Yates (1978), comparing four different solutions, concluded that the addition of corticosteroid (Lederspan) produced a significant advantage in the restoration of mobility. In view of the medicolegal issues Australian doctors tend to use either no corticosteroid or a soluble short-acting corticosteroid. Cyriax insisted that the addition of a corticosteroid to the anaesthetic was of no assistance.

Indications

1. Hyperacute lumbago
2. Nerve root pain with or without neurological signs
3. Intractable backache
4. Severe back pain in last two months of pregnancy
5. Diagnostic trial
6. Trial procedure prior to surgery.

Corrigan and Maitland (1983), and the authors, have achieved the best results in patients with relatively severe sciatica with or without neurological signs. The more severe the pain, the greater the chance of success. However, the success rate is lower for hyperacute lumbago where there is intense lumbar pain with marked muscular spasm. Older patients, even those in their seventies and eighties, can achieve excellent results, especially with sciatica.

The 'ideal' patient

- Middle aged.
- Recent onset (two to six weeks) of pain.
- Low back pain with sciatica.
- No neurological signs.
- No intervertebral foraminal encroachment.

Precautions

- Strict asepsis.
- A no-touch technique wherever possible.
- Ensure dural sac is not pierced – a shorter needle is preferable (for example, 4 cm or 5 cm rather than 7.5 cm or 10 cm).
- Ensure no injection occurs into a vein.
- Constantly check for CSF and blood by aspiration.
- Give the injection slowly.
- Anticipate side effects.
- Have an assistant to monitor blood pressure and pulse.
- Have resuscitation facilities available.
- Rest the patient for 30 minutes after the injection, gradually proceeding from lying to sitting to standing and then moving about.

The physiological effects of the caudal injection

The injected fluid ascends cranially for a distance proportional to the force and volume injected, running up the neural canal and along the external aspect of the lower lumbar nerve roots. It does not enter any joint.

Its precise mode of action is not known but it will produce anaesthesia in the following:

- dura mater
- nerve sheaths
- structures innervated by the sinuvertebral nerve
- anterior and posterior nerve roots
- the posterior longitudinal ligament
- the ganglia of the sympathetic chain and the visceral afferent fibres accompanying the sympathetic fibres.

Contra-indications

- Patients who are hypersensitive to local anaesthetic.
- Localised skin infection.

Local anaesthetic used

Half strength standard solution (without adrenaline or epinephrine) of any of the local anaesthetics such as lignocaine/lidocaine 0.5%, procaine 0.5% or bupivacaine 0.25%. This usually anaesthetises the nociceptive (pain-sensitive) nerve fibres and leaves the motor nerve fibres intact. The recommended volume is 15–20 ml.

Cyriax claimed that procaine was the best anaesthetic but bupivacaine is generally the preferred solution.

Anatomical landmarks

The epidural space lies between the two layers of the dura mater, namely the outer (periosteal) layer and the inner layer, termed the dura. It extends continuously from the foramen magnum to the sacral hiatus and contains a plexus of veins. The dural sac usually ends at the S2 level but sometimes aberrations occur and it may extend almost to the sacral hiatus, a fact which must always be borne in mind. The spinal cord usually ends opposite the L1–L2 disc and the nerve roots continue as far down to the sacrum and the cauda equina.

The opening of the sacral hiatus is normally covered by a strong ligament which at times can feel quite firm and gritty, especially in the older patient.

The hiatus, which is a triangular opening near the end of the posterior sacrum, lies at the top of the two sacral cornua.

Identifying the sacral hiatus

The sacral hiatus can be identified as follows:

- Palpate the two sacral cornua and mark the hiatus at the top end of the hollow formed by the cornua.
- It lies directly beneath the upper limit of the intergluteal fold.
- It tends to correspond to the proximal interphalangeal joint with the tip of the index finger resting on the tip of the coccyx.
- It lies at the caudal apex of an equilateral triangle drawn with the horizontal base between the posterior superior iliac spines (opposite S2). This apex is usually situated over the sacral hiatus (Figure 28.6).

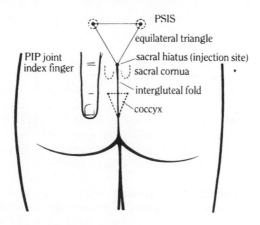

Figure 28.6 Identify the sacral hiatus by four methods:
(1) palpating the sacral cornua.
(2) noting the upper limit of the intergluteal fold.
(3) measuring the tip of the coccyx to the PIP of the index finger.
(4) drawing an equilateral triangle with the base being the line between the postero-superior iliac spines.

Injection procedure

- Mark the sacral hiatus after its identification.
- Lie the patient prone with a pillow under the symphysis pubis to slightly flex the hips (or with the operating table 'broken').
- Relax the glutei by inversion of the ankles (feet in pigeon toe position).
- Clean and drape the area, avoiding spirit running onto the anus. Using a 25 G or a 23 G needle, anaesthetise the skin and subcutaneous tissue **(this is very important)**.
- Select a spinal tap cannula: 21, 22 or 23 G × 50 mm (choose a 90 mm cannula if the patient is very obese).
- Insert the cannula at 20 degrees to the vertical, to reach bone.
- Withdraw slightly and lower a further 40 to 45 degrees towards the intergluteal cleft (Figure 28.7).
- Insert the needle upwards (cranially) keeping strictly to the midline. The angle to the skin should be about 25 to 30 degrees: if too superficial, the needle will pass above the hiatus.
- When the ligament is pierced there is a sensation of 'giving'.
- Angle the needle slightly downwards as you insert it for about 2 cm. Avoid proceeding any further because of the risk of piercing the dura – the needle must not reach S2 (Figure 28.8).

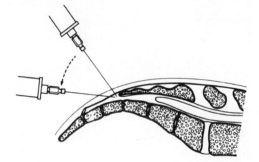

Figure 28.7 The caudal epidural: the method of introducing the needle into the sacral hiatus.

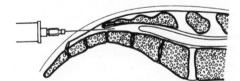

Figure 28.8 The caudal epidural: the needle should lie free in the space and fall short of the end of the dural sac.

- The needle is rotated through 90 degrees twice – check for a backflow of cerebrospinal fluid (CSF) or blood:
  - if blood is obtained, partly withdraw the needle and reinsert it, keeping as far posterior as possible to avoid the greater concentration of veins anteriorly;
  - if CSF is withdrawn, abandon the procedure.
- Inform the patient that the procedure is surprisingly comfortable but that some heaviness will be felt in the back of the legs and that pain may be initially exacerbated.
- Inject the fluid carefully and slowly over a five-minute period (at least) with at least three aspiration checks for blood.
- The plunger of the syringe should move with relative ease. If the needle lies between periosteum and bone, the injection meets resistance (Figure 28.9) and the needle requires replacement.

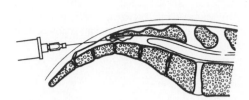

Figure 28.9 The caudal epidural: the needle is jammed under the periosteum and meets resistance.

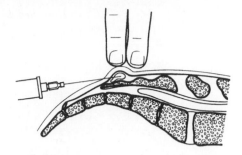

Figure 28.10 The caudal epidural: palpating for fluid extravasating posterior to the sacrum.

- As the injection proceeds, place a palpating hand just above the sacral hiatus. A swelling developing over the presacral tissues can be palpated and indicates that the needle lies posterior to the sacrum (Figure 28.10). The needle has to be reinserted and a greater angle to the skin is obviously required. The appearance of the procedure is shown in Figure 28.11.

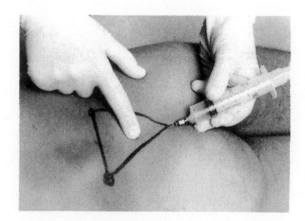

Figure 28.11 The caudal epidural: the appearance of the procedure.

- Ask the patient to report any unusual symptoms such as giddiness or lightheadedness, which is actually reasonably common but indicates a need for caution. Monitor the pulse and blood pressure during the procedure and stop the injection if an adverse reaction develops.

Side effects

Side effects include syncopal feelings as the spinal canal volume adjusts; lightheadedness and a 'detached' feeling; drowsiness; numbness over the sacral area; muscular weakness (with motor involvement); and bradycardia. (For bradycardia, give intravenous atropine if the pulse rate is less that 50 per minute.)

Toxic reaction and its management

Occasional twitching may occur, for which no treatment is required. For convulsions, intravenous diazepam should be administered. If hypotension is present, elevate the legs, give oxygen and a volume expander such as Hartmann's solution, inject a pressor agent such as ephedrine intravenously.

Follow up

Inform the patient that it may take at least a week for the injection to be effective, especially for sciatic pain. The injection may be repeated in one week if there is some improvement. Cyriax and others recommend two injections in many instances but generally at least 50 to 60 per cent of patients show significant improvement and one injection is sufficient. The injection can be repeated many times if improvement is followed by relapse. If no improvement occurs surgical intervention for radicular pain should be considered.

29
The lumbosacral spine: case histories and management problems

---

Contents
☐ Lumbar spine: manual therapy
☐ Case histories
☐ Answers to management problems: lumbar spine

The following ten case histories of patients with low back pain are presented for discussion in courses on manual therapy for back pain. However, readers may choose to answer the problems independently. For each patient, make the appropriate decisions according to the following plan:

1. Provisional diagnosis
2. Level of the lesion
3. Degree of irritability (low, moderate or high)
4. Management plan
5. Select the appropriate manual therapy (if any) from the mobilisation, muscle energy and manipulation techniques as listed.
   A. Select the appropriate technique or techniques of first choice for that particular patient.
   B. Select the second line technique or techniques should the patient fail to respond to the initial treatment.

The main techniques are summarised in list form and are also presented in a coded format.

LMo = lumbar mobilisation
LMa = lumbar manipulation
LMET = lumbar muscle energy therapy

LUMBAR SPINE: MANUAL THERAPY

Summary of techniques

Mobilisation techniques

1. Accessory rotation: initial range
2. Accessory rotation: mid range   LMo 1
3. Accessory rotation: end range

4. Anterior directed central gliding	LMo 2
5. Anterior directed unilateral gliding	LMo 3
6. Transverse directed rotational gliding	LMo 4
7. Longitudinal distraction gliding = traction	LMo 5

Manipulation techniques

1. Non-specific rotation: method A	
2. Non-specific rotation: method B	LMa 1
3. Rotation in flexion	LMa 2
4. Rotation in extension	LMa 3
5. Specific rotation	LMa 4
6. Rotation in sitting position	LMa 5
7. Manipulation under general anaesthesia	LMa 6

Muscle energy techniques

1. MET for restricted flexion: method A	LMET 1
2. MET for restricted flexion: method B	LMET 2
3. MET for restricted extension	LMET 3

Injection techniques

1. Trigger point injection
2. Epidural anaesthesia

CASE HISTORIES

Case 1

A 30-year-old male (teacher) presents within two days of the sudden onset of right-sided low back pain after bending over to lift his baby from the floor. The pain is aggravated by sitting and by movements towards the right side which provoke sharp pain persisting for two to three hours.

Inspection

Guarded movement, spasm in paravertebral muscles, slight left lateral deviation.

Palpation

Tenderness in right paraspinal area L3–L4.

Movements

Restricted and painful flexion, extension and R lateral flexion.

Dural signs

SLR normal, end stage slump test positive.

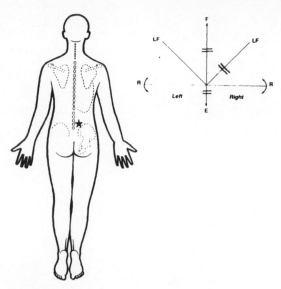

X-ray

Normal.

Questions

1. Provisional diagnosis.
2. Spinal level of lesion.
3. Irritability (low, moderate or high).
4. Management plan.
5. Selection of manual therapy techniques:
   A. First line techniques
   B. Second line techniques.

Case 2

A 28-year-old female (housewife) presents with a six week history of low back pain (central and to the left). It came on gradually after a day of spring cleaning when she moved furniture around the house. The pain comes on after two to three hours of housework but settles soon after resting. Bending forwards to make the beds aggravates the pain which is a deep dull ache.

Inspection

Normal movement, normal back appearance.

Palpation

Tender over L4 spinous process and unilateral L4–L5 (L).

Movements

Restricted and tender flexion and (L) lateral flexion; other movements free.

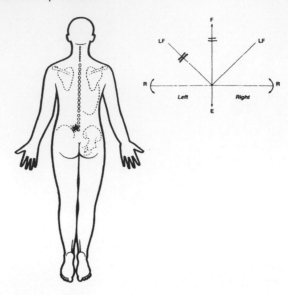

Dural signs

Nil.

X-ray

Normal.

Questions

1. Provisional diagnosis.
2. Spinal level of lesion.
3. Irritability (low, moderate or high).
4. Management plan.
5. Selection of manual therapy techniques:
   A. First line techniques
   B. Second line techniques.

Case 3

A 45-year-old female (dressmaker) presents with a three hour history of pain in the backs of both thighs and anaesthesia in the perineal area, thighs and buttocks. There is associated incontinence of urine and weakness of the legs making walking very difficult. The problem followed a manipulation for a recent episode of low back pain with left-sided sciatica when a 'firm thrust was applied to the low lumbar area with her leg pulled up behind her'. Soon after this she described loss of feeling in the 'pelvic area'.

Inspection

Walks supported; dribbling of urine from a flaccid urethra.

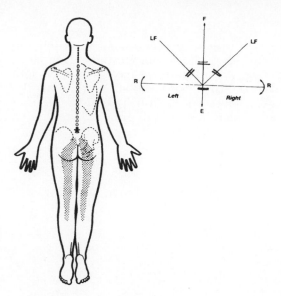

Palpation

Tender over L5 and L5–S1 interspace (central).

Movements

(Tested carefully) restriction of all lumbar movements.

Dural signs

Positive.

Neurological

Loss of sensation to pinprick and touch around the vulva and anus; absent left ankle jerk.

X-ray

Normal.

Questions

1. Provisional diagnosis.
2. Spinal level of lesion.
3. Irritability (low, moderate or high).
4. Management plan.
5. Selection of manual therapy techniques:
   A. First line techniques
   B. Second line techniques.

Case 4

A 21-year-old carpenter presents with a five day history of central and right-sided low back pain after lifting a heavy timber frame. It varies in severity from mild to moderate, when it radiates into the upper right buttock. He has attempted to return to work but after two hours the pain forces him to stop and it takes one to two hours to settle to a comfortable level. He is free of pain in bed at night.

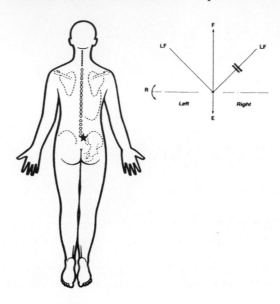

Inspection

Slightly restricted movements.

Palpation

Tender over L5 and unilateral L5–S1 (R); no muscle spasm.

Movements

Restricted R lateral flexion.

Dural signs

Nil.

X-ray

Normal.

Questions

1. Provisional diagnosis.
2. Spinal level of lesion.

3. Irritability (low, moderate or high).
4. Management plan.
5. Selection of manual therapy techniques:
   A. First line techniques
   B. Second line techniques.

Case 5

A 38-year-old motor mechanic presents with a five day history of left-sided low back pain with pain and paraesthesia radiating down the leg especially in the outer aspect of the leg and ankle and into the sole of the foot. The pain developed several hours after lifting a motor. The problem is aggravated by sitting, coughing, sneezing, and straining at the toilet. It is relieved by resting and lying down.

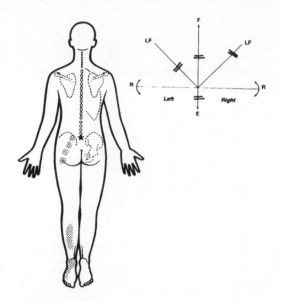

Inspection

Scoliosis to the right; loss of lumbar lordosis.

Palpation

Tender over spinous process L5; muscle spasm paravertebral.

Movements

Restricted and painful flexion, extension and bilateral lateral flexion (more so to the left).

Dural signs

Positive: SLR 30° on left, slump test positive at level 2.

Neurological

Reduced power eversion left foot; diminished sensation over little toe; sluggish L ankle jerk; difficulty walking on toes (left).

X-ray

Normal.

Questions

1. Provisional diagnosis.
2. Spinal level of lesion.
3. Irritability (low, moderate or high).
4. Management plan.
5. Selection of manual therapy techniques:
   A. First line techniques
   B. Second line techniques.

Case 6

A 57-year-old male (farmer) presents with several months of gener-alised low back pain and stiffness. The deep ache is bilateral and occasionally radiates into the upper buttocks. It is worse after long periods of gardening and car travel but restricted activity helps his pain and stiffness.

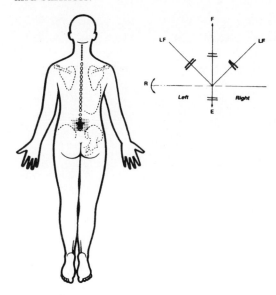

Inspection

Flattened lumbar lordosis, moves stiffly.

Palpation

Deep tenderness centrally over L3, L4, L5 spinous processes and bilaterally at these levels.

Movements

All movements restricted.

Dural signs

Nil.

X-ray

Degenerative changes including disc narrowing especially at L4, L5 and S1 levels.

Questions

1. Provisional diagnosis.
2. Spinal level of lesion.
3. Irritability (low, moderate or high).
4. Management plan.
5. Selection of manual therapy techniques:
   A. First line techniques
   B. Second line techniques.

Case 7

A 25-year-old female, 26 weeks pregnant, presents with central and right-sided low back pain for the past six weeks. The pain is aggravated by activity and relieved by rest. At times it is severe (after standing for long periods); rest settles the pain after 30 minutes.

Inspection

Guarded movements when arising from chair.

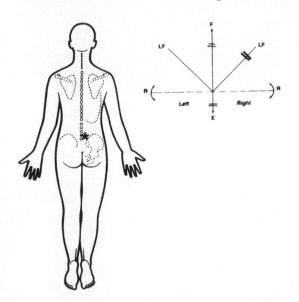

Palpation

Tender over L4 centrally and L4–L5 unilaterally (R).

Movements

Limited flexion, extension and lateral flexion to right.

Other joint tests

Normal, including sacro-iliac joint.

Dural signs

Nil.

Questions

1. Provisional diagnosis.
2. Spinal level of lesion.
3. Irritability (low, moderate or high).
4. Management plan.
5. Selection of manual therapy techniques:
   A. First line techniques
   B. Second line techniques.

Case 8

A 34-year-old male (salesman) presents with a three hour history of agonising right-sided low back pain of sudden onset after twisting around in his car to grab his brief case from the back seat. He has a recent history of nagging low back pain. There is no radiation of pain.

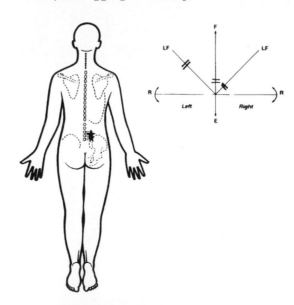

Inspection

Severe limitation of movement, marked scoliosis to right, marked muscle spasm.

Palpation

Generalised spasm, very tender L4–L5 unilateral on R.

Movements

Limited flexion, lateral flexion R and L, especially to R.

Dural signs

Unable to test.

X-ray

Normal.

Questions

1. Provisional diagnosis.
2. Spinal level of lesion.
3. Irritability (low, moderate or high).
4. Management plan.
5. Selection of manual therapy techniques:
   A. First line techniques
   B. Second line techniques.

Case 9

A 38-year-old male (bricklayer) presents with a three week history of left-sided low back pain with radiation into the left leg which varies considerably. It is aggravated by working for long periods, although he can continue working.

Inspection

Walks normally, difficulty turning on couch.

Palpation

Tenderness over L5–S1 (left side).

Movements

Normal movements/provocation (quadrant) test positive on left.

Dural signs

SLR to 75°, slump test negative.

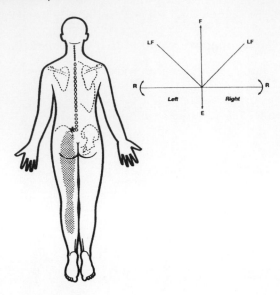

Neurological

Normal.

X-ray

Normal.

Questions

1. Provisional diagnosis.
2. Spinal level of lesion.
3. Irritability (low, moderate or high).
4. Management plan.
5. Selection of manual therapy techniques:
    A. First line techniques
    B. Second line techniques.

Case 10

A 22-year-old female, six months post partum, presents complaining of central low back pain with radiation into both buttocks since childbirth. The pain is aggravated by lifting her baby and activity. At times the pain is intense.

Inspection

Movements slightly guarded.

Palpation

Tender over L5, upper sacrum and L5–S1 interspace.

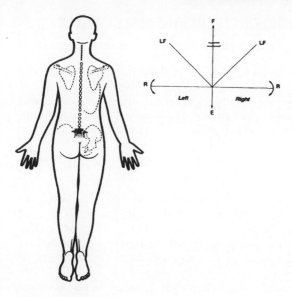

Movements

Limited flexion.

Other joints

Sacro-iliac joints slightly positive to compression.

Dural signs

Slump test positive to level 5.

Neurological

Normal.

X-ray

Sacralisation L5, minor narrowing L5–S1 disc space.

Questions

1. Provisional diagnosis.
2. Spinal level of lesion.
3. Irritability (low, moderate or high).
4. Management plan.
5. Selection of manual therapy techniques:
   A. First line techniques
   B. Second line techniques.

ANSWERS TO MANAGEMENT PROBLEMS: LUMBAR SPINE

Although these management strategies highlight the physical aspects of patient management, the authors emphasise the importance of considering the whole person and considering their anxieties and personal problems. Giving appropriate reassurance and providing empathy and responsible care is essential.

Case 1

1, 2. The provisional diagnosis is possibly apophyseal joint dysfunction at the right L3–L4 level and/or on 1V disc disruption. It is most likely to be an apophyseal joint lesion. Nerve root compression due to an L3–L4 disc prolapse is not common and this fact renders a clinical diagnosis of a disc prolapse at this level more difficult.

3. This patient demonstrates high irritability, which is not uncommon in the first few days of an acute back injury.

4. Conservative management is appropriate at this stage with bed rest for two days; basic analgesics such as aspirin, codeine or paracetamol/acetaminophen; coping guidelines for acute back pain (Chapter 28). The patient should return for review in about three days.

5. Manipulative techniques are not appropriate for this patient in the presence of muscle spasm and high irritability. Furthermore, it is likely that this acute problem may subside quickly with rest. Some simple back extension exercises (if possible) may help but exercises are usually ill advised for severe acute pain.

    Mobilisation techniques can be used but gentle stage 1 techniques may be the only ones tolerated:

    First line:　　LMo 1　Rotation (stage 1 – initial range)
    Second line:　LMo 3　ADG unilateral (if tolerated)
    　　　　　　　LMo 4
    　　　　　　　LMo 5

    Muscle energy therapy techniques could also be used.
    On review, as the irritability subsides, manipulation may be possible.

Case 2

1, 2. The provisional diagnosis is apophyseal joint dysfunction at the L4–L5 level or an MID at this level.

3. The patient has low irritability and perhaps is unfortunate that the problem has not disappeared spontaneously.

4. Management should consist of patient education advice about lifting and daily activities, the use of mild analgesics for pain and exercises, especially flexion and extension exercises.

5. Mobilisation or manipulation could be used for this patient but in view of the low irritability and chronicity of the problem, manipulation would be the logical choice.

    The first line techniques would be LMa 3 (rotation in extension) and LMa 4 (specific rotation) at L4–L5 with the patient lying on the right side.

    The second line techniques would be LMa 5 (rotation in sitting).

Case 3

This patient has cauda equina compression caused by a large L5–S1 intervertebral disc sequestration. This followed an inappropriate direct thrust into hyperextension manipulation over the prolapsed L5–S1 disc.

The patient requires urgent referral to a neurosurgeon or an orthopaedic surgeon for decompression of the spinal segment and discectomy.

Case 4

1, 2. The provisional diagnosis is apophyseal joint dysfunction at the L5–S1 level (right side) or an MID at this level and/or possible internal disruption of the intervertebral disc including prolapse.
3. This patient has moderate irritability and a good prognosis can be anticipated.
4. Management should include the usual advice about analgesics, relative rest, coping strategies, exercise and prevention.
5. The patient has moderate irritability but no muscle spasm. Either mobilisation or manipulation could be used. In view of the moderate irritability, however, mobilisation would be the preferable first line technique namely LMo 1 (accessory rotation) and LMo 2 or LMo 3.

    Any of the muscle energy therapy techniques could be used.

    The second line techniques are LMa 4 (specific rotation) and LMa 5 (rotation in sitting).

Case 5

1, 2. This patient has an L5–S1 intervertebral disc prolapse causing S1 nerve root compression.
3. The patient has a high irritability problem.
4. A protracted course can be anticipated, for example, six to twelve weeks. A trial of conservative treatment would be appropriate, involving:
    - relative rest in bed (firm base essential)
    - analgesics – try simple analgesics initially – for example, aspirin, paracetamol (acetaminophen), codeine or a combination of these. Avoid strong narcotics if possible.
    - NSAIDs – for example, diclofenac, naproxyn, indomethacin, piroxicam

- tranquilliser/muscle relaxant – for example, diazepam
- swimming and exercise prescription (following improvement and when these exercises are manageable).
  If the patient is not responding or his circumstances demand more active treatment, an epidural anaesthetic injection is appropriate.

5. The first line manual techniques for this patient include LMo 1 (initial range accessory rotation), and LMo 5 (traction) but these have to be given with care and are likely to have modest results only.

   Spinal manipulation is absolutely contra-indicated.

Case 6

1, 2. This patient has lumbar spondylosis or generalised osteoarthritis of his lumbar spine, especially from the mid to lower levels.   The intervertebral disc degeneration is part of the overall degenerative pathology.

3. There is low irritability.

4. The general management of lumbar spondylosis includes basic analgesics (depending on patient response and tolerance), stronger NSAIDs (observing the usual precautions), warmth, an appropriate balance between light activity and rest, exercises and hydrotherapy. Trials of electrotherapy such as TENS and alternative treatments such as acupuncture might be worthwhile.

5. The first line techniques are mobilisation, particularly LMo 2 (central anterior directed gliding), LMo 3 (unilateral anterior directed gliding) and LMo 1 (accessory rotation). These patients may obtain a worthwhile response to regular mobilisation and exercises.

   As a rule manipulation should not be used, mainly because it is less effective in the presence of chronic inflammation. However, if mobilisation improves the pain and mobility, general manipulations such as LMa 1 (non-specific rotation) and LMa 5 (rotation in sitting) can be of considerable benefit.

Case 7

1, 2. This patient probably has apophyseal joint dysfunction at the right L4–L5 level or an MID. Dysfunction of the apophyseal and sacro-iliac joints can be a problem during pregnancy.

3. Moderate irritability is present.

4. Management includes the usual advice of combining sensible restricted activity with appropriate rest. The use of drugs and radiological investigation has to be tempered during pregnancy but mild analgesics and antenatal exercises should help the problem.

5. Manual therapy can be used during the second trimester but techniques involving only side lying and sitting should be used.

   Mobilisation is the best first line technique but it is mainly restricted to rotational methods (LMo 1) through all the ranges as tolerated.

Manipulation, which is an appropriate second line technique (if the patient does not respond to mobilisation), includes LMa 1 (non-specific rotation techniques), LMa 4 (specific rotation) and LMa 5 (rotation in sitting). The manipulation techniques should be as gentle as possible.

Case 8

1, 2. The patient has probably sustained acute dysfunction of the L4–L5 apophyseal joint on his right side. Other possibilities are an intervertebral disc prolapse, but the suddenness of the attack makes dysfunction of the apophyseal joint the likely diagnosis.
3.   This is a case of extremely high irritability.
4.   Management of this severe problem includes suitable analgesia which may include admission to hospital for injections of strong analgesics and muscle relaxants. The application of ice packs (or sometimes heat) can be beneficial.
5.   Manual therapy has limited application and spinal manipulation through such intense muscle spasm is contra-indicated.

Because the painful site is localised, a trigger point injection of 8 ml of local anaesthetic is appropriate. Massage and a muscle energy technique could be used, but the most appropriate technique is rotational mobilisation (LMo 1), starting with stage 1 and attempting to work through to stage 3.

Many of these dramatic problems can settle completely within a few days, so initial symptomatic, conservative management is recommended.

Case 9

1, 2. This patient has apophyseal joint dysfunction at the L5–S1 level on the left side with referred pain.
3.   There is low irritability.
4.   This patient requires the usual advice about back care and prevention.
5.   This patient appears to be an ideal case for manual therapy.

First line techniques are the mobilisations:

LMo 1 – rotation (stage 3)
LMo 3 – anterior directed unilateral gliding

Second line techniques are the manipulations:

LMa 4 – specific (L5–S1) rotation
LMa 5 – rotation in sitting

Case 10

1, 2. The diagnosis in this patient is somewhat controversial. The finding of sacralisation of L5 may not be of any significance.

This clinical pattern could be due to dysfunction of the sacro-iliac joints or an L5–S1 disc disruption.

3.   Moderate irritability is present.
4.   The usual advice about back care should be given, and a prescription for extension exercises, especially advising swimming.
5.   First line manual therapy is mobilisation, namely LMo 2 (central gliding).

Second line techniques are manipulation techniques, specifically directed at L5–S1 and the sacro-iliac joints.

Bibliography

Abrahams, V. C. (1979) The physiology of neck muscles: their role in head movement and maintenance of posture. *Cand. J. Physiol. Pharmacol.*, **55**, 332–338.

American Medical Association (1984) *Guides to the Evaluation of Permanent Impairment.* Chicago.

Barraclough, D. and Mitchell, H. (1982) Management of low back pain. *Current Therapeutics*, **4**, 41–45.

Bartelink, D. L. (1957) Clinical effects of disc prolapse. *J. Bone Joint Surg.*, **39B**, 718–722.

Benn, C. T. and Wood, P. H. N. (1975) Pain in the back. An attempt to estimate the size of the problem. *Rheumatol. Rehabit.*, **14**, 121–128.

Berquist-Ulmann, M. and Larson, U. (1977) Back pain; controlled clinical trial. *Acta. Orthop. Scand. Supplement*, 170.

Bertelen, S. (1969) Neurovascular compression syndromes of the neck and shoulder. *Acta. Chir. Scand.*, **135**, 137–148.

Bogduk, N. (1976) The anatomy of the lumbar intervertebral disc syndrome. *Med. J. Aust.*, **1**, 878.

Bogduk, N. (1979) The lumbar zygapophyseal joints: their anatomy and clinical significance. Proceedings of low back pain symposium. *Manip. Ther. AA.*

Bogduk, N. (1980). The anatomy and pathology of lumbar back disability. A paper – 'Course on Rehabilitation of Disability of the Back', University of Sydney, March, 29–30.

Bogduk, N. (1983) The innervation of the lumbar spine. *Spine*, **8**, 286–293.

Bogduk, N. (1984) The rationale for patterns of neck and back pain. *Patient Management*, **8**, 13–21.

Bogduk, N. (1985) Low back pain. *Aust. Fam. Physician*, **14**, 1168–1172.

Bogduk, N. (1986). The anatomy and pathophysiology of whiplash. *Clinical Biomechanics*, **1**, 92–101.

Bogduk, N. (1988) Neck pain: an update. *Aust. Fam. Physician*, **17**, 75–80.

Bogduk, N. and Cherry, D. (1985) Epidural corticosteroid agents for sciatica. *Med. J. Aust.*, **2**, 402–406.

Bogduk, N., Colman, R. R. S. and Winer, C. E. R. (1977) An anatomical assessment of the 'percutaneous rhizolysis' procedure. *Med. J. Aust.*, **1**, 397–399.

Bogduk, N. and Jull, G. A. (1985) The theoretical pathology of acute locked back: a basis for manipulative therapy. *Man. Med.*, **1**, 78–82.

Bogduk, N. and Twomey, L. T. (1987) *Clinical Anatomy of the Lumbar Spine.* Melbourne, Churchill Livingstone.

Bourdillon, J. F. (1973) *Spinal Manipulation*, 2nd edn. London, Heinemann.

Bradley, K. C. (1974) The anatomy of backache. *Aust. NZ. J. Surg.*, **44**, 227.

Bradley, K. C. (1985) The posterior primary rami of segmental nerves. In: *Aspects of Manipulative Therapy*, Glasgow, E. F., Twomey, L. T., Scull, E. R. et al (eds) 2nd edn. pp. 59–63. Melbourne, Churchill Livingstone.

Browne, C. (1986) Common regional pain syndromes: meeting the diagnostic challenge. *Patient Management*, **10**, 20–34.

Buswell, J. S. (1982). Low back pain: a comparison of two treatment programmes. *NZ. J. Physiotherapy*, **10** (2), 13–17.

Buswell, J. S. (1985) An approach to research in manual therapy. In: *Aspects of Manipulative Therapy*, Glasgow, E. F. Twomey, L. T. Scull, E. R. et al. (eds) 2nd edn, pp. 123–127. Melbourne, Churchill Livingstone.

Cady, L. D. Bischoff, D. P., O'Connell, E. R. et al. (1979) Strengths and fitness and subsequent back injuries in firefighters. *J. Occup. Med.*, **21**, 269–272.

Cailliet, R. (1986) *Low Back Pain Syndrome*. Philadelphia, F A Davis, pp. 25–36.

Charnley, J. (1951) Orthopaedic signs in the diagnosis of disc protrusion. *Lancet*, **27**, 186.

Coombs, E. N. (1961) A comparison between epidural anaesthesia and bed rest in sciatica. *Br. Med. J.*, **1**, 20.

Corrigan, A. B., Carr G. and Tugwell, S. (1982) Intraspinal corticosteroid injections. *Med. J. Aust.*, **1**, 224–225.

Corrigan, B. and Maitland, G. D. (1983) *Practical Orthopaedic Medicine*. London, Butterworths.

Corrigan, B. and March, L. (1984) Cervical spine dysfunction: a pain in the neck. *Patient Management*, **8**, 43–45.

Coxhead, C. E., Inskip, H., and Meade, T. W. et al. (1981) Multi-centre trial of physiotherapy in the management of sciatic symptoms. *Lancet*, **1**, 1065–1068.

Coyer, A. B. and Curwen, I. H. M. (1955) Lower back pain treated by manipulation. *Br. Med. J.*, **1**, 705–707.

Crock, H. V. (1970) Reappraisal of intervertebral disc lesions. *Med. J. Aust.*, **1**, 983.

Currier, D. P. (1979) *Elements of Research in Physical Therapy*. Baltimore, Williams & Wilkins.

Cyriax, J. H. (1975) Manipulation in the treatment of low back pain. *Br. Med. J.*, **2**, 334.

Cyriax, J. H. (1980) *Textbook of Orthopaedic Medicine*, Vol 2. 10th edn. London, Baillière Tindall.

Cyriax, J. H. (1982) *Textbook of Orthopaedic Medicine*, Vol 1. 8th edn. London, Baillière Tindall.

Cyriax, J. H. and Cyriax, P. J. (1983) *Illustration Manual of Orthopaedic Medicine*. London, Butterworths.

De Palma, A. and Rothman, R. H. (1970) *The Intervertebral Disc*. Philadelphia, Saunders, pp. 134–138.

Deyo, R. A., Diehl, A. K. and Rosenthal, M. (1986) How many days of bed rest for acute low back pain? A randomised clinical trial. *N. Engl. J. Med.*, **315**, 1064–1070.

Deyo, R. A. (1983) Conservative therapy for low back pain: distinguishing useful from useless therapy. *JAMA*, **250**, 1057–1062.

Dilke, T. F. W., Burry, H. C. and Grahame, R. (1975) Extradural corticosteroid injection in management of lumbar nerve root compression. *Br. Med. J.*, **2**, 161–164.

Dillane, J. B., Fry, J. and Kalton, G. (1966) Acute back syndrome – a study from general practice. *Br. Med. J.*, **2**, 82–84.

Dixon, A. J. (1973) Progress of problems on back pain research. *Rheumatol Rehabilitation*, **12**, 165–175.

Dvorak, J. and Dvorak, V. (1984) *Manual Medicine*. Stuttgart, New York: Georg, Thieme, Verlag and Thieme-Stratton Inc.

Dvorak, J. and Dvorak, V. (1984) *Manual Medicine Diagnostic*. Stuttgart, New York: Georg, Thieme, Verlag and Thieme-Stratton Inc.

Doran, D. M. L. and Newell, D. J. (1975) Manipulation in treatment of low back pain: a multi-centre study. *Br. Med. J.*, **2**, 161–165.

Easter Seal Society (1982) *The Easter Seal Guide to Children's Orthopaedics.* Toronto, The Easter Seal Society, pp. 64–67.

Edwards, B. C. (1969) Low back pain and pain resulting from lumbar spine conditions: a comparison of treatment results. *Aust. J. Physiother.,* **25**, 104–110.

Elvey, R. (1983) Treatment of conditions accompanied by signs of abnormal brachial plexus tension. In: Jull, G. (ed). Proceedings of neck and shoulder symposium, *Manipulative Therapists Association of Australia.* Brisbane, MTAA, pp. 53–65.

Elvey, R. L. (1985) Brachial plexus tension tests and the pathoanatomical origin of arm pain. In: *Aspects of Manipulative Therapy,* Glasgow, E. F. Twomey, L. T., Scull, E. R. et al. (eds). Melbourne, Churchill Livingstone, pp. 117–122.

Elvey, R. L. (1986) The investigation of arm pain. In: *Modern Manual Therapy of the Vertebral Column.* Grieve, G. P. (ed). London, Churchill Livingstone, pp. 530–535.

Elvey, R. L., Quinter, J. and Thomas A. N. (1986) A clinical study of RSI. *Aust. Fam. Physician,* **15**, 1314–1322.

Evans, D. P. (1978). Lumbar spinal manipulation on trial – clinical assessment. *Rheumatol. Rehabilitation,* **17**, 46–53.

Evans, D. P. (1982) *Backache: Its Evolution and Conservative Treatment.* Lancaster, MTP Press Ltd.

Evans, W. (1930) Intra-sacral epidural injections in the treatment of sciatica. *Lancet,* **2**, 1225.

Farrell, J. P. and Twomey, L. T. (1982) Acute low back pain: comparison of two conservative treatment approaches. *Med. J. Aust.,* **1**, 160–164.

Ferguson, D. (1983) Occupational factors in back strain. Seminar manual of occupational injuries. *RACS,* **173**, 133–139.

Fisk, J. W. (1977). *A Practical Guide to Management of the Painful Neck and Back.* Springfield, Charles C Thomas.

Fisk, J. W. (1979) A controlled trial of manipulation in a selected group of patients with low back pain favouring one side. *NZ. Med. J.,* **90**, 288–291.

Fisk, J. W. (1980) Manipulation in physical medicine: when should it be attempted. *Patient Management,* **2**, 57–63.

Fordyce, W. E. (1973) Operant conditioning in the treatment of chronic pain. *Arch. Phys. Med. Rehabil.,* **54**, 399–406.

Fox, E. J. and Melzack, R. (1976) Transcutaneous electrical stimulation and acupuncture: comparison of treatment of low back pain. *Pain,* **1**, 141–148.

Francis, J. (1973) Subcutaneous lumbar rhizolysis. *Med. J. Aust.,* **2**, 749–750.

Frymoyer, J. W. et al. (1980) Epidemiologic studies of low back pain. *Spine,* **5**(5), 419–423.

Ganong, W. F. (1981) *Review of Medical Physiology,* 10th edn. Los Altos, Lange, pp. 74–92.

Ganora, A. (1984) Chronic back pain: diagnosis, treatment and rehabilitation. *Patient Management,* **8**, 55–77.

Gilbert, J. R. et al. (1985) Clinical trial of common treatments for low back pain in family practice. *Br. Med. J.,* **291**, 791–794.

Gilbert, J. R. (1986) Management of low back pain in family practice: a critical review. *Can. Fam. Physician,* **32**, 1855–1861.

Grahame, R. (1980) Clinical trials in low back pain. *Clin. Rheum. Dis.,* **6**, 143–156.

Grieve, G. P. (1981) *Common Vertebral Joint Problems.* Edinburgh, Churchill Livingstone.

Guymer, A. J. (1986) Proprioceptive neuromuscular facilitation for vertebral joint conditions. In: *Modern Manual Therapy of the Vertebral Column.* Grieve, G. P. (ed), pp. 622–639. London, Churchill Livingstone.

Hadler, N. M. (1986) Regional back pain. *N. Engl. J. Med.,* **315**, 1090–1092.

Harley, C. (1984) Manipulative techniques. *Update*, **2**, 29–35.

Hazleman, B. and Bulgen, D. (1979) Low back pain. *Med. Journ.*, **13**, 869–875.

Hart, F. B. (1985) *Practical Problems in Rheumatology*. London, Martin Dunitz, pp. 55–76.

Hay, M. C. (1976) Anatomy of the lumbar spine. *Med. J. Aust.*, **1**, 874–876.

Henderson, I. (1985) Low back pain and sciatica: evaluation and surgical management. *Aust. Fam. Physician*, **14**, 1149–1159.

Hirsch, C. (1966) Aetiology and pathogenesis of low back pain. *Israel J. Med. Sci.*, **2** (3), 362–370.

Hoehler, F. K., Tobis, J. S. and Buerger, A. A. (1981) Spinal manipulation for low back pain. *JAMA*, **245**, 1835–1838.

Hoppenfeld, S. (1976) *Physical Examination of the Spine and Extremities*. New York, Appleton-Century-Crofts.

Hoppenfeld, S. (1977) *Orthopaedic Neurology*. Philadelphia, J. B. Lippincott.

Horal, J. (1969) The clinical appearance of low back pain disorders in Gotenberg, Sweden. *Acta. Orthop. Scand.*, Suppl. 118.

Houston, J. R. (1975) A study of subcutaneous 'rhizolysis' in the treatment of chronic backache. *J. Roy. Coll. Gen. Practit.*, **23**, 692.

Hult, L. (1954) The Munkfors investigation. *Acta. Orthop. Scand.*, Suppl. 16.

Ireland, D. (1986) The hand (part 2). *Aust. Fam. Physician*, **15**, 1502–1513.

Jacobs, D. (1984) Intraspinal injection of depot corticosteroids. *Med. J. Aust.*, **140**, 49.

Jayson, D. (1976) *The Lumbar Spine and Back Pain*. London, Grune and Stratton.

Jayson, M. I. V. (1979) Back pain: some new approaches. *Med. J. Aust.*, **1**, 513–516.

Jeans, T. (1979) Relief of chronic pain by brief intense TENS – a double blind study, Proc. 2nd World Congress, PAIN.

Kaltenborn, F. (1976) *Mobilisation of the Spinal Column*. NZ. Uni. Press.

Kane, W. I. and Moe, J. H. (1970) A scoliosis prevalence survey in Minnesota. *Clin. Orthop.*, **69**, 216–218.

Kendall, P. H. and Jenkins, S. M. (1968) Exercises for backache: a double blind controlled study. *Physiotherapy*, **54**, 154–157.

Kenna, C. (1984) The whiplash syndrome. *Aust. Fam. Physician*, **13**, 256–258.

Kenna, C. (1985) The physical examination of the back. *Aust. Fam. Physician*, **11**, 1244–1254.

Kenna, C. (1985) Spinal manipulation for doctors: a workshop course. Melbourne, RACGP.

Kenna, C. (1986) Examination of the neck: part two. *Aust. Fam. Physician*, **15**, 1204–1212.

Kenna, C. (1987) Whiplash. *Aust. Fam. Physician*, **16**, 727–734.

Kenna, C. and Murtagh, J. (1986) Examination of the neck: part one. *Aust. Fam. Physician*, **15**, 1015–1021.

King, J. S. and Lagger, R. (1976) Sciatica viewed as referred pain syndrome. *Surg. Neurol.*, **5**, 46–48.

King, J. S. (1977) Randomised trial of the Rees and Shealy methods for the treatment of low back pain. In: *Approaches to the Validation of Manipulative Therapy*. Buerger, A. A. & Tobis, J. S. (eds), p. 70 Springfield, Illinois, Thomas.

Kraus, H., and Nagler, W. (1983) Evaluation of an exercise program for back pain. *Am. Fam. Physician*, **28**(3), 153–158.

Lancet, (1978) Editorial 2 May pp. 977–979.

Lazorthes, G. (1971) *Le Système Nerveux Périphérique*. Paris, Masson Ed.

Lee, D. (1986) Principles and practice of muscle energy and functional techniques. In: *Modern Manual Therapy of the Vertebral Column*, Grieve, G. P. (ed). pp. 640–655, London, Churchill Livingstone.

Lettvin, M. (1977) *The Back Book*. London, Souvenir Press.

Lewit, K. (1975). Blocking MACP. *Manipulation News*, **7**, 12–14.

Lewit, K. (1977) *Manuelle Medizin im Rahmen der Medizinischen Rehabilitation*. Johann Ambrosius Barth, Leipzig.

Lewit, K. (1985) *Manipulative Therapy in Rehabilitation of the Motor System*. London, Butterworths.

Lidstrom, A., and Zachrisson, M. (1970) Physical therapy on low back pain and sciatica. *Scand. J. Rehabil. Med.*, **2**, 37–39.

Lippit, A. B. (1979) The facet joint and its role in spinal pain: management with facet joint injections. *Spine*, **4**, 441–446.

Little, T. (1981) Chronic pain: modern concepts in management. *Aust. Fam. Physician*, **4**, 265–269.

McGuckin, N. (1986) The T4 syndrome. In: *Modern Manual Therapy of the Vertebral Column*, Grieve, G. D. (ed). London, Churchill Livingstone, pp. 370–376.

McKenzie, R. A. (1979) Extension exercise: is it helpful in recurrent low back pain? *Mod. Medicine Aust.*, **3**, 10–67.

McKenzie, R. A., (1970) Prophylaxis in recurrent low back pain. *NZ. Med. J.*, **89**, 22–23.

McKenzie, R. A. (1981) *The Lumbar Spine: Mechanical Diagnosis and Therapy*. Lower Hutt, Spinal Publications.

McKenzie, R. A. (1983) *treat Your Own Back*. Lower Hutt, Spinal Publications.

McKenzie, R. A. (1983). *Treat Your Own Neck*. Lower Hutt, Spinal Publications.

MacNab, I. (1977) *Backache*. Baltimore, Williams and Wilkins.

MacNab, I. (1979) Management of low back pain. *Curr. Pract. Orthop. Surg.*, **5**, 241.

MacNab, I. (1971) The whiplash syndrome. *Orthop. Clin. North. Am.*, **2**, 402.

McQueen, A. (1987) Surgical relief for the painful shoulder. *Aust. Fam. Physician*, **16**, 766–770.

Maigne, R. (1986) Manipulation of the spine. In: *Manipulation, Traction and Massage*, Basmajian, J. V. (ed), Paris, RML, pp. 71–96.

Maitland, G. D. (1977) *Peripheral Manipulation*, 2nd edn, London, Butterworths.

Maitland, G. D. (1977) *Spinal Manipulation*, 2nd edn, London, Butterworths.

Maitland, G. D. (1979) Movement of pain sensitive structures in the vertebral canal in a group of physiotherapy students. Proceedings of Inaugural Congress, *Manipulative Therapists Association of Australia*, Sydney, pp. 37–51.

Maitland, G. D. (1979) *Musculo-skeletal Examination and Recording Guide*. Adelaide, Lauderdale Press.

Marshall, L. (1978) *Your Back*. Melbourne, Sun Books.

Matthews, J. A. and Hickling, J. (1975) Lumbar traction: a double blind controlled study for sciatica. *Rheum. Rehabil.*, **14**, 222.

Mehta, M. (1973) Intractable pain. Saunders, London, p. 147.

Mehta, M., Melzack, R. and Wall, P. (1965) Pain mechanisms: a new theory. *Science*, **150**, 971.

Mennell, J., McM. (1986) Trigger points in referred spinal pain. In: *Modern Manual Therapy of the Vertebral Column*, Grieve G. P. (ed). London, Churchill Livingstone, pp. 250–258.

Mitchell, F. L., Moran, P. S. and Pruzzo, N. A. (1979) *An Evaluation and Treatment Manual of Osteopathic Muscle Energy Procedures*. Valley Park, Mitchell Moran and Associates.

Mixter, W. J. and Barr, J. S. (1934) Rupture of the intervertebral disc with involvement of the spinal canal. *N. Engl. J. Med.* **211**, 210–215.

Mooney, V. and Robertson, J. (1976) The facet syndrome. *Clin. Orthop.*, **115**, 149–156.

Mooney, V. and Cairns, D. (1978) Management in the patient with chronic low back pain. *Orthop. Clin. North Am.*, **9**, 543.

Moran, H. (1984) Injection techniques for common arm disorders. *Aust. Fam. Physician*, **13**, 108–111.

Moritz, U. (1979) Evaluation of manipulation and other manual therapy: criteria for measuring the effect of treatment. *Scand. J. Rehab. Med.*, **11**, 173–179.

Morrison, M. C. T. (1975) Manipulation for backache. *Othopaedics, Oxford*, **8**, 19–29.

Morrison, M. C. T. (1984) The best back to manipulate? *Ann. R. Coll. Surgeons Eng.*, **86**, 52–53.

Murtagh, J. E. (1974) Acute back pain. *Aust. Fam. Physician*, **3**, 266–275.

Murtagh, J. E. (1974) CHECK programme. RACGP, Unit 25, Unit 26.

Murtagh, J. E. (1979) CHECK programme. RACGP, Unit 89.

Murtagh, J. E. (1982) CHECK programme. RACGP, Unit 127.

Murtagh, J. E. (1983) Examination and diagnosis of low backache. *Aust. Fam. Physician*, **12**, 322–328.

Murtagh, J. E. (1985) CHECK programme. RACGP, Unit 167.

Murtagh, J. E. (1985) Patient education: exercises for your back. *Aust. Fam. Physician*, **14**, 1225.

Murtagh, J. E. (1986) *Back Pain*. Melbourne, Pitman.

Murtagh, J. E. (1987) Patient education: exercises for your neck. *Aust. Fam. Physician*, **16**, 485.

Murtagh, J. E. (1987) Patient education: exercises for your thoracic spine. *Aust. Fam. Physician*, **16**, 1310.

Murtagh, J. E. (1994) *General Practice*. Sydney, McGraw Hill, p. 280.

Murtagh, J. E., Findlay, D. and Kenna, C. (1985) Low back pain. *Aust. Fam. Physician*, **14**, 1214–1224.

Nachemson, A. L. (1976) The lumbar spine: an orthopaedic challenge. *Spine*, **1**(1), 59–71.

Nachemson, A. L. and Jayson, M. (ed). (1980) *The Lumbar Spine and Back Pain*, 2nd edn, Tunbridge Wells, Pitman Medical.

Parker, G. B., Tupling, H. and Pryor, D. S. (1978) A controlled trial of cervical manipulation for migraine. *Aust. NZ. J. Med.*, **8**, 589–593.

Paterson, J. K. and Burn, L. (1985) *An Introduction to Medical Manipulation*. Lancaster, MTP Press Ltd.

Pedersen, P. A. (1981) Prognostic indicators in low back pain. *J. R. Coll. Gen. Pract.*, **31**, 209–216.

Piterman, L. (1985) Industrial lower back injuries in primary care: a five year retrospective study. A research paper submitted for Master Medicine (Primary Medical Care), Melbourne University.

Piterman, L. and Dunt, D. (1987) Occupational lower back injuries in a primary medical care setting: a five year follow up study. *Med. J. Aust.* **147**, 276–279.

Porter, R. W. (1983) *Understanding Back Pain. Patient Handbook 13*. Edinburgh, Churchill Livingstone.

Rasmussen, G. G. (1977) Manipulation in the treatment of low back pain; randomised clinical trial. 5th International Congress, FIMM, Copenhagen.

Rathburn, J. B. and MacNab, I. (1970) The microvascular pattern of the rotator cuff. *J. Bone. Joint. Surg.*, **52B**, 528–540.

Rees, S. (1976) Disconnective neurosurgery. Multiple bilateral percutaneous rhizolysis (facet rhizotomy). In: *Current Controversies in Neurosurgery*. Morley, T. P. (ed). Philadelphia, Saunders, p. 80.

Rees, W. S. (1975) Multiple bilateral percutaneous rhizolysis. *Med. J. Aust.*, **1**, 536–537.

Rees, W. S. (1975) Multiple bilateral percutaneous rhizolysis of segmental nerves in the treatment of the intervertebral disc syndrome. *Ann. Gen. Pract.*, **16**, 126–129.

Reilly, P. and Littlejohn, G. (1990) Current thinking on fibromyalgia syndrome. *Aust. Fam. Physician*, **19**, 1505–1536.

Richardson, A. T. (1975) The painful shoulder. *Proc. R. Soc. Med.*, **68**, 731.

Rosenblatt, J. (1983) Caudal epidural anaesthesia. *Aust. Fam. Physician*, January, 40.

Rowe, M. L. (1969) Low back pain in industry – a position paper. *J. Occup. Med.*, **11**, 161.

Ryan, M. D. and Taylor, K. F. (1981) Management of lumbar nerve root pain by intrathecal and epidural injections of depot methyl prednisolone acetate. *Med. J. Aust.*, **2**, 532–534.

Rymer, W. Z., Houk S. C. and Crago, P. E. (1979) Mechanisms of the clasp knife reflex studies in an animal model. *Exp. Brain. Res.*, **37**, 93–113.

Schaeffer, H. R. (1976) A neurosurgeon looks at spinal conditions (letter). *Med. J. Aust.*, **1**, 676.

Schmoril, G. and Junghans, H. (1956) *Clinique et Radiologie de la Colonne Vertebrale Normale et Pathologique.* Paris, Dion Ed, pp. 99–102.

Selby, D. K. (1982) Conservative care of non specific low back pain. *Orthop. Clin. North. Am.*, **13**, 427–437.

Selecki, B. R., Ness, T. D., Limbers, P. et al. (1973) Low back pain: a joint neurosurgical and orthopaedic project. *Med. J. Aust.*, **2**, 889–893.

Shealy, C. N. (1973) *Role of Spinal Facets in Back and Sciatic Pain.* New York, American Association for the Study of Headache.

Sheon, R., Moskowitz, R. W. and Goldberg, V. M. (1987) *Soft Tissue Rheumatic Pain*, 2nd edn, Philadelphia, Lea & Febiger.

Simons, D. G. and Travell, J. C. (1983) Myofascial origins of low back pain – 1. Principles of diagnosis and treatment. *Postgrad. Med.*, **73**, 66–108.

Sims-Williams, H. and Jaysom, M. (1978) Controlled trial of mobilisation and manipulation for patients with low back pain in general practice. *Br. Med. J.*, **2**, 1338–1340.

Sims-Williams, H. and Jaysom, M. (1979) Controlled trial of mobilisation and manipulation for low back pain hospital patients. *Br. Med. J.*, **2**, 1318.

Smythe, H. A. and Moldofsky, H. (1977) Two contributions to understanding of the 'fibrositis' syndrome. *Bull. Rheum. Dis.*, **28**, 928–931.

Stilwell, D. L. (1973) The nerve supply of the vertebral column and its associated structures in the monkey. *Anat. record*, **125**, 139.

Stephens, J. (1984) Idiopathic adolescent scoliosis. *Aust. Fam. Physician*, **13**, 180–184.

Stoddard, A. (1969) *Manual of Osteopathic Practice.* London, Hutchinson, p. 240.

Swift, T. R. and Nichols, F. T. (1984) The droopy shoulder syndrome. *Neurol.*, **34**, 212–215.

Tanner, J. (1987) *Beating Back Pain.* London, Dorling Kindersley.

Travell, J. G. (1949) Rapid relief for acute 'stiff neck' by ethyl chloride spray. *Amer. Med. Wom. Assoc.*, **4**, 89.

Travell, J. G. (1952) Ethyl chloride spray for painful muscle spasm. *Arch. Phys. Med.*, **33**, 291.

Travell, J. G. and Rinzler, S. H. (1952) The myofascial genesis of pain. *Postgrad. Med.*, **11**, 423–424.

Travell, J. and Simons, D. G. (1983) *Myofascial Pain and Dysfunction. The Trigger Point Manual.* Baltimore, Williams & Wilkins, p. 186.

Visher, T. L. (1985) *The Painful Shoulder.* Basel, Documenta Geigy.

Waddell, G. et al. (1980) Non-organic physical signs in low back pain. *Spine*, **5**, 117–125.

Welfing, J. (1969) *Painful Shoulder.* Basel, Documenta Geigy.

White, A. H., Derby, R. and Wynne, G. (1980) Epidural injections for diagnosis and treatment of low back pain. *Spine*, **5**, 78–86.

Wiesel, S. W., Feffer, H. L. and Rothman, R. H. (1984) Industrial low back pain: a prospective evaluation of a standardised diagnostic and treatment protocol. *Spine*, **9**, 199–203.

Wilkinson, M. (1971) *Cervical Spondylosis*, 2nd edn, London, Heinemann.

Winer, C. E. R. (1985) A survey of controlled clinical trials of spinal manipulation. In: *Aspects of Manipulative Therapy*, Glasgow, E. F., Twomey, L. T., Scull, E. R. et al., 2nd edn, Melbourne, Churchill Livingstone, pp. 97–108.

Wyke, B. (1980) The neurology of low back pain. In: *The Lumbar Spine and Back Pain*. Jayson, M. I. V. (ed), London, Pitman Medical, pp. 265–339.

Yates, D. A. H. (1978) A comparison of the types of epidural injection commonly used in the treatment of low back pain and sciatica. *Rheum. Rehabil.*, **17**, 282.

Index

Printed and bound by CPI Group (UK) Ltd, Croydon, CR0 4YY

10/10/2024

01043166-0002